Advances in Cholestatic Liver Diseases

Editor

CYNTHIA LEVY

CLINICS IN LIVER DISEASE

www.liver.theclinics.com

Consulting Editor
NORMAN GITLIN

February 2016 • Volume 20 • Number 1

ELSEVIER

1600 John F. Kennedy Boulevard • Suite 1800 • Philadelphia, Pennsylvania, 19103-2899

http://www.theclinics.com

CLINICS IN LIVER DISEASE Volume 20, Number 1
February 2016 ISSN 1089-3261, ISBN-13: 978-0-323-42991-7

Editor: Kerry Holland
Developmental Editor: Meredith Clinton

Clinics in Liver Disease (ISSN 1089-3261) is published quarterly by Elsevier Inc., 360 Park Avenue South, New York, NY 10010-1710. Months of issue are February, May, August, and November. Business and Editorial Offices: 1600 John F. Kennedy Blvd., Ste. 1800, Philadelphia, PA 19103-2899. Customer Service Office: 3251 Riverport Lane, Maryland Heights, MO 63043. Periodicals postage paid at New York, NY and additional mailing offices. Subscription prices are $275.00 per year (U.S. individuals), $100.00 per year (U.S. student/resident), $453.00 per year (U.S. institutions), $395.00 per year (international individuals), $200.00 per year (international student/resident), $562.00 per year (international instituitions), $340.00 per year (Canadian individuals), $200.00 per year (Canadian student/resident), and $562.00 per year (Canadian institutions). Foreign air speed delivery is included in all *Clinics* subscription prices. All prices are subject to change without notice. **POSTMASTER:** Send address changes to *Clinics in Liver Disease*, Elsevier Health Sciences Division, Subscription Customer Service, 3251 Riverport Lane, Maryland Heights, MO 63043. **Customer Service: Telephone: 1-800-654-2452 (U.S. and Canada); 314-447-8871 (outside U.S. and Canada). Fax: 314-447-8029. E-mail: journalscustomer service-usa@elsevier.com (for print support); journalsonlinesupport-usa@elsevier.com (for online support).**

Reprints. For copies of 100 or more of articles in this publication, please contact the Commercial Reprints Department, Elsevier Inc., 360 Park Avenue South, New York, NY 10010-1710. Tel.: 212-633-3874; Fax: 212-633-3820; E-mail: reprints@elsevier.com.

Clinics in Liver Disease is covered in *MEDLINE/PubMed (Index Medicus)*, Science Citation Index Expanded, Journal Citation Reports/Science Edition, and Current Contents/Clinical Medicine.

Contributors

CONSULTING EDITOR

NORMAN GITLIN, MD, FRCP (LONDON), FRCPE (EDINBURGH), FAASLD, FACP, FACG
Formerly, Professor of Medicine, Chief of Hepatology, Emory University; Currently, Consultant, Atlanta Gastroenterology Associates, Atlanta, Georgia

EDITOR

CYNTHIA LEVY, MD
Associate Professor of Medicine, Division of Hepatology, University of Miami Miller School of Medicine, Miami, Florida

AUTHORS

SUE V. BEATH, BSc, MB.BS
The Liver Unit, Birmingham Children's Hospital, Birmingham; Honorary Senior Lecturer, University of Birmingham, West Midlands, United Kingdom

KIRSTEN MURI BOBERG, MD, PhD
Section of Gastroenterology, Department of Transplantation Medicine, Division of Cancer Medicine, Surgery and Transplantation and Norwegian PSC Research Center, Oslo University Hospital, Rikshospitalet; Institute of Clinical Medicine, University of Oslo, Rikshospitalet, Oslo, Norway

CHRISTOPHER L. BOWLUS, MD
Professor, Division of Gastroenterology and Hepatology, University of California Davis School of Medicine, Sacramento, California

ROGER W. CHAPMAN, MD, FRCP, FAASLD
Translational Gastroenterology Unit, John Radcliffe Hospital, Headington; Nuffield Department of Medicine, University of Oxford, Oxford, United Kingdom

CHRISTOPHE CORPECHOT, MD
Hepatology Department, Reference Center for Chronic Inflammatory Biliary Diseases (MIVB), French Network for Childhood and Adult Rare Liver Diseases (FILFOIE), Saint-Antoine Hospital, Assistance Publique - Hôpitaux de Paris (APHP); Inserm UMR_S938, Faculty of Medicine Pierre et Marie Curie, Paris, France

EMMA L. CULVER, BSc, MBChB, PhD, MRCP
Translational Gastroenterology Unit, John Radcliffe Hospital, Headington; Nuffield Department of Medicine, University of Oxford, Oxford, United Kingdom

FRANK CZUL, MD
University of Miami Miller School of Medicine, Miami, Florida

JESSICA K. DYSON, MBBS
Institute of Cellular Medicine, Newcastle University, Medical School, Framlington Place, Newcastle upon Tyne, United Kingdom

BERTUS EKSTEEN, MBChB, FRCP(London), PhD
Division of Gastroenterology and Hepatology, Snyder Institute for Chronic Diseases, University of Calgary, Calgary, Alberta, Canada

ANNAROSA FLOREANI, MD
Department of Surgery, Oncology and Gastroenterology, University of Padova, Padova, Italy

TRINE FOLSERAAS, MD, PhD
Section of Gastroenterology, Department of Transplantation Medicine, Division of Cancer Medicine, Surgery and Transplantation and Norwegian PSC Research Center, Oslo University Hospital, Rikshospitalet; Institute of Clinical Medicine, University of Oslo, Rikshospitalet, Oslo, Norway

MARIA TERESA GERVASI, MD
Department of Obstetrics and Gynecology, Azienda Ospedaliera, Padova, Italy

DAVID SETH GOLDBERG, MD, MSCE
Assistant Professor of Medicine, Division of Gastroenterology, University of Pennsylvania, Philadelphia, Pennsylvania

GIDEON M. HIRSCHFIELD, MBChB, PhD, FRCP (UK)
National Institute for Health Research (NIHR) Birmingham Liver Biomedical Research Unit (BRU), Centre for Liver Research, University of Birmingham, Birmingham, United Kingdom

PIETRO INVERNIZZI, MD, PhD
Liver Unit and Center for Autoimmune Liver Diseases, Humanitas Clinical and Research Center, Milan, Italy; Division of Rheumatology, Allergy, and Clinical Immunology, University of California Davis, Davis, California

DAVID E.J. JONES, MD, PhD
Professor, Institute of Cellular Medicine, Newcastle University, Medical School, Framlington Place, Newcastle upon Tyne, United Kingdom

LAURA JOPSON, MBChB
Institute of Cellular Medicine, Newcastle University, Medical School, Framlington Place, Newcastle upon Tyne, United Kingdom

DEIRDRE A. KELLY, MD
Consultant Paediatric Hepatologist, The Liver Unit, Birmingham Children's Hospital, Birmingham, West Midlands, United Kingdom

VANDANA KHUNGAR, MD, MSc
Assistant Professor of Medicine, Division of Gastroenterology, University of Pennsylvania, Philadelphia, Pennsylvania

CYNTHIA LEVY, MD
Associate Professor of Medicine, Division of Hepatology, University of Miami Miller School of Medicine, Miami, Florida

ANA LLEO, MD, PhD
Liver Unit and Center for Autoimmune Liver Diseases, Humanitas Clinical and Research Center, Rozzano, Milan, Italy

SIMONA MARZORATI, PhD
Liver Unit and Center for Autoimmune Liver Diseases, Humanitas Clinical and Research Center; Department of Electronics, Information and Bioengineering, Politecnico di Milano, Milan, Italy

GIORGINA MIELI-VERGANI, MD, Phd, FRCP, FRCPCH, FAASLD
Professor of Paediatric Hepatology, Paediatric Liver, GI and Nutrition Centre, King's College Hospital, London, United Kingdom

SOUVIK SARKAR, MD
Assistant Professor, Division of Gastroenterology and Hepatology, University of California Davis School of Medicine, Sacramento, California

WOUTER L. SMIT, MSc
Academic Medical Center, University of Amsterdam, Amsterdam, The Netherlands; Nuffield Department of Medicine, University of Oxford, Oxford, United Kingdom

PALAK J. TRIVEDI, BSc (Hons), MBBS, MRCP (UK)
Academic Clinical Lecturer and Specialist Registrar in Hepatology and Gastroenterology, National Institute of Health Research (NIHR) Birmingham Liver Biomedical Research Unit, Institute of Immunology and Immunotherapy, University of Birmingham, Birmingham, United Kingdom

DIEGO VERGANI, MD, PhD, FRCPath, FRCP, FAASLD
Institute of Liver Studies, King's College Hospital, London, United Kingdom

Contents

> Dysregulation of the key genetic, immunologic, and microbiome com-
> pounds of the gut-liver axis is the basis for inflammatory bowel disease
> (IBD) and primary sclerosing cholangitis (PSC). This creates opportunities
> to accelerate therapies that have been traditionally developed for IBD to be
> used in PSC to the benefit of both diseases. Shared genetic susceptibility
> loci has yielded important clues into the pathogenesis of PSC-IBD. Under-
> standing of the critical links between PSC and IBD are essential in
> designing clinical care pathways for these complex patients.

> The immune-mediated hepatobiliary diseases, primary biliary cirrhosis
> and primary sclerosing cholangitis are relatively rare, and account for a
> significant amount of liver transplant activity and liver-related mortality
> globally. Precise disease mechanisms are yet to be described, although
> a contributory role of genetic predisposition is firmly established. In addi-
> tion to links with the major histocompatibility complex, a number of asso-
> ciations outside this region harbor additional loci which underscore the
> fundamental role of breaks in immune tolerance and mucosal immunoge-
> nicity in the pathogenesis of autoimmune biliary disease. We provide an
> overview of these key discoveries before discussing putative avenues
> of therapeutic exploitation based on existing findings.

> Primary biliary cirrhosis (PBC) and primary sclerosing cholangitis (PSC)
> are the most common chronic cholestatic liver diseases (CLD) in adults,
> and are associated with immune mechanisms. PBC is considered a
> model autoimmune disease, and more than 90% of patients present
> very specific autoantibodies against mitochondrial antigens. Whether
> PSC should be considered an autoimmune, or merely immune-
> mediated disease, is still under debate. This review addresses the
> clinical relevance of autoantibodies in CLD and their pathogenic mech-
> anisms, and it illustrates the technology available for appropriate auto-
> antibody detection.

risk of recurrence after transplant are linked to the severity of bowel disease.

All patients with primary biliary cirrhosis (PBC) and abnormal liver biochemistry should be considered for specific therapy. Ursodeoxycholic acid (UDCA) is the only FDA-approved drug for treating PBC. Approximately 40% of patients with PBC respond incompletely to treatment with UDCA, thus having increased risk of death or need for liver transplantation. No second-line therapies for patients with inadequate response to UDCA therapy have been approved. This review provides a current perspective on potential new approaches to treatment in PBC, and highlights some of the challenges we face in evaluating and effectively implementing those treatments.

Fatigue is a significant problem for patients with primary biliary cirrhosis and although experienced less by patients with primary sclerosing cholangitis, a minority still report significant fatigue. Fatigue is the symptom with the greatest impact on quality of life, particularly when associated with social dysfunction. The pathogenesis of fatigue in cholestatic liver disease is complex, poorly understood, and probably has central and peripheral components. Managing fatigue in cholestatic liver disease presents a challenge for clinicians given the complexity and its numerous associations. This article presents a structured approach to managing fatigue in cholestatic liver disease to improve fatigue severity and quality of life.

Methods of liver fibrosis assessment have changed considerably in the last 20 years, and noninvasive markers have now been recognized as major first-line tools in the management of patients with chronic viral hepatitis infection. But what about the efficiency and utility of these surrogate indices for the more uncommon chronic cholestatic liver diseases, namely primary biliary cirrhosis and primary sclerosing cholangitis? This article provides clinicians with a global overview of what is currently known in the field. Both diagnostic and prognostic aspects of noninvasive markers of fibrosis in cholestatic liver diseases are presented and discussed.

When cholestasis occurs in patients receiving total parenteral nutrition, it is the result of many pathogenic pathways converging on the hepatic acinus. The result may be a temporary rise in liver function tests. The resulting fibrosis, portal hypertension, and jaundice are hallmarks of type 3 intestinal-associated liver disease to which children are more susceptible than adults. The key to prevention is in identifying high-risk scenarios, meticulous monitoring, and personalized prescription of parenteral nutrition solutions combined with an active approach in reducing the impact of inflammatory events when they occur by prompt use of antibiotics and line locks.

Intrahepatic cholestasis of pregnancy (ICP) is characterized by maternal pruritus, and elevated serum transaminases and bile acids. Genetic defects in at least 6 canalicular transporters have been found. Association studies stress the variability of genotypes, different penetrance, and influence of environmental factors. Serum autotaxin is a sensitive, specific, and robust diagnostic marker. Elevated maternal bile acids correlate with fetal complications. Long-term sequelae for mothers include the gallstone risk and chronic liver disease. There is an association between ICP and hepatitis C. Current treatment is ursodeoxycholic acid, owing to benefits on pruritus, liver function, safety, and decreased rates of adverse effects.

Liver transplantation (LT) is an established lifesaving therapy for patients with cholestatic liver diseases, including primary cholestatic diseases, namely primary sclerosing cholangitis and primary biliary cirrhosis, as well as secondary forms of cholestatic liver disease, including those with cholestatic complications of LT needing a retransplant. Patients with cholestatic liver diseases can be transplanted for complications of end-stage liver disease or for disease-specific symptoms before the onset of end-stage liver disease. These patients should be regularly assessed. Patient survival after LT for cholestatic liver diseases is generally better than for other indications.

CLINICS IN LIVER DISEASE

THE CLINICS ARE AVAILABLE ONLINE!
Access your subscription at:
www.theclinics.com

Preface

Advances in Cholestatic Liver Diseases

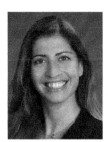

Cynthia Levy, MD
Editor

The past decades have seen major advances in the understanding of cholestatic liver diseases, now finally starting to translate into better diagnosis and management of these conditions. In this issue of *Clinics in Liver Disease*, we discuss how such advances can be applied to clinical practice. First, Dr Eksteen provides an excellent overview of the implications of gut-liver axis in the pathogenesis of primary sclerosing cholangitis (PSC) and how this knowledge can be used to target newer therapies. Drs Trivedi and Hirschfield follow with a summary of recent genetic discoveries in both primary biliary cirrhosis (PBC) and PSC, and Drs Marzorati, Invernizzi, and Lleo explain how to interpret autoantibodies in cholestatic diseases.

IgG4-related sclerosing cholangitis has emerged as one of the main differential diagnoses with PSC. Drs Smit, Culver, and Chapman present a comprehensive summary of current understanding of the pathophysiology, natural history, diagnosis, and treatment of IgG4-related sclerosing cholangitis. Patients with PSC can present in a variety of ways. For instance, they may have normal versus elevated IgG4, with normal or abnormal serum alkaline phosphatase, with or without inflammatory bowel disease, with or without dominant strictures! Drs Sarkar and Bowlus discuss the various clinical phenotypes of PSC and suggest a management approach based on the clinical presentation. One of the greatest challenges in the management of patients with PSC lies on the significantly increased risk of malignancies, including cholangiocarcinoma, gallbladder neoplasia, and colorectal neoplasia. Drs Folseraas and Boberg focus on the epidemiology of these malignancies and discuss available and upcoming strategies for early detection. Then, to complete the discussion on multiple phenotypes and challenges in the management of PSC, Drs Mieli-Vergani and Vergani address the peculiarities of sclerosing cholangitis in children.

In terms of therapeutics, the area with greatest advances has been PBC. Dr Czul and I present a broad discussion on the reliability of surrogate markers, such as serum alkaline phosphatase and total bilirubin, as well as their use in clinical practice to

Clin Liver Dis 20 (2016) xiii–xiv
http://dx.doi.org/10.1016/j.cld.2015.10.013   liver.theclinics.com
1089-3261/16/$ – see front matter © 2016 Published by Elsevier Inc.

monitor response and determine prognosis. Results of recent phase 3 trials are discussed, and we provide the reader with up-to-date management recommendations. In addition to the treatment of the specific disease, managing extrahepatic manifestations is of utmost importance. Fatigue is a common and significant symptom affecting many patients with cholestatic diseases, especially PBC. Drs Jopson, Dyson, and Jones explain the pathophysiology of fatigue in PBC/PSC and provide very concise, easy-to-use, key points for its proper management.

As we continue to move away from liver biopsy to diagnose or stage patients with cholestatic diseases, the need for reliable, noninvasive markers of prognosis increases. Dr Corpechot offers the reader a state-of-the-art summary on the status of vibration-controlled transient elastography in the assessment of patients with cholestatic diseases. The following two articles address areas where major growth in the understanding of pathogenesis led to improved overall diagnosis and/or management: intestinal failure-associated liver disease, comprehensively addressed by Drs Beath and Kelly, and intrahepatic cholestasis of pregnancy, reviewed by Drs Floreani and Gervasi. Finally, despite all of these advances, liver transplantation is still required for many patients with cholestatic liver diseases. Drs Khungar and Goldberg address indications for liver transplantation, waitlist mortality, overall results, disease recurrence, and more!

I would like to sincerely thank all the contributors for taking time off from their extremely busy schedules to share their knowledge and passion in this issue of *Clinics in Liver Disease*, and the editorial board at Elsevier, especially Kerry Holland and Meredith Clinton, for their amazing work ethic and diligence.

Cynthia Levy, MD
Division of Hepatology
University of Miami Miller Medical School
1500 Northwest 12th Avenue, Suite 1101
Miami, FL 33136, USA

E-mail address:
clevy@med.miami.edu

The Gut-Liver Axis in Primary Sclerosing Cholangitis

Bertus Eksteen, MBChB, FRCP(London), PhD

KEYWORDS

- Primary sclerosing cholangitis • Inflammatory bowel disease • Vedolizumab
- Cholangiocarcinoma • Genetics • Microbiome • Pouchitis

KEY POINTS

- Inflammatory bowel disease (IBD) occurs in at least 70% of cases of primary sclerosing cholangitis (PSC).
- IBD and PSC have shared genetic susceptibility loci (FUT2; IL-2; MST-1).
- Aberrant expression of gut adhesion molecules in PSC ($\alpha 4\beta 7$, MAdCAM-1) is a key feature of the gut-liver axis and provides significant opportunities for drug therapy in PSC.

INTRODUCTION

Primary sclerosing cholangitis (PSC) is a progressive immune-mediated liver disease that results in progressive fibro-stenotic strictures and destruction of the biliary tree. The cause of PSC is unknown and is not only associated with high rates of progression to liver cirrhosis and end-stage liver disease but also a significant risk of cholangiocarcinoma and gall bladder carcinoma. PSC has always been regarded as a rare disease but as awareness of PSC (particularly in the inflammatory bowel disease [IBD] community) has grown and combined with improved access to noninvasive means of imaging the biliary tree, it has become clear that PSC is not a rare disease and accounts for roughly 10% of all liver transplants performed each year. PSC remains an orphan disease for which there is yet no effective treatment apart from liver transplantation, which provides a temporary solution, as this disease often recurs after successful liver transplantation.

The author has nothing to disclose.
Division of Gastroenterology and Hepatology, Health Research and Innovation Centre (HRIC), Snyder Institute for Chronic Diseases, University of Calgary, 4AC66 – 3280 Hospital Drive Northwest, Calgary, Alberta T2N 4N1, Canada
E-mail address: b.eksteen@ucalgary.ca

Clin Liver Dis 20 (2016) 1–14
http://dx.doi.org/10.1016/j.cld.2015.08.012   liver.theclinics.com
1089-3261/16/$ – see front matter © 2016 Elsevier Inc. All rights reserved.

EPIDEMIOLOGY OF PRIMARY SCLEROSING CHOLANGITIS AND INFLAMMATORY BOWEL DISEASE

The most striking feature of PSC is its close association with IBD and highlights the importance of the gut-liver axis. It is clear that between 5.0% and 7.5 % of individuals with IBD will eventually develop PSC and at least 70% of patients with PSC will develop IBD. The association can be continuous, with simultaneous presentation of IBD and PSC with remission of liver inflammation after successful treatment of IBD in some cases, or discontinuous, as PSC can arise many years after initial diagnosis of IBD or even in some instances, after a curative surgery for ulcerative colitis (UC) has been performed. Conversely it is recognized that IBD can arise de novo after a successful liver transplant for PSC despite high levels of immunosuppression.[1,2]

In developed countries, there has been an increase in IBD, which led to similar increases in the incidence of PSC. The clinical presentation of PSC has evolved through time from a largely fibrotic cholestatic disease that affects the large bile ducts and high rates of end-stage liver disease to often milder phenotypes associated with modest liver inflammation and small duct involvement in the setting of IBD (**Fig. 1**). This heterogeneity is explained in part by the recent findings of multiple disease susceptibility genes in PSC and geographically highly variable gut microbiome patterns in PSC and IBD. The male-to-female ratio has been in the order of 7:1 but this has evolved with the most recent studies suggesting a 2:1 ratio. This is reflective of the evolution of IBD, which has also seen an increase in female sufferers. It is also clear that PSC has a specific presentation in children and young adults as well as a delayed phenotype of mild nonprogressive disease beyond the sixth decade of life.

The incidence of PSC is variable and is extrapolated from IBD data. A recent systematic review reports significant variation geographically with a mean incidence of 1.3 per 100,000 patient years, which is likely an underestimation due to underreporting bias of PSC or IBD. In some populations, this is reported to be as high as 7 cases per 100,000 population. This variation is reflective of the variation in UC, the incidence of which similarly ranges from 40 to 225 cases per 100,000 population. This is likely an underestimation, as there is a significant association between PSC and Crohn disease, as well as a failure to capture PSC as a diagnosis in administrative databases because of a lack of a specific disease code.[3] The prevalence of PSC ranges from 16.2 per 100,000 to 20.9 per 100,000 in Western populations. It is likely that both the incidence and prevalence of PSC is grossly underestimated, as PSC can present as a subclinical disease with normal liver tests, thus avoiding diagnosis, and in 20% to 30% of individuals will not occur with coexisting IBD. Another confounding factor is

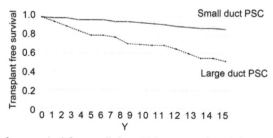

Fig. 1. Transplant-free survival for small-duct PSC compared with large-duct disease. (*Data from* Bjornsson E, Olsson R, Bergquist A, et al. The natural history of small-duct primary sclerosing cholangitis. Gastroenterology 2008;134(4):975–80.)

the availability of biliary imaging and variability in local protocols to assess newly diagnosed patients with IBD for coexisting PSC. Most of the published data in PSC is related to Northern European and North American populations. However, it is clear that Southern European and Asian populations suffer with less coexisting IBD (approximately 30%–50%) and that the ratio of UC to Crohn colitis varies significantly. Initial reports suggested that more than 90% of IBD in PSC consisted of UC, but more recent data derived from the Immunochip cohort suggests that Crohn colitis now accounts for one-third of the IBD in patients with PSC.[4,5]

CLINICAL FEATURES OF PRIMARY SCLEROSING CHOLANGITIS AND INFLAMMATORY BOWEL DISEASE

IBD is the most dominant disease associated with PSC and occurs in roughly 70% of PSC sufferers at a ratio of 6:1 UC to Crohn disease. IBD in PSC often precedes the diagnosis of PSC by a mean of 7 years and typically presents as a pancolitis. This can be asymptomatic due to relative rectal sparing and predominantly right-sided inflammation. Thirty percent of individuals with PSC appear not to suffer from IBD. It is unclear whether these individuals truly have no gut inflammation or whether this is a failure to detect subclinical inflammation by standard means, as virtually all patients with PSC will describe some degree of changes in their bowel habit and diarrhea at some stage.

It appears that the strongest association between PSC and IBD comes from colonic rather than ileal disease (**Table 1**). More than 70% of individuals will have backwash ileitis as a feature of a disease and have a distribution that favors the proximal colon with relative rectal sparing.[6] Although cases of isolated small bowel Crohn disease or perianal Crohn disease have been described in PSC, this is particularly unusual. The range of IBD disease activity is very variable in PSC with most individuals at presentation suffering from mild or asymptomatic IBD. Increasingly, it is not uncommon for PSC and IBD to be diagnosed simultaneously due to heightened awareness to test for PSC at IBD diagnosis. A proportion of individuals with PSC will proceed to end-stage liver disease and liver transplantation only to develop de novo IBD following transplantation. This disease can often be aggressive and unresponsive to immunosuppressive drugs, as it already occurs in the presence of potent immunosuppressive drugs required for the liver allograft. It is also not uncommon to have a curative panproctocolectomy for UC and to develop PSC subsequently.

Table 1		
Features of IBD in 71 patients with PSC and IBD (PSC-IBD) and compared with 142 patients with UC alone		
IBD Features	**PSC-IBD, %**	**UC, %**
Pancolitis	87	54
Rectal Sparing	52	6
Ileitis	51	7
Pouchitis	71	30

Abbreviations: IBD, inflammatory bowel disease; PSC, primary sclerosing cholangitis; UC, ulcerative colitis.

Adapted from Loftus EV Jr, Harewood GC, Loftus CG, et al. PSC-IBD: a unique form of inflammatory bowel disease associated with primary sclerosing cholangitis. Gut 2005;54(1):92.

The link with IBD is, however, significantly different at the age extremes of the disease. Individuals in their teenage and young adult years often suffer with very active IBD and require intense immunosuppression or the initiation of biological therapies that target tumor necrosis factor alpha (TNF-α). No direct effects have been demonstrated to suggest that anti–TNF-α treatment directly affects the liver but rather indirectly by controlling IBD. It is not uncommon for these young individuals treated with these drugs to see improvements in their liver transaminases, whereas older patients with PSC often have mild IBD, which often requires very little therapy to maintain remission.

Pouchitis is a particular concern in PSC, as almost 100% of individuals with PSC will develop pouchitis following a total proctocolectomy and the formation of an ileal pouch anal anastomosis (IPAA). Great variation is reported in different studies as to the response to standard therapy, with most studies suggesting that one-third to two-thirds of individuals will eventually develop refractory pouchitis. A large study of more than 1000 individuals with IPAA surgery demonstrated pouchitis rates of 61% at 5 years and 79% at 10 years for individuals with PSC, which was roughly double the rates seen in individuals with only UC[7] (Fig. 2).

In addition to increased risks of pouchitis, individuals with PSC and IBD do suffer with high rates of colorectal neoplasia that is predicted to be 20% to 25% lifetime risk (Fig. 3). The current guidelines for surveillance in these individuals requires an annual colonoscopy with 4-quadrant biopsies every 10 cm to detect mucosal dysplasia. This may be improved with the use of high-definition colonoscopy or dye spray techniques to highlight flat neoplastic lesions or dysplastic glands for targeted biopsies. A further technique that is promising is the use of confocal laser endomicroscopy, which allows a microscopic assessment of the colonic mucosa to detect very early changes in gland pattern as occurs with dysplasia but is not widely used outside of research-based protocols. The risk of colorectal cancer remains after liver transplantation, and hence surveillance is indicated after successful liver transplantation. Some studies have suggested that ursodeoxycholic acid or 5-aminosalicylate preparations can lower the risk of PSC-associated colorectal cancer.[11] However, in a recent study of high-dose ursodeoxycholic acid, there were suggestions that this drug might increase the development of neoplasia.[12] For many individuals who suffer with either refractory IBD or dysplasia, a panproctocolectomy would be indicated and, given the high rates of pouchitis, a standard end ileostomy would be the preferred surgery. This is, however, not entirely without complications, as peristomal varices can occur in individuals with advancing liver disease and increasing portal hypertension.

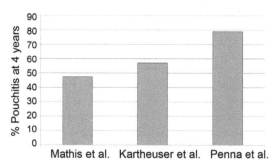

Fig. 2. Rates of pouchitis in PSC patients 4 years following pouch surgery. (Data from Refs.[8–10])

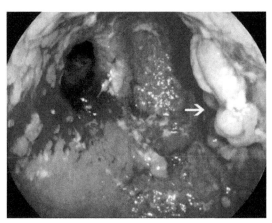

Fig. 3. Endoscopic picture of severe right-sided colitis with a patent ileocecal valve and ileitis and a colonic neoplasm (*arrow*).

PRIMARY SCLEROSING CHOLANGITIS AND INFLAMMATORY BOWEL DISEASE AFTER LIVER TRANSPLANTATION

Liver transplantation is a lifeline for many patients with PSC but is not a durable cure for PSC, as it recurs in 20% to 25% of recipients over a 5-year to 10-year period after liver transplantation with cadaveric organs and possibly at even higher rates using living related organs. As an example, a cohort of 230 PSC recipients with a median follow-up time of 82.5 months found a rate of recurrent PSC (rPSC) of 23.5%, with a time to developing rPSC of 4.1 years. A study in 2004 analyzed 3309 patients transplanted for PSC from the United Network for Organ Sharing (UNOS) database and found a higher retransplantation rate and a lower survival when compared with PBC (Primary Biliary Cirrhosis) recipients from the same study population at 7 years after transplantation.[13] Recent studies suggest that PSC is second only to hepatitis C as a leading cause for recurrent disease and subsequent graft loss but is likely to be overtaken by recurrent fatty liver as part of the obesity epidemic.[14]

The risk of recurrent disease appears to be closely linked to gut inflammation and IBD with some studies suggesting that a high IBD activity peritransplant is associated with recurrent disease.[15] A further study has demonstrated that a curative colectomy for IBD before transplantation was associated with very low rates of recurrent PSC, suggesting an important interaction between the gut and the liver in this disease[16] (**Fig. 4**). As these individuals will continue to have a high risk of colorectal cancer,

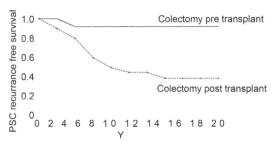

Fig. 4. PSC after transplant-free survival. (*Adapted from* Alabraba E, Nightingale P, Gunson B, et al. A re-evaluation of the risk factors for the recurrence of primary sclerosing cholangitis in liver allografts. Liver Transpl 2009;15(3):330–40.)

it might not be unreasonable in some individuals with difficult to control IBD to consider a colonic resection before transplantation, as this would place them at low risk of recurrent PSC and also obviate the need for frequent endoscopic screening thereafter. As PSC severity is poorly correlated with MELD (model of end-stage liver disease) or Child Pugh scores and the relative scarcity of the cadaveric organs, living related liver donation is increasingly used as a mechanism to provide allografts for these individuals. This has been associated with excellent results despite the higher risk of biliary complications. However, there is some suggestion that these individuals might be at higher risk of recurrent disease, which may be indicative of shared PSC susceptibility genes between siblings and potential risks of PSC within their immediate family.

Further risk factors for rPSC include male sex, long warm graft ischemia time, a history of acute cellular rejection, the use of extended donor criteria, cadaveric grafts, and human leukocyte antigen DRB1*08 (HLADRB1* 08). No medical therapy has been shown to prevent PSC recurrence or stop disease progression. The data that colectomy before transplantation is associated with less rPSC suggests a critical role of the inflamed colon in recurrent disease pathogenesis with the hope that the widespread use of potent biological therapies for IBD might result in a "chemical colectomy" to reduce rPSC. Currently, the only option for recurrent PSC is retransplantation, but is associated with increased mortality and higher rates of complications than the initial transplant.[17]

PATHOGENESIS
Shared Primary Sclerosing Cholangitis and Inflammatory Bowel Disease Genetic Susceptibility

HLA remains the strongest genetic link to PSC, but the relationship of PSC to other immune-mediated diseases is possibly best appreciated by genome-wide association studies that have defined 16 non-HLA risk loci for PSC by comparing more than 3700 PSC cases of European ancestry to 25,000 population controls, which are summarized in (**Table 2**). These data demonstrate significant overlap with other autoimmune diseases, including UC, Crohn disease, celiac disease, type 1 diabetes, sarcoidosis, psoriasis, and rheumatoid arthritis. This is consistent with clinical observations, as patients with PSC often suffer with other autoimmune conditions and act to highlight shared pathways that can be exploited to the benefit of related immune-mediated diseases but also highlights heterogeneity, which might explain differing disease presentations and clinical outcomes. Much work still need to be done to determine the biological effects of these genetic risk loci.[18]

Interleukin-2/Interleukin-2 Receptor α Pathway

These risk loci are commonly shared between multiple autoimmune diseases, including PSC and IBD, and has an important part in the gut-liver axis. Interleukin (IL)-2 has a central place in regulation and programming of the adaptive immune system. Mice deficient in the IL-2 receptor α gene readily develop biliary inflammation that resembles PBC and enterocolitis. Specific studies in PSC to assess the impact of this risk locus are lacking. However, supportive evidence comes from previous studies that demonstrated impaired T-cell responses and reduced levels of IL-2 expression following mitogen stimulation of liver-derived lymphocytes from patients with PSC. In parallel, decreased expression of IL-2 receptor was observed in these T cells.[18,21]

Table 2
Genetic risk loci associated with PSC based on published genome-wide association studies and Immunochip data

Chromosome	Lead SNP	Risk Allele	Common Allele	Nearby Gene Loci
1	rs3748816	A	C	MMEL1, TNFRSF14
2	rs6720394	G	A	BCL2L11
2	rs7426056	A	C	CD28
2	rs3749171	A	G	GPR35
3	rs3197999	A	C	MST1
4	rs13140464	C	T	IL2, IL21
6	rs56258221	G	A	BACH2
10	rs4147359	A	C	IL2RA
11	rs7937682	G	T	SIK2
12	rs11168249	G	T	HDAC7
12	rs3184504	A	G	SH2B3, ATXN2
18	rs1788097	A	G	CD226
18	rs1452787	G	A	TCF4
19	rs60652743	A	G	PRKD2, STRN4
21	rs2836883	G	T	PSMG1

Abbreviations: PSC, primary sclerosing cholangitis; SNP, single nucleotide polymorphism.
Data from Refs.[18–20]

Macrophage-Stimulating–1 Pathway

The RS3197999 macrophage-stimulating *(MST)-1* locus has the strongest non-HLA genetic linkage to PSC ($P<2.4 \times 10^{-26}$) and is a shared with UC and Crohn disease. *MST-1* is widely expressed in the liver and by the biliary epithelium and associated with macrophage differentiation skewed toward an M2 (anti-inflammatory) phenotype. It is also reported to alter leukocyte trafficking by modulating integrin-mediated adhesion. The risk locus for PSC predicts a hypofunctional MSP1 (macrophage-stimulating protein 1) with reduced receptor affinity and hence could affect PSC either by direct alteration of its function within the liver or by a lack of regulatory/tolerogenic effects on recruited leukocyte subsets, such as macrophages.[22]

Fucosyltransferase 2 Pathway

The RS601338 locus encodes galactoside 2-α-L-fucosyltransferase 2 *(FUT-2)*, which is intimately involved in protein glycosylation on mucosal surfaces, which includes ABH blood antigens and the Ca19 to 9 pathway. This polymorphism gives rise to a truncated FUT-2 enzyme, which results in the inability to synthesize ABH antigens on mucosal surfaces and in salivary glands and is commonly referred to as a nonsecretor. Similarly *FUT2* polymorphisms are associated with different baseline levels of secreted Ca19 to 9 in the serum. FUT-2 locus is shared between PSC and Crohn disease. The exact role is PSC is not known but appears to alter the mucosal milieu and the composition of the commensal microbiome in the biliary tree. FUT-2 homozygous risk allele carriers have reduced biliary Proteobacteria and increased populations of firmicutes.[20,23]

Salt-Inducible Kinase-2 Pathway

The RS79376A2 locus that confers risk for PSC is located in an intronic site of the *SIK-2* gene, which encodes salt-inducible kinase (SIK)-2 and is suggested to affect regulation of the gene product by as yet undefined mechanisms. SIK-2 can influence both IL-10 in macrophages and NUR-77, which functions as an important transcription factor in leukocytes. IL-10 is critical in maintaining immunologic tolerance, whereas IL-10 deficiency is associated with early-onset IBD. Similarly, IL-10–deficient mice developed severe colitis and provided a rationale that led to evaluation of IL-10 as a potential treatment for IBD. In strong linkage disequilibrium with the SIK-2 locus is RS11168249, which is situated within the HDAC7 gene, which encodes histone deacetylase 7. This molecule is implicated in the negative selection of T cells in the thymus, a critical process in determining the development of central immune tolerance. HDAC7 is likely to play a central role in PSC, as it is also linked to an intronic site in the PRKD-2 gene, which encodes serine threonine protein kinase D2. PRKD-2 phosphorylates HDAC-7 during T-cell receptor engagement with thymocytes, which lead to the exclusion of HDA-7 from the nucleus and eventual negative selection of immature T cells through apoptosis. The convergence of these 3 risk alleles to a single T-cell selection pathway suggests that a loss of central tolerance is at least in part involved in the pathogenesis of PSC and IBD but does require biological validation.[18]

Entero-Hepatic Immune Dysregulation in Primary Sclerosing Cholangitis and Inflammatory Bowel Disease

The most attractive hypothesis for development of PSC is one in which the entero-hepatic immune system develops cross-reactive immunity to an antigen (autoantigen or enteric microbiome) in the setting of reduced tolerance, which leads to immune-mediated gut and biliary inflammation. This is in part supported by the strong association with the HLA, which hints at specific but as of yet undefined antigen recognition in PSC. Evidence of immune activation in support of such a theory comes from observations in which total immunoglobulin (Ig)G levels are often raised in PSC in the absence of overlapping autoimmune hepatitis and the presence of specific antibodies such as antineutrophil cytoplasmic antibodies directed against PR3 (proteinase 3).

The strongest evidence linking the gut and liver comes from cellular immunology. The biliary epithelium not only functions by contributing to bile secretion but is an active participant in directing innate and adaptive liver immunity. Biliary epithelium secretes IgA and expresses multiple pattern recognition receptors, such as Toll-like receptors (TLRs) and nucleotide oligomerization domain (NOD)-like receptors to aid in the detection of invading pathogens through pathogen-associated molecular patterns, such as lipopolysaccharide.[24] This results in the secretion of proinflammatory cytokines, such as IL-6, TNF-α, and IL-1 ß, to drive proinflammatory responses. As part of this process, chemokines, such as CXCL12, CXCL16, CXCL9 to CXCL11, and CCL20, are secreted to attract proinflammatory leukocytes, including Th1 and Th17 T cells to the liver.[25–27] Biliary epithelium also expresses the integrin ligands, intercellular adhesion molecule 1 and vacular cell adhesion molecule 1 (VCAM-1), which furthers contributes to the adhesion, accumulation, and persistence of inflammatory leukocytes in the peribiliary space to take part in biliary inflammation in PSC.[28] Although proinflammatory CD8 recruitment to the biliary tree dominates during PSC, biliary epithelium also secretes CCL28, which serves as an attractant for immune-regulatory T cells that express the chemokine receptor CCR10 to try to limit biliary inflammation[29] and B cells.

The biliary epithelium can skew the nature of the inflammation by secretion of IL-6 and CCL20, which preferentially attract IL-17–producing CD4 cells (Th17) and creates a positive feedback loop to expand these proinflammatory cells in situ.[26] Expression of VCAM-1 not only helps effector T cells to adhere to the biliary epithelium and biliary structures, but also provides a survival signal to these T cells to ensure their persistence and thus chronic inflammation.[28] Much of these processes are generic to the biliary epithelium and can be found in related biliary conditions, such as PBC.[30]

However, what sets PSC apart from other liver diseases is that in addition to these generic proinflammatory recruitment pathways to the biliary epithelium, there is aberrant expression of gut-specific adhesion molecules, such as the chemokine receptor CCL25 and the integrin ligand, mucosal vascular addressin cell adhesion molecule 1 (MAdCAM-1). Normally, these molecules are highly restricted to the gut, where they drive selective recruitment of gut-specific T and B cells that express the CCL25 receptor, CCR9, and the integrin combination, $\alpha 4\beta 7$, which binds to MAdCAM-1. These 2 molecules are preferentially imprinted on T and B cells in mesenteric lymph nodes by CD103 expressing gut dendritic cells under the control of retinoic acid.[31] This provides a mechanism whereby gut dendritic cells that have been exposed to enteric pathogens can program specific T and B cells to selectively target the gut. In PSC, this normally closely regulated mechanism of gut tropism becomes aberrant and CD8 T cells derived from the gut are able to be recruited to the liver and potentially perpetuate biliary inflammation. The opposite is also true in that vascular adhesion protein 1 (VAP-1) is normally expressed in the uninflamed liver and during IBD is rapidly upregulated in the gut, hence providing a mechanism whereby T and B cells potentially traffic between the gut and the liver in PSC and IBD.[32] This provides an important rationale of how gut and liver inflammation might be linked and provides important adhesion molecule targets that could be exploited as future therapies for individuals with PSC and IBD.[33,34]

THERAPEUTIC TARGETING OF THE GUT-LIVER AXIS IN PRIMARY SCLEROSING CHOLANGITIS AND INFLAMMATORY BOWEL DISEASE
Altering the Microbiome

The role of the gut microbiota is increasingly being recognized as critically important in IBD disease pathogenesis through both direct interactions with the enteric immune system and indirectly via activation of pathogen recognition receptors, such as the TLRs and NOD-like receptors by bacterial motifs such as LPS (lipopolysaccharide).[35] This represents a modifiable therapeutic target that has seen significant successes, such as the use of antibiotic or probiotic treatments for pouchitis or fecal microbial transplants to treat UC.[36] Given the close relationship between PSC and IBD, similar interactions with the microbiome have been proposed and explored in case series and prospective trials. Tetracycline, metronidazole, vancomycin, and azithromycin (often in combination with ursodeoxycholic acid [UDCA]) have all been shown in case reports to significantly reduce hepatic inflammation as measured by aspartate transaminase, alanine transaminase, and/or alkaline phosphatase.[37]

This has led to 3 prospective studies. Eighty patients with PSC were randomized to 36 months of UDCA (15 mg/kg per day) plus metronidazole or UDCA alone.[38] The investigators reported superiority of metronidazole and UDCA over UDCA alone with significant improvements in alkaline phosphatase, Mayo PSC risk score, and histologic stage and grade. Similarly, 16 patients with PSC treated with minocycline for 1 year had significant decreases in alkaline phosphatase.[39] Unfortunately, 25% of the patients withdrew from the study due to intolerance to minocycline. The most notable study to date has been a double blind, randomized pilot study of 35 PSC cases randomized to low-dose vancomycin (125 mg 4 times a day), high-dose vancomycin (250 mg 4 times a day), low-dose metronidazole (250 mg 3 times a day), or high-dose metronidazole (500 mg 3 times a day). Low-dose and high-dose vancomycin groups were superior to metronidazole and achieved significant decreases in serum alkaline phosphatase levels at 12 weeks.[40] The beneficial effects of oral vancomycin are particularly encouraging in pediatric patients. A prospective series of 14 pediatric cases has reported significant decreases in alkaline phosphatase and disease symptoms in almost all cases. Prospective validation of these results in large randomized trials is required to fully establish the utility of antibiotics in PSC and correct patient selection.

Immunosuppression and Anti-Tumor Necrosis Factor α Therapy

The use of immunosuppressive drugs in PSC has been largely disappointing. Despite evidence of altered autoimmunity in PSC, the use of immunosuppressive drugs in PSC has had little impact with no evidence of long-term efficacy or delay in progression to end-stage PSC or complications. Most studies using immunosuppressive drugs were performed as uncontrolled pilot studies and have included the use of azathioprine, cyclosporine, tacrolimus, methotrexate, and corticosteroids. Tacrolimus, azathioprine, and corticosteroids did show modest improvements in liver biochemistry, but these effects were either not sustained or the outcomes assessed over prolonged periods to assess progression to cirrhosis.[41] A criticism is that most of these studies included advanced PSC with significant fibrosis with potentially minimal active inflammation to target.

Targeted Entero-Hepatic Therapies for Primary Sclerosing Cholangitis and Inflammatory Bowel Disease

Gut adhesion molecules are very attractive targets for pharmaceutical intervention in IBD, and given their entero-hepatic expression in PSC, there is the possibility that these anti-inflammatory IBD compounds could yield significant benefits in PSC.

The first molecule to successfully target gut-specific adhesion and provided a paradigm for this strategy in treating IBD was natalizumab, which targeted the α4 integrin[42] (**Fig. 5**); α4 can associate with either β1, which binds to VCAM-1, or β7, which binds to MAdCAM-1. This drug proved efficacious in patients with moderate to severe Crohn disease. Unfortunately, some individuals treated with natalizumab developed progressive multifocal leukoencephalopathy, which is a rare, fatal demyelinating disease of the brain caused by reactivation of John Cunningham (JC) virus. Reactivation of JC virus is thought to be related to the α4β1 inhibitory effects of natalizumab.

Subsequently, much work has been done to selectively target α4β7 specifically without interfering of α4β1 to limit unwanted systemic immunosuppression.[43] Several compounds have emerged as potential candidates in IBD. This includes etrolizumab (Genentech), which selectively targets β7, and PF-00547659 (Pfizer) as a selective inhibitor of MAdCAM-1, the ligand for α4β7. The most successful new drug in this class

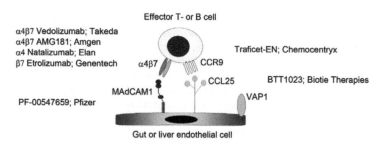

Fig. 5. Key adhesion molecules involved in T-cell or B-cell recruitment in PSC-IBD and therapeutic compounds under investigation.

is vedolizumab, which has been developed by Millennium Pharmaceuticals and Takeda. This molecule selectively targets the combination of $\alpha4\beta7$ as a heterodimer with minimal effects individually on $\alpha4$ or $\beta7$. Its potential utility in IBD came from studies in Cotton-top tamarins, in which rapid and dramatic improvements were seen at 24 and 72 hours after treatment. This resulted in significant improvements in gut histology and reduction in mucosal T-cell infiltration.[44]

Vedolizumab has subsequently shown clinical efficacy in randomized placebo-controlled studies as an induction and maintenance therapy in moderate to severe UC (Gemini 1 study),[45] moderate to severe Crohn disease (Gemini 2),[46] and in patients with moderate to severe Crohn disease who had previously failed other treatments (Gemini 3).[47] It was given approval by the Food and Drug Administration in May 2014 and ongoing safety data are being collected in the Gemini Long-Term Safety study, which is a 7-year study that aims to report in 2016. Most adverse events have been headache, nasopharyngitis, nausea, arthralgia, upper respiratory infections, and fatigue. Serious infections tended to occur more frequently in Crohn disease rather than UC.

Chemokine receptor inhibitors, as well as atypical adhesion molecules such as VAP-1, also have been developed. CCR9 has been selectively targeted in IBD by Traficent-EN (Chemocentryx); however, this study failed to achieve its endpoints. Less specific inflammatory chemokine receptors, such as CCR2 and CCR5, are in development. VAP-1 is currently the focus of a pilot study in PSC using the inhibitor, BTT1023 (Biotie Therapies; NCT02239211).

SUMMARY

Dysregulation of the key genetic, immunologic, and microbiome compounds of the gut-liver axis is the basis for IBD and PSC. This creates opportunities to accelerate therapies that have been traditionally developed for IBD to be used in PSC to the benefit of both diseases. Understanding of the critical links between PSC and IBD is essential in designing clinical care pathways for these complex patients.

REFERENCES

1. Chapman R, Fevery J, Kalloo A, et al. Diagnosis and management of primary sclerosing cholangitis. Hepatology 2010;51(2):660–78.
2. Eaton JE, Talwalkar JA, Lazaridis KN, et al. Pathogenesis of primary sclerosing cholangitis and advances in diagnosis and management. Gastroenterology 2013;145(3):521–36.
3. Molodecky NA, Myers RP, Barkema HW, et al. Validity of administrative data for the diagnosis of primary sclerosing cholangitis: a population-based study. Liver Int 2011;31(5):712–20.
4. Molodecky NA, Soon IS, Rabi DM, et al. Increasing incidence and prevalence of the inflammatory bowel diseases with time, based on systematic review. Gastroenterology 2012;142(1):46–54.e42 [quiz: e30].
5. Molodecky NA, Kareemi H, Parab R, et al. Incidence of primary sclerosing cholangitis: a systematic review and meta-analysis. Hepatology 2011;53(5):1590–9.
6. Loftus EV Jr, Harewood GC, Loftus CG, et al. PSC-IBD: a unique form of inflammatory bowel disease associated with primary sclerosing cholangitis. Gut 2005; 54(1):91–6.
7. Rahman M, Desmond P, Mortensen N, et al. The clinical impact of primary sclerosing cholangitis in patients with an ileal pouch-anal anastomosis for ulcerative colitis. Int J Colorectal Dis 2011;26(5):553–9.

8. Mathis KL, Dozois EJ, Larson DW, et al. Ileal pouch-anal anastomosis and liver transplantation for ulcerative colitis complicated by primary sclerosing cholangitis. Br J Surg 2008;95(7):882–6.

9. Penna C, Dozois R, Tremaine W, et al. Pouchitis after ileal pouch-anal anastomosis for ulcerative colitis occurs with increased frequency in patients with associated primary sclerosing cholangitis. Gut 1996;38(2):234–9.

10. Kartheuser AH, Dozois RR, LaRusso NF, et al. Comparison of surgical treatment of ulcerative colitis associated with primary sclerosing cholangitis: ileal pouch-anal anastomosis versus Brooke ileostomy. Mayo Clin Proc 1996; 71(8):748–56.

11. Pardi DS, Loftus EV Jr, Kremers WK, et al. Ursodeoxycholic acid as a chemopreventive agent in patients with ulcerative colitis and primary sclerosing cholangitis. Gastroenterology 2003;124(4):889–93.

12. Eaton JE, Silveira MG, Pardi DS, et al. High-dose ursodeoxycholic acid is associated with the development of colorectal neoplasia in patients with ulcerative colitis and primary sclerosing cholangitis. Am J Gastroenterol 2011;106(9):1638–45.

13. Maheshwari A, Yoo HY, Thuluvath PJ. Long-term outcome of liver transplantation in patients with PSC: a comparative analysis with PBC. Am J Gastroenterol 2004; 99(3):538–42.

14. Rowe IA, Webb K, Gunson BK, et al. The impact of disease recurrence on graft survival following liver transplantation: a single centre experience. Transpl Int 2008;21(5):459–65.

15. Joshi D, Bjarnason I, Belgaumkar A, et al. The impact of inflammatory bowel disease post-liver transplantation for primary sclerosing cholangitis. Liver Int 2013; 33(1):53–61.

16. Alabraba E, Nightingale P, Gunson B, et al. A re-evaluation of the risk factors for the recurrence of primary sclerosing cholangitis in liver allografts. Liver Transpl 2009;15(3):330–40.

17. Kim WR, Wiesner RH, Poterucha JJ, et al. Hepatic retransplantation in cholestatic liver disease: impact of the interval to retransplantation on survival and resource utilization. Hepatology 1999;30(2):395–400.

18. Liu JZ, Hov JR, Folseraas T, International PSC Study Group. Dense genotyping of immune-related disease regions identifies nine new risk loci for primary sclerosing cholangitis. Nat Genet 2013;45(6):670–5.

19. Ellinghaus D, Folseraas T, Holm K, et al. Genome-wide association analysis in primary sclerosing cholangitis and ulcerative colitis identifies risk loci at GPR35 and TCF4. Hepatology 2013;58(3):1074–83.

20. Folseraas T, Melum E, Rausch P, et al. Extended analysis of a genome-wide association study in primary sclerosing cholangitis detects multiple novel risk loci. J Hepatol 2012;57(2):366–75.

21. Melum E, Franke A, Schramm C, et al. Genome-wide association analysis in primary sclerosing cholangitis identifies two non-HLA susceptibility loci. Nat Genet 2011;43(1):17–9.

22. Karlsen TH, Franke A, Melum E, et al. Genome-wide association analysis in primary sclerosing cholangitis. Gastroenterology 2010;138(3):1102–11.

23. Wannhoff A, Hov JR, Folseraas T, et al. FUT2 and FUT3 genotype determines CA19-9 cut-off values for detection of cholangiocarcinoma in patients with primary sclerosing cholangitis. J Hepatol 2013;59(6):1278–84.

24. Matsushita H, Miyake Y, Takaki A, et al. TLR4, TLR9, and NLRP3 in biliary epithelial cells of primary sclerosing cholangitis: relationship with clinical characteristics. J Gastroenterol Hepatol 2015;30(3):600–8.

25. Heydtmann M, Lalor PF, Eksteen JA, et al. CXC chemokine ligand 16 promotes integrin-mediated adhesion of liver-infiltrating lymphocytes to cholangiocytes and hepatocytes within the inflamed human liver. J Immunol 2005;174(2): 1055–62.
26. Oo YH, Banz V, Kavanagh D, et al. CXCR3-dependent recruitment and CCR6-mediated positioning of Th-17 cells in the inflamed liver. J Hepatol 2012;57(5): 1044–51.
27. Curbishley SM, Eksteen B, Gladue RP, et al. CXCR3 activation promotes lymphocyte transendothelial migration across human hepatic endothelium under fluid flow. Am J Pathol 2005;167(3):887–99.
28. Afford SC, Humphreys EH, Reid DT, et al. Vascular cell adhesion molecule 1 expression by biliary epithelium promotes persistence of inflammation by inhibiting effector T-cell apoptosis. Hepatology 2014;59(5):1932–43.
29. Eksteen B, Miles A, Curbishley SM, et al. Epithelial inflammation is associated with CCL28 production and the recruitment of regulatory T cells expressing CCR10. J Immunol 2006;177(1):593–603.
30. Trivedi PJ, Adams DH. Mucosal immunity in liver autoimmunity: a comprehensive review. J Autoimmun 2013;46:97–111.
31. Eksteen B, Mora JR, Haughton EL, et al. Gut homing receptors on CD8 T-cells are retinoic acid dependent and not maintained by liver dendritic or stellate cells. Gastroenterology 2009;137(1):320–9.
32. Lalor PF, Tuncer C, Weston C, et al. Vascular adhesion protein-1 as a potential therapeutic target in liver disease. Ann N Y Acad Sci 2007;1110:485–96.
33. Adams DH, Eksteen B. Aberrant homing of mucosal T cells and extra-intestinal manifestations of inflammatory bowel disease. Nat Rev Immunol 2006;6(3):244–51.
34. Eksteen B, Grant AJ, Miles A, et al. Hepatic endothelial CCL25 mediates the recruitment of CCR9+ gut-homing lymphocytes to the liver in primary sclerosing cholangitis. J Exp Med 2004;200(11):1511–7.
35. Jostins L, Ripke S, Weersma RK, et al. Host-microbe interactions have shaped the genetic architecture of inflammatory bowel disease. Nature 2012;491(7422): 119–24.
36. Moayyedi P, Surette MG, Kim PT, et al. Fecal microbiota transplantation induces remission in patients with active ulcerative colitis in a randomized controlled trial. Gastroenterology 2015;149(1):102–9.e6.
37. Tabibian JH, Talwalkar JA, Lindor KD. Role of the microbiota and antibiotics in primary sclerosing cholangitis. Biomed Res Int 2013;2013:389537.
38. Farkkila M, Karvonen AL, Nurmi H, et al. Metronidazole and ursodeoxycholic acid for primary sclerosing cholangitis: a randomized placebo-controlled trial. Hepatology 2004;40(6):1379–86.
39. Silveira MG, Torok NJ, Gossard AA, et al. Minocycline in the treatment of patients with primary sclerosing cholangitis: results of a pilot study. Am J Gastroenterol 2009;104(1):83–8.
40. Tabibian JH, Weeding E, Jorgensen RA, et al. Randomised clinical trial: vancomycin or metronidazole in patients with primary sclerosing cholangitis—a pilot study. Aliment Pharmacol Ther 2013;37(6):604–12.
41. Talwalkar JA, Gossard AA, Keach JC, et al. Tacrolimus for the treatment of primary sclerosing cholangitis. Liver Int 2007;27(4):451–3.
42. Ghosh S, Goldin E, Gordon FH, et al. Natalizumab for active Crohn's disease. N Engl J Med 2003;348(1):24–32.
43. Lobaton T, Vermeire S, Van Assche G, et al. Review article: anti-adhesion therapies for inflammatory bowel disease. Aliment Pharmacol Ther 2014;39(6):579–94.

44. Podolsky DK, Lobb R, King N, et al. Attenuation of colitis in the cotton-top tamarin by anti-alpha 4 integrin monoclonal antibody. J Clin Invest 1993;92(1):372–80.
45. Feagan BG, Rutgeerts P, Sands BE, et al. Vedolizumab as induction and maintenance therapy for ulcerative colitis. N Engl J Med 2013;369(8):699–710.
46. Sandborn WJ, Feagan BG, Rutgeerts P, et al. Vedolizumab as induction and maintenance therapy for Crohn's disease. N Engl J Med 2013;369(8):711–21.
47. Sands BE, Feagan BG, Rutgeerts P, et al. Effects of vedolizumab induction therapy for patients with Crohn's disease in whom tumor necrosis factor antagonist treatment had failed. Gastroenterology 2014;147(3):618–27.e3.

The Immunogenetics of Autoimmune Cholestasis

Palak J. Trivedi, MBBS, MRCP (UK), Gideon M. Hirschfield, MBChB, PhD, FRCP (UK)*

KEYWORDS

- Autoimmunity • Autoimmune liver disease • Mucosal immunity
- Primary sclerosing cholangitis • Primary biliary cirrhosis

KEY POINTS

- The strongest genetic associations in primary biliary cirrhosis (PBC) and primary sclerosing cholangitis (PSC) occupy distinct regions of the major histocompatibility complex (MHC).
- Most non-MHC associations overlap with other autoimmune diseases, with putative risk loci indicating altered immunoregulatory pathways, aberrant microbial handling and dysregulated mucosal immunity generally.
- Less than 20% of the expected heritability is explained by currently available genome-wide studies.
- Epigenetics have provided insight into sex predisposition as well as overexuberant chemokine-mediated lymphocyte recruitment in the pathogenesis of immune-mediated liver disease.
- Recognition of definitive immune regulatory mechanisms and pathway defects may facilitate approaches to risk stratification as well as in the identification of ostensible therapeutic avenues.

INTRODUCTION

Chronic cholestatic liver diseases encompass a range of disorders affecting the hepatobiliary system and arise secondary to a variety of causes, including molecular defects caused by genetic variation or drugs, structural changes due to congenital

Dr G.M. Hirschfield is a coinvestigator for UK-PBC (www.uk-pbc.com) supported by a Stratified Medicine Award from the UK Medical Research Council (MR/L001489/1) and Principal Investigator for UK-PSC, an NIHR Rare Disease Translational Collaboration. Dr P.J. Trivedi has received funding from the NIHR Biomedical Research Unit and is recipient of a Wellcome Trust Clinical Research Fellowship (099907/Z/12/Z). The views expressed are those of the authors(s) and not necessarily those of the National Health System, the National Institute for Health Research, or the Department of Health.
National Institute of Health Research (NIHR) Birmingham Liver Biomedical Research Unit, Institute of Immunology and Immunotherapy, University of Birmingham, Wolfson Drive, Birmingham B15 2TT, UK
* Corresponding author. Centre for Liver Research, Institute of Biomedical Research, University of Birmingham, Birmingham B15 2TT, UK.
E-mail address: g.hirschfield@bham.ac.uk

disorders, or autoreactive bile duct injury.[1] In clinical practice, the latter is most often applied in reference to primary biliary cirrhosis (PBC) and primary sclerosing cholangitis (PSC), themselves part of the broader spectrum of immune-mediated liver disease.[2] Support of an autoimmune cause is provided by strong genetic links with human leukocyte antigen (HLA), the presence of high circulating autoantibody titers, and a clear increased frequency of concomitant autoimmune disease in affected individuals as well as associated family members.

However, unlike many classic autoimmune syndromes, PBC and PSC do not typically respond to immunosuppressive therapy; with the development of newer therapeutic interventions being significantly mired by gaps in understanding disease etiopathogenesis. Nevertheless, recent developments have begun to dissect the impact of certain genetic polymorphisms not only on predisposition but also varying phenotypic presentations, susceptibility to progressive disease, and putative therapeutic avenues based on the rational targeting of immune pathways presumed relevant to disease initiation.

Genetic exploration of rare diseases frequently establish major genes that regulate pathogen-specific immune responses, and genome-wide association studies (GWAS) have been increasingly productive for recognizing common variants within a given population. However, identifying the exact genes that result in statistical associations is often not possible to determine, and often many plausible candidates at a given susceptibility locus are proposed.[3] Conversely, if only one candidate susceptibility gene is identified, the associated causative variant is often unknown.[4]

EPIDEMIOLOGIC CONSIDERATIONS: HERITABILITY AND FAMILIAL CLUSTERING

Although PBC and PSC represent relatively rare disease entities, systematic reviews of disease frequency suggest an increasing incidence and prevalence globally.[5] Moreover, both conditions continue to pose a significant burden on health care services, accounting for approximately 25% of all first liver transplantations in the Western world.[6] For PBC, clustering of cases has been reported in certain geographic areas, for instance, in coastal First Nations of British Columbia where disease prevalence is as high as 25% within generations of well-characterized multiplex families.[7] Studies of monozygotic twins provide further support of a genetic predisposition, with a reported 63% concordance rate, among the highest reported for any autoimmune disease.[8] Moreover, a family history seems to be one of the strongest identified risk factors for disease development (odds ratio: 10.7), with approximately 6% of the patients having an affected first-degree relative.[9] Conversely, population studies from Australia estimate a prevalence of PBC between 19.1 per million among birth natives relative and 183 per million among those migrating to the continent from Europe.[10,11] Although these data support an inherent genetic predisposition to disease development, the incidence seems to decrease in consecutive generations of descendants of European migrants possibly indicating the impact of environmental influences.[12]

Heritable aspects of PSC are also evinced through family studies, wherein disease prevalence in first-degree relatives of affected patients is 100-times greater than that observed across unrelated comparator populations.[13] Clinical associations between PSC and colonic inflammatory bowel disease (IBD) are well described,[14] and the risk of developing PSC and/or ulcerative colitis (UC) is also significantly increased in families of afflicted individuals compared with controls.[15]

Despite the evidence of familial aggregation, neither PBC nor PSC display classic Mendelian inheritance. Rather, they exhibit a complex and possibly dynamic gene-gene/gene-environment interaction contributing to disease manifestation at various levels. Therefore, some of the currently proposed genes may influence disease risk by determining how a given individual responds to a particular environmental antigen. Others may act in concert and express the consequence of variation in a stepwise manner and be responsible for diverse clinical phenotypes depending on the coexistence of genetic variability in distinct immune pathways (**Fig. 1**).

HUMAN LEUKOCYTE ANTIGEN ASSOCIATIONS

The highly polymorphic major histocompatibility complex (MHC) has been implicated in the etiopathogenesis of human autoimmunity for decades, with strong albeit distinct HLA signals recently confirmed for autoimmune liver disease through GWAS.[1,16] Comprehension of how HLA impacts cholestatic disease mechanistically is somewhat limited, although the fact that an association has been identified in the first instance suggests a defect in the direction and precision of antigen-specific immune responses.

In PBC, several single-nucleotide polymorphisms (SNPs) mapping within or near genes across the HLA region meet the significance threshold for genome-wide association ($P < 5 \times 10^{-8}$), with peak signals mapping between *HLA-DQA1* and *HLA-DQB1*.[17–20] PBC-specific associations have also been reported for *HLA-DRB1*08*,

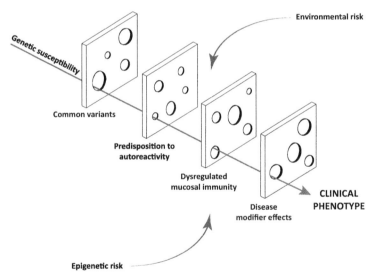

Fig. 1. Aggregation of genetic risk in complex diseases. PBC and PSC represent complex diseases, in which the cause is attributed to presence of ostensible genetic risk factors that exhibit a poorly understood interaction with coexisting environmental influences. Individual susceptibility factors are frequently nonpathogenic in isolation, and currently identified genetic variants frequently occur in the healthy population to a certain degree. However, in an individual who is immunologically primed, the cumulative loss of an unfortunately high burden of protective factors gives rise to breaks in immune tolerance (indicated by *holes*) that predispose to autoimmunity (eg, dysregulated *IL-2* or *IL-12* signaling pathways) in addition to pathogenic responses to the commensal microbiome (eg, *CARD-9* variants) that result in a clinically identifiable presentation. Additional modifier genes or epigenetic influences may also exist, which influence the rate of progression and variant clinical phenotypes (eg, *Fut-2* polymorphisms).

HLA-DRB1*11, HLA-DRB1*14, and HLA-DPB1*03:01, with most corresponding amino acids forming residues in the antigen-binding pocket of the MHC molecule suggesting defective antigen presenting capacity. However, HLA associations vary geographically, with increased PBC susceptibility demonstrated for HLA-DRB1*08:01 in European patients and HLA-DRB1*08:03 – DQB1*06:01 and HLA-DRB1*04:05 – DQB1*04:01 haplotypes implicated in Japanese patients with PBC.[21] A novel association with the HLA-DRB1*0901 – DQB1*0303 haplotype and progression to cirrhosis and liver transplantation have also been suggested in Japan, whereas HLA-DRB1*13:02 – DQB1*06:04 and HLA-DRB1*11:01 – DQB1*03:01 seem protective.[22]

Pathologically, PBC is characterized by highly conserved humoral and cellular autoreactive immune responses to the mitochondrial pyruvate dehydrogenase complex E2 (PDC-E2).[23,24] This loss of tolerance has been attributed to the aberrant expression of molecular mimics of PDC-E2 on the cell surface of biliary epithelial cells (BEC), which behave as immunodominant epitopes and bind with HLA-DRB4.[25] However, interactions between other HLA haplotypes and PDC-E2 have not yet determined.

Variation within the MHC region also represents the most significant genetic risk factor for PSC, with proposed SNPs in near-perfect linkage disequilibrium with HLA-B*08:01 as well as more complex associations described for HLA-DRB1*03:01, HLA-DRB1*13:01, HLA-DQA1*01:03, and HLA-DQA1*01:01.[26–28] Simultaneously, strong protective influences of the HLA-DRB1*04 – DQB1*03:02 and HLA-DRB1*07:01 – DQB1*03:03 haplotypes have been documented. Further insight into risk-related alleles in the class-II region of patients has been provided by fine mapping of HLA-DRB1 genotypes[29]; and 3-dimensional modeling of the corresponding protein chain has identified key amino acids influencing the range of peptides incorporated into the binding pocket of the MHC.

Despite a striking coexistence with colonic inflammation (in ~80% of cases), most of the HLA associations in PSC are distinct from those identified in IBD, with the exception of a recently identified link to HLA-DRB1*15:01 that is seen to overlap with that of UC (increased risk) and Crohn disease (decreased risk) as well as a multitude of organ-specific autoimmune disease.[30] The negative prognostic impact of colitis in PSC has been consistently demonstrated in well-characterized patient cohorts and population-based series,[31,32] with more variable stratification capabilities reported for those patients having elevated serum immunoglobulin G4 (IgG4) levels.[33,34] Nevertheless, patients with PSC and high serum IgG4 also exhibit an increased frequency of HLA-DRB1*15, the presence of which may, therefore, signify a common high-risk phenotype. Conversely, individuals who manifest the small duct variant of PSC in the absence of concomitant IBD harbor several distinct HLA associations, possibly implying a distinct cholangiopathic entity.[28,35]

T-CELL SIGNALING

In keeping with an immune-mediated cause, PBC and PSC display several immunopathogenic traits common to human autoimmune disease, including overexuberant effector and cytotoxic T-cell responses to pathogen stimulation,[36–38] in parallel to a relative loss of immunoregulatory leukocyte functions.[39,40]

Pathologically, PBC is characterized by a progressive lymphocytic cholangitis centered on smaller intrahepatic bile ducts, and consistent with involvement of the adaptive immune system the infiltrate is predominated by T cells. Large-scale genetic studies have underscored the impact of adaptive regulatory immune pathways;

in PBC, this is perhaps best highlighted by interleukin 12 (IL-12) and downstream Janus Kinase (JAK) and Signal Transducer and Activator of Transcription (STAT) signaling.[17,37,41] IL-12 is central in generating effector type-1 helper T-cell (T_h1) responses directed toward clearance of intracellular pathogens, and interferon γ (IFNγ) release suppresses IL-23–driven induction of IL-17–producing helper T-lymphocytes (T_h17).[42] Additionally, impaired expression of the IL-12 receptor subunit IL-12Rβ2 has been shown to facilitate regulatory T-cell (T_{reg}) suppressive functions in the context of a proinflammatory environment. *IL-12A* and *IL-12RB2* variants confer an augmented risk of autoimmunity in many human conditions and have been recently validated in a meta-analysis of several PBC GWAS.[17–19,43–46] The significance of this observation is elegantly illustrated in experimental cholangiopathy models, wherein mice that lack the p40 subunit of IL-12 (*IL12p40*$^{-/-}$) exhibit dramatic reductions in histologic cholangitis and a significant decrease in the levels of intrahepatic, proinflammatory cytokines.[47] Many other loci associated with PBC suggest that Toll-like receptor signaling upstream of IL-12 production may also play a role in disease. For instance, IFN regulatory factor-5 interacts with nuclear factor κB (NFκB), which consequently induces expression of several effector T-cell cytokines, including IL-12. Furthermore, variants at the *IL12A* locus have been reported to affect the risk of PBC recurrence following liver transplantation.[48] Several additional genetic variants involved in key T-cell signaling have been suggested by candidate association studies but not yet emerged as risk loci in PBC GWAS. The classic example here is cytotoxic T-lymphocyte–associated protein-4, which encodes a protein expressed on T-cells and competitively binds to costimulatory molecules CD80 and CD86, thereby ameliorating effector signaling through CD28.[49]

Of interest, *CD28* has emerged as a risk locus in PSC and encodes a T-cell costimulatory molecule necessary for activation and proliferation. A recently published study by Liaskou and colleagues[50] has demonstrated that in PSC, CD4$^+$ T lymphocytes lacking CD28 can be induced by tumor necrosis factor α (TNFα) and infiltrate the peribiliary region where they induce BEC apoptosis through secretion of proinflammatory cytokines in addition to granzyme and perforin-mediated injury. Of note, CD28 is required for IL-2 production, which in turn is required for both the induction (activation of effector T cells) and termination of inflammatory immune responses (induction of T_{reg}).

TUMOR NECROSIS FACTOR α SIGNALLING

TNFα is an activating factor for several intracellular pathways that determine the fate of epithelial cells, including hepatocytes and BEC.[51] Interactions between specific members of the TNF pathway lead to the induction of apoptosis as well as activation of NFκB signaling; and in PBC, GWAS have identified 3 loci containing genes in TNFα signaling pathways.[18,20,52] Macrophages from patients with PBC when stimulated with apoptotic bodies from BEC produce high levels of TNFα, with serum levels of TNFα reflecting the severity of intrahepatic damage.[23,53]

A prominent role for TNFα in the immunopathogenesis of PSC has also been suggested through induction of immunopathogenic T-cell phenotypes[50] as well as indirectly through the hepatic endothelial induction of mucosal chemokines and adhesion molecules that are normally gut restricted in an NFκB-dependent manner.[54] Moreover, PSC genetic risk associations include the 1p36 locus that encompasses the gene encoding TNF-superfamily receptor TNFRSF14, a protein expressed on CD4$^+$ and CD8$^+$ T cells, B cells, monocytes, neutrophils, dendritic cells, and mucosal epithelium, which behaves as a molecular switch modulating lymphocyte activation.[55]

MUCOSAL IMMUNE ACTIVATION IN LIVER AUTOIMMUNITY

T_h17 cells are abundant in the intestinal lamina propria where they are induced by commensal bacteria and provide protection against invading pathogens.[56,57] In mice, peripheral T_h17-cells can be redirected from the periphery to the small intestine via chemokine recruitment through CCR6-CCL20 interactions; and in humans, CCL20 is expressed on inflamed bile ducts, suggesting that the same chemokine pathway might promote accumulation in the inflamed liver.[58] Of interest, the recent PBC GWAS meta-analysis by Cordell and colleagues[46] identified CCL20 as a plausible candidate gene, which, given the role of this chemokine axis in the formation and function of gut lymphoid tissues, suggests a pivotal role of the mucosal immune system in the initiation or perpetuation of lymphocytic cholangitis.[59]

The chemokine receptor CXCR5 has also been identified as a risk locus in PBC[18] and is involved in the migration of both T lymphocytes and B lymphocytes to sites of antibody production along a chemokine gradient (ligand CXCL13). CXCR5 is constitutively expressed on mature B lymphocytes and induced on T-follicular helper cells (T_{Fh}) in response to antigen and is critical to formation of intestinal lymphoid follicles.[60] Emerging evidence also indicates that CXCR5 deficiency is associated with defective germinal center responses within the liver, the critical location for driving B-lymphocyte differentiation.[61] This observation is of particular interest given that patients with PBC exhibit an increased frequency of T_{FH} cells in vivo that correlates with increased B-cell activation, disease severity, and biochemical response to ursodeoxycholic acid.[61] IL-7 is another key player for both T and B lymphocyte development and is also necessary for sustaining peripheral T-cell populations. Receptor induction occurs on T-cell positive selection in the thymus and directs thymic $CD8^+$ lineage specification and peripheral naïve T-cell homeostasis, whilst simultaneously having a role in myeloid cell differentiation.[62,63] IL-7R expression is generally reduced on T_{reg} compared with other T-cell subsets, and IL-7 signaling plays an important role in the imprinting of a gut-tropic ($\alpha4\beta7$-integrin positive) phenotype[64] —a noteworthy observation given that mucosal lymphocytes purportedly drive proinflammatory responses in autoimmune cholestasis.[59,65]

Genetic links to mucosal immunity are even more evident in PSC (**Fig. 2**).[59] The importance IL-2/IL-2Rα polymorphisms, suggested through associations at the 4q27 and 10p15 loci, respectively,[26] is supported by the fact that mice lacking IL-2Rα develop autoantibodies and a T-cell–mediated cholangitis together with colitis.[66] Moreover, liver-derived lymphocytes from patients with PSC show reduced expression of the IL-2 receptor and an impaired proliferative response to pathogen stimulation in vitro.[67] IL-2 can contribute to termination of inflammatory immune responses by promoting the development, survival, and function of T_{reg}. Loss of IL2Rα signaling function in PSC is supported by the observation that patients who harbor variant polymorphisms exhibit reduced circulating populations of T_{reg}.[39]

An immunosuppressive role for histone deacetylase (HDAC)-7, a gene implicated in the negative selection of T cells in the thymus and development of tolerogenic immune responses,[26] is supported by a genetic association at 12q13 in PSC GWAS in which the most associated polymorphism was located within an intron encoding serine-threonine protein kinase (PRK)-D2 (19q13). When T-cell receptors of thymocytes are engaged, PRKD2 phosphorylates HDAC7 resulting in loss of its gene regulatory functions. This gives rise to apoptosis and negative selection of immature T cells. Notably, this negative selection takes place owing to a loss of HDAC7-mediated repression of the leukocyte transcription factor Nur77.[26] Nur77 expression parallels that of IL-10 and is heavily influenced by salt-inducible kinase (SIK)-2 polymorphisms, the latter of

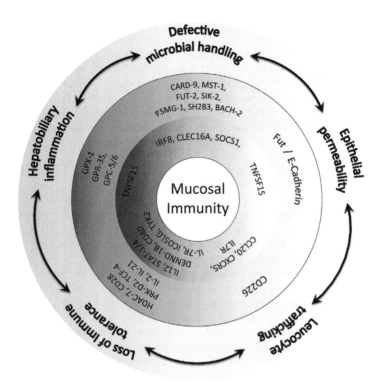

Fig. 2. Mucosal genetics in autoimmune cholestatic liver disease. The strongest genetic associations in autoimmune cholestatic liver disease are within the MHC. However, a significant proportion of non-HLA associations and epigenetic influences underscore the importance of mucosal immunogenicity in the pathogenesis of autoimmune cholangitis. These associations include defective microbial handling and immunopathogenic responses to the commensal microbiome, defects in epithelial (eg, intestinal or biliary) barrier function, dysregulated leukocyte trafficking and homing to sites of injury, loss of intestinal and hepatobiliary tolerogenic responses, and consequently direct tissue inflammation. The outer (*green*) ring in this diagram indicates the putative mucosal pathway, with PSC risk genes identified by the middle (*blue*) ring and PBC risk genes the inner (*red*) ring.

which is also proposed as a genetic risk-locus in PSC. Of note, *IL-10* variants are an established susceptibility factor for early onset ulcerative colitis,[68] and exposing $Il10^{-/-}$ mice to a diet high in saturated fat has been shown to induce specific changes in the bile acid pool that consequently leads to alterations in the gut microbiome and increased susceptibility to IBD[69] – linking multiple putative risk loci to a common mucosal pathway in PSC. Further impression of impaired mucosal tolerance is suggested through a genetic association at 18q21, which contains transcription factor-4; congenital deficiency of which not only results in partial blockade of early B- and T-cell development but also attenuated development of plasmacytoid dendritic cells (pDC) in murine models.[70]

Caspase-recruitment domain (CARD)-9 is an important downstream mediator of signaling from mucosal pattern-recognition receptors (PRR), and genetic associations suggest a link between defective intestinal mucosal microbial handling and the development of PSC.[71] $Card9^{-/-}$ mice seem more susceptible to experimentally-induced colitis and typified by defective IFNγ and T$_h$17 responses, as well as reduced transcription of the mucosal chemokine CCL20; signifying the critical importance of CARD9 in the maintenance of epithelial immunostasis.[72] Another one of the strongest non-HLA associations in PSC is macrophage-stimulating (*MST*)-1, which is also associated with UC and Crohn disease. MST-1 is expressed by BEC and involved in regulating innate immune responses to bacterial ligands, as well as modulating lymphocyte trafficking in lymphoid tissues through integrin- and selectin-mediated adhesion.[73–75] Glutathione peroxidase (GPX)-1 is an antioxidant enzyme located close to MST-1, and polymorphisms in *GPX-1* may also confer an increased disease susceptibility to PSC.[29] Moreover, *Gpx1/2*$^{-/-}$ mice develop a chronic ileocolitis with an increased frequency of colonic malignancy.[76]

Variants in *Fut-2*, an enzyme encoding galactoside 2-alpha-L-fucosyltransferase-2, have also been suggested to confer increased susceptibility to PSC (as well as Crohn's disease), although fall short of reaching significance at a genome-wide level.[77,78] Fucosyltransferase variants alter the recognition and binding of various pathogens to carbohydrate receptors on the mucosal surface and are associated with changes in the commensal phyla in affected patients with PSC characterized by elevated *Firmicutes* and reduced *Proteobacteria*. These aforementioned microbial changes are akin to that observed in *FUT-2* mutations associated with Crohn's colitis and again links defective immune responses to the gut microbiota in PSC. Moreover, variants in *FUT-2* have been described as a risk factor for the development of dominant biliary stenosis in PSC, a putative surrogate of adverse clinical outcomes.[34,79]

An increased lifetime risk of hepatobiliary carcinoma as well as colorectal malignancy is well recognized in PSC[32] and previous studies have indicated that the latter is associated with altered fucosylation of the adhesion molecule E-cadherin.[80] A recent study in mice has illustrated that congenital E-cadherin deletion results in spontaneous periportal inflammation and periductal fibrosis, in addition to an enhanced susceptibility to hepatobiliary cancer, akin to clinical PSC, implying that cholangitis and oncogenesis are a direct result of defective pathogen sensing.[81]

IMMUNO-EPIGENETIC INFLUENCES

Less than 20% of the heritability of autoimmune cholestatic liver diseases have been uncovered by GWAS, and it is likely that some of the missing risk is attributable to environmental triggers or nonhereditary genetic influences. As a female preponderant disease, the frequency of preferential X-chromosome monosomy on peripheral lymphocytes seems to increase with age, at a rate significantly greater compared with normal and non-PBC liver disease-matched controls.[82,83] Of further interest is the increased rate of Y-chromosome loss in men with PBC,[84] suggesting that X-linked alleles or haplotypes predispose to autoimmunity as a result of haploinsufficiency irrespective of sex.

Support of this hypothesis has recently been provided by the Milan PBC Epigenetic Study Group who report striking demethylation of the *CXCR3* promoter that inversely correlated with receptor expression in peripheral blood CD4$^+$ T cells.[85] This finding is of particular significance given that CXCR3 is highly expressed on T_h1 and T_h17 liver-infiltrating CD4$^+$ cells, and the cognate ligands (CXCL9–11) are known to be upregulated on the damaged bile ducts in PBC liver.[86] A further epigenetic observation is reduced methylation of the CD40-ligand promoter regions among patients with PBC compared with controls,[87] which is of particular interest given the importance of CD40 in T- and B-cell interactions. Of note, elevated circulating levels of CD40 have been detected in the serum of patients with systemic autoimmune diseases[88] and ectopic B-cell expression reportedly associated with intestinal inflammation.[89]

Table 1
Conceivable therapeutic targets arising from genetic and epigenetic studies

Pathway	Intervention and Rationale	Expedients	Precedents
IL-12/IL-23	*PBC* IL-12 drives differentiation of activated, naïve T-cells to IFNγ-producing Th1 cells, contributing to loss of tolerance in several models of autoimmunity. Murine models of cholangiopathy also exhibit a milder hepatobiliary phenotype in the absence of functional IL-12. IL-23 (which shares a common p40 subunit with IL-12) is also essential for differentiation of Th17 responses, CD8-mediated IL-17 release and implicated in the breakdown of immune self-tolerance.	Anti-IL-12/23 (ustekinumab) Anti-IL-17A (secukinumab/ixekizumab) Anti-IL17RA (brodalumab)	Crohn disease[93] Psoriasis Psoriasis[94] Uveitis Ankylosing spondylitis Crohn disease[94]
NFκB	*PBC and PSC* Nuclear transcription factor with pleiotropic effects, including regulation of expression of human endothelial adhesion molecules responsible for leukocyte recruitment (eg, VAP-1 and MAdCAM-1), as well as pathways involved in T-cell activation (eg, CD80/CD86).	Anti-CD80 (abatacept) Anti-α4β7 – cognate integrin for MAdCAM-1 (vedolizumab)	Intestinal inflammation[95,96]
CD40–CD40L	*PBC* CD40–CD40L interactions are critical for T-cell–B-cell interactions and elevated circulating CD40 levels recognized in a host of human autoimmune diseases. CD40 antagonists have been shown to be effective in inducing remission from experimentally induced colitis, hematological malignancies and autoimmune encephalitis.	Anti-CD40 (dacetuzumab/lucatumumab)	Multiple sclerosis[97] (preclinical) Chronic lymphatic leukemia, non-Hodgkin lymphoma, multiple myeloma[98]
CXCR3–CXCL9/10/11	*PBC* CXCR3 expression is upregulated on liver-infiltrating Th1 and Th17 cells in early stage PBC and the corresponding ligands secreted in larger quantities by inflamed (versus noninflamed) BEC.	Anti-CXCL10 (MDX-1100)	Rheumatoid arthritis[99]

(continued on next page)

Table 1
(continued)

Pathway	Intervention and Rationale	Expedients	Precedents
CXCR5–CXCL13	*PBC* This chemokine axis guides both B- and T-cell positioning along CXCL13 chemokine gradients and facilitates migration to germinal centers.	Anti-CXCL13 (MAb 5261)	(Preclinical development)[100]
CCL20–CCR6	*PBC* Responsible for the recruitment and positioning of T-cells (predominantly T_h17 cells) around inflamed BEC.	Anti-CCR6	(Preclinical development)
ORMDL3	*PBC* Represents one of several putative risk genes at the 17q12–21 locus and regulates eosinophil trafficking and coexpression of $\alpha4$ integrins. ORMDL3 is also observed to predict response to corticosteroids in childhood asthma.[101,102]	May help to identify corticosteroid response in selected patients	–
GPR35	*PSC* Expressed by intestinal epithelial cells in the intestine and in multiple leukocyte subtypes. Specific activation of GPR35 has been demonstrated to significantly reduce IL-4 release from natural killer T cells. PRKD2 polymorphisms are associated with early onset IBD.[103,104]	Anti-GPR35	Antibody recently developed; clinical applications not yet specified[105]
PRKD2/HDAC7/ Nur77/SIK2	*PSC* A serine-threonine protein kinase, which phosphorylates HDAC7; this gives rise to nuclear exclusion and loss of gene regulatory functions, ultimately resulting in apoptosis and negative selection of immature T cells due to a loss of HDAC7-mediated repression of Nur77, which is regulated by SIK2.	Anti-PRKD2	(Preclinical development)[106]

THERAPEUTIC CONSIDERATIONS AND FUTURE OUTLOOK

The combined output from GWAS and associated works thus far provides explanation for less than 20% of disease heritability in PBC and PSC.[1] Therefore, clinical merits of genomic studies will only be fully realized when genetic and epigenetic data can link to the gut microbiome and environmental influences that collectively occupy the complex orchestra of disease pathogenesis, akin to that which has been described for celiac disease.[90]

Simultaneously, a stratified approach to therapy is hoped to arise that focuses on carefully selected patient populations and structured care delivery.[34] For instance, specific transcriptional signatures enriched for genes involved in memory T-cell generation and receptor-signaling (including IL-7) have been described in UC and Crohn's disease that accurately predict colectomy risk from the point of diagnosis; it is plausible that such bioindicators also exist in immune-mediated liver diseases given the overlapping defects in mucosal immunogenicity.[91] A further, major aim of genetic studies in PBC and PSC has been in the identification of ostensible avenues for future therapeutic exploration. The wealth of overlapping susceptibility loci that are shared with other autoimmune diseases has been extensively discussed in several recent articles,[1,3,4,92] which collectively imply a common genetic architecture underlying immune-mediated tissue injury. This hypothesis needs to be tested and confirmed but, if correct, suggests novel approaches to treatment in which regulatory pathways are enhanced or effector responses suppressed by preventing the activation and recruitment of immunopathogenic cell populations (**Table 1**).

Presently, there is a large shortfall between the available genetic information to date and permeation into clinical practice, a providence that PBC and PSC share with other complex diseases studied on a genome-wide scale. Nevertheless, the advances to date in understanding genetics of chronic cholestasis speak broadly to the ultimate goal of all such studies: to guide treatment that is biologically driven and mechanistically linked.

REFERENCES

1. Hirschfield GM, Chapman RW, Karlsen TH, et al. The genetics of complex cholestatic disorders. Gastroenterology 2013;144(7):1357–74.
2. Trivedi PJ, Hirschfield GM. Review article: overlap syndromes and autoimmune liver disease. Aliment Pharmacol Ther 2012;36(6):517–33.
3. Karlsen TH, Kaser A. Deciphering the genetic predisposition to primary sclerosing cholangitis. Semin Liver Dis 2011;31(2):188–207.
4. Folseraas T, Liaskou E, Anderson CA, et al. Genetics in PSC: what do the "risk genes" teach us? Clin Rev Allergy Immunol 2014;48(2–3):154–64.
5. Boonstra K, Beuers U, Ponsioen CY. Epidemiology of primary sclerosing cholangitis and primary biliary cirrhosis: a systematic review. J Hepatol 2012;56(5): 1181–8.
6. Charman S, Copley L, Tovikkai C, et al. UK Liver Transplant Audit (NHS Blood and Transplant). 2012. Available at: https://www.rcseng.ac.uk/surgeons/research/surgical-research/docs/liver-transplant-audit-report-2012. Accessed July 21, 2015.
7. Arbour L, Rupps R, Field L, et al. Characteristics of primary biliary cirrhosis in British Columbia's First Nations population. Can J Gastroenterol 2005;19(5):305–10.
8. Selmi C, Mayo MJ, Bach N, et al. Primary biliary cirrhosis in monozygotic and dizygotic twins: genetics, epigenetics, and environment. Gastroenterology 2004; 127(2):485–92.

9. Corpechot C, Chrétien Y, Chazouillères O, et al. Demographic, lifestyle, medical and familial factors associated with primary biliary cirrhosis. J Hepatol 2010; 53(1):162–9.

10. Sood S, Gow PJ, Christie JM, et al. Epidemiology of primary biliary cirrhosis in Victoria, Australia: high prevalence in migrant populations. Gastroenterology 2004;127(2):470–5.

11. Watson RG, Angus PW, Dewar M, et al. Low prevalence of primary biliary cirrhosis in Victoria, Australia. Melbourne Liver Group. Gut 1995;36(6):927–30.

12. Trivedi PJ, Cullen S. Etiopathogenesis of primary biliary cirrhosis: an overview of recent developments. Hepatol Int 2013;7(1):28–47.

13. Bergquist A, Lindberg G, Saarinen S, et al. Increased prevalence of primary sclerosing cholangitis among first-degree relatives. J Hepatol 2005;42(2):252–6.

14. Trivedi PJ, Chapman RW. PSC, AIH and overlap syndrome in inflammatory bowel disease. Clin Res Hepatol Gastroenterol 2012;36(5):420–36.

15. Bergquist A, Montgomery SM, Bahmanyar S, et al. Increased risk of primary sclerosing cholangitis and ulcerative colitis in first-degree relatives of patients with primary sclerosing cholangitis. Clin Gastroenterol Hepatol 2008;6(8):939–43.

16. De Boer YS, van Gerven NMF, Zwiers A, et al. Genome-wide association study identifies variants associated with autoimmune hepatitis type 1. Gastroenterology 2014;147(2):443–52.e5.

17. Hirschfield GM, Liu X, Xu C, et al. Primary biliary cirrhosis associated with HLA, IL12A, and IL12RB2 variants. N Engl J Med 2009;360(24):2544–55.

18. Mells GF, Floyd JAB, Morley KI, et al. Genome-wide association study identifies 12 new susceptibility loci for primary biliary cirrhosis. Nat Genet 2011;43(4): 329–32.

19. Liu X, Invernizzi P, Lu Y, et al. Genome-wide meta-analyses identify three loci associated with primary biliary cirrhosis. Nat Genet 2010;42(8):658–60.

20. Nakamura M, Nishida N, Kawashima M, et al. Genome-wide association study identifies TNFSF15 and POU2AF1 as susceptibility loci for primary biliary cirrhosis in the Japanese population. Am J Hum Genet 2012;91(4):721–8.

21. Invernizzi P. Human leukocyte antigen in primary biliary cirrhosis: an old story now reviving. Hepatology 2011;54(2):714–23.

22. Umemura T, Zen Y, Hamano H, et al. Immunoglobin G4-hepatopathy: association of immunoglobin G4-bearing plasma cells in liver with autoimmune pancreatitis. Hepatology 2007;46(2):463–71.

23. Lleo A, Bowlus CL, Yang G-X, et al. Biliary apotopes and anti-mitochondrial antibodies activate innate immune responses in primary biliary cirrhosis. Hepatology 2010;52(3):987–98.

24. Lleo A, Selmi C, Invernizzi P, et al. Apotopes and the biliary specificity of primary biliary cirrhosis. Hepatology 2009;49(3):871–9.

25. Shimoda S, Van de Water J, Ansari A, et al. Identification and precursor frequency analysis of a common T cell epitope motif in mitochondrial autoantigens in primary biliary cirrhosis. J Clin Invest 1998;102(10):1831–40.

26. Liu JZ, Hov JR, Folseraas T, et al. Dense genotyping of immune-related disease regions identifies nine new risk loci for primary sclerosing cholangitis. Nat Genet 2013;45(6):670–5.

27. Karlsen TH, Franke A, Melum E, et al. Genome-wide association analysis in primary sclerosing cholangitis. Gastroenterology 2010;138(3):1102–11.

28. Naess S, Björnsson E, Anmarkrud JA, et al. Small duct primary sclerosing cholangitis without inflammatory bowel disease is genetically different from large duct disease. Liver Int 2014;34(10):1488–95.

29. Melum E, Franke A, Schramm C, et al. Genome-wide association analysis in primary sclerosing cholangitis identifies two non-HLA susceptibility loci. Nat Genet 2011;43(1):17–9.
30. Okada Y, Yamazaki K, Umeno J, et al. HLA-Cw*1202-B*5201-DRB1*1502 haplotype increases risk for ulcerative colitis but reduces risk for Crohn's disease. Gastroenterology 2011;141(3):864–71.e1–5.
31. Rudolph G, Gotthardt D, Kloeters-Plachky P, et al. PSC with dominant bile duct stenosis, IBD is associated with an increase of carcinomas and reduced survival. J Hepatol 2010;53(2):313–7.
32. Boonstra K, Weersma RK, van Erpecum KJ, et al. Population-based epidemiology, malignancy risk, and outcome of primary sclerosing cholangitis. Hepatology 2013;58(6):2045–55.
33. Mendes FD, Jorgensen R, Keach J, et al. Elevated serum IgG4 concentration in patients with primary sclerosing cholangitis. Am J Gastroenterol 2006;101(9): 2070–5.
34. Trivedi PJ, Corpechot C, Pares A, et al. Risk stratification in autoimmune cholestatic liver diseases: Opportunities for clinicians and trialists. Hepatology 2015. [Epub ahead of print].
35. Berntsen NL, Klingenberg O, Juran BD, et al. Association between HLA haplotypes and increased serum levels of IgG4 in patients with primary sclerosing cholangitis. Gastroenterology 2015;148(5):924–7.e2.
36. Katt J, Schwinge D, Schoknecht T, et al. Increased Th17 response to pathogen stimulation in patients with primary sclerosing cholangitis. Hepatology 2013; 58(3):1084–93.
37. Yang C-Y, Ma X, Tsuneyama K, et al. IL-12/Th1 and IL-23/Th17 biliary microenvironment in primary biliary cirrhosis: implications for therapy. Hepatology 2014; 59(5):1944–53.
38. Hudspeth K, Pontarini E, Tentorio P, et al. The role of natural killer cells in autoimmune liver disease: a comprehensive review. J Autoimmun 2013;46: 55–65.
39. Sebode M, Peiseler M, Franke B, et al. Reduced FOXP3(+) regulatory T cells in patients with primary sclerosing cholangitis are associated with IL2RA gene polymorphisms. J Hepatol 2014;60(5):1010–6.
40. Rong G, Zhou Y, Xiong Y, et al. Imbalance between T helper type 17 and T regulatory cells in patients with primary biliary cirrhosis: the serum cytokine profile and peripheral cell population. Clin Exp Immunol 2009;156(2): 217–25.
41. Yao Y, Yang W, Yang Y-Q, et al. Distinct from its canonical effects, deletion of IL-12p40 induces cholangitis and fibrosis in interleukin-2Rα(-/-) mice. J Autoimmun 2014;51:99–108.
42. Korn T, Bettelli E, Oukka M, et al. IL-17 and Th17 cells. Annu Rev Immunol 2009; 27:485–517.
43. Filipe-Santos O, Bustamante J, Chapgier A, et al. Inborn errors of IL-12/23- and IFN-gamma-mediated immunity: molecular, cellular, and clinical features. Semin Immunol 2006;18(6):347–61.
44. Barrett JC, Clayton DG, Concannon P, et al. Genome-wide association study and meta-analysis find that over 40 loci affect risk of type 1 diabetes. Nat Genet 2009;41(6):703–7.
45. Barrett JC, Hansoul S, Nicolae DL, et al. Genome-wide association defines more than 30 distinct susceptibility loci for Crohn's disease. Nat Genet 2008;40(8): 955–62.

46. Cordell HJ, Han Y, Mells GF, et al. International genome-wide meta-analysis identifies new primary biliary cirrhosis risk loci and targetable pathogenic pathways. Nat Commun 2015, in press.

47. Yoshida K, Yang G-X, Zhang W, et al. Deletion of interleukin-12p40 suppresses autoimmune cholangitis in dominant negative transforming growth factor beta receptor type II mice. Hepatology 2009;50(5):1494–500.

48. Carbone M, Mells GF, Alexander GJ, et al. Calcineurin inhibitors and the IL12A locus influence risk of recurrent primary biliary cirrhosis after liver transplantation. Am J Transplant 2013;13(4):1110–1.

49. Juran BD, Atkinson EJ, Larson JJ, et al. Carriage of a tumor necrosis factor polymorphism amplifies the cytotoxic T-lymphocyte antigen 4 attributed risk of primary biliary cirrhosis: evidence for a gene-gene interaction. Hepatology 2010; 52(1):223–9.

50. Liaskou E, Jeffery LE, Trivedi PJ, et al. Loss of CD28 expression by liver-infiltrating T cells contributes to pathogenesis of primary sclerosing cholangitis. Gastroenterology 2014;147(1):221–32.e7.

51. Tacke F, Luedde T, Trautwein C. Inflammatory pathways in liver homeostasis and liver injury. Clin Rev Allergy Immunol 2009;36(1):4–12.

52. Kar SP, Seldin MF, Chen W, et al. Pathway-based analysis of primary biliary cirrhosis genome-wide association studies. Genes Immun 2013;14(3):179–86.

53. Neuman M, Angulo P, Malkiewicz I, et al. Tumor necrosis factor-alpha and transforming growth factor-beta reflect severity of liver damage in primary biliary cirrhosis. J Gastroenterol Hepatol 2002;17(2):196–202.

54. Liaskou E, Karikoski M, Reynolds GM, et al. Regulation of mucosal addressin cell adhesion molecule 1 expression in human and mice by vascular adhesion protein 1 amine oxidase activity. Hepatology 2011;53(2):661–72.

55. Steinberg MW, Shui J-W, Ware CF, et al. Regulating the mucosal immune system: the contrasting roles of LIGHT, HVEM, and their various partners. Semin Immunopathol 2009;31(2):207–21.

56. Atarashi K, Nishimura J, Shima T, et al. ATP drives lamina propria T(H)17 cell differentiation. Nature 2008;455(7214):808–12.

57. Puel A, Döffinger R, Natividad A, et al. Autoantibodies against IL-17A, IL-17F, and IL-22 in patients with chronic mucocutaneous candidiasis and autoimmune polyendocrine syndrome type I. J Exp Med 2010;207(2):291–7.

58. Esplugues E, Huber S, Gagliani N, et al. Control of TH17 cells occurs in the small intestine. Nature 2011;475(7357):514–8.

59. Trivedi PJ, Adams DH. Mucosal immunity in liver autoimmunity: a comprehensive review. J Autoimmun 2013;46:97–111.

60. Marchesi F, Martin AP, Thirunarayanan N, et al. CXCL13 expression in the gut promotes accumulation of IL-22-producing lymphoid tissue-inducer cells, and formation of isolated lymphoid follicles. Mucosal Immunol 2009;2(6): 486–94.

61. Wang L, Sun Y, Zhang Z, et al. CXCR5+ CD4+ T follicular helper cells participate in the pathogenesis of primary biliary cirrhosis. Hepatology 2015;61(2): 627–38.

62. Zhang W, Sharma R, Ju S-T, et al. Deficiency in regulatory T cells results in development of antimitochondrial antibodies and autoimmune cholangitis. Hepatology 2009;49(2):545–52.

63. Oertelt S, Lian Z-X, Cheng C-M, et al. Anti-mitochondrial antibodies and primary biliary cirrhosis in TGF-beta receptor II dominant-negative mice. J Immunol 2006;177(3):1655–60.

64. Cimbro R, Vassena L, Arthos J, et al. IL-7 induces expression and activation of integrin α4β7 promoting naive T-cell homing to the intestinal mucosa. Blood 2012;120(13):2610–9.
65. Tsuda M, Ambrosini YM, Zhang W, et al. Fine phenotypic and functional characterization of effector cluster of differentiation 8 positive T cells in human patients with primary biliary cirrhosis. Hepatology 2011;54(4):1293–302.
66. Wakabayashi K, Lian Z-X, Moritoki Y, et al. IL-2 receptor alpha(-/-) mice and the development of primary biliary cirrhosis. Hepatology 2006;44(5):1240–9.
67. Bo X, Broome U, Remberger M, et al. Tumour necrosis factor alpha impairs function of liver derived T lymphocytes and natural killer cells in patients with primary sclerosing cholangitis. Gut 2001;49(1):131–41.
68. Moran CJ, Walters TD, Guo C-H, et al. IL-10R polymorphisms are associated with very-early-onset ulcerative colitis. Inflamm Bowel Dis 2013;19(1):115–23.
69. Devkota S, Wang Y, Musch MW, et al. Dietary-fat-induced taurocholic acid promotes pathobiont expansion and colitis in Il10-/- mice. Nature 2012;487(7405):104–8.
70. Reizis B. Regulation of plasmacytoid dendritic cell development. Curr Opin Immunol 2010;22(2):206–11.
71. Hara H, Saito T. CARD9 versus CARMA1 in innate and adaptive immunity. Trends Immunol 2009;30(5):234–42.
72. Sokol H, Conway KL, Zhang M, et al. Card9 mediates intestinal epithelial cell restitution, T-helper 17 responses, and control of bacterial infection in mice. Gastroenterology 2013;145(3):591–601.e3.
73. Raab M, Wang H, Lu Y, et al. T cell receptor "inside-out" pathway via signaling module SKAP1-RapL regulates T cell motility and interactions in lymph nodes. Immunity 2010;32(4):541–56.
74. Katagiri K, Katakai T, Ebisuno Y, et al. Mst1 controls lymphocyte trafficking and interstitial motility within lymph nodes. EMBO J 2009;28(9):1319–31.
75. Häuser F, Deyle C, Berard D, et al. Macrophage-stimulating protein polymorphism rs3197999 is associated with a gain of function: implications for inflammatory bowel disease. Genes Immun 2012;13(4):321–7.
76. Lee D-H, Esworthy RS, Chu C, et al. Mutation accumulation in the intestine and colon of mice deficient in two intracellular glutathione peroxidases. Cancer Res 2006;66(20):9845–51.
77. Folseraas T, Melum E, Rausch P, et al. Extended analysis of a genome-wide association study in primary sclerosing cholangitis detects multiple novel risk loci. J Hepatol 2012;57(2):366–75.
78. Rausch P, Rehman A, Künzel S, et al. Colonic mucosa-associated microbiota is influenced by an interaction of Crohn disease and FUT2 (secretor) genotype. Proc Natl Acad Sci U S A 2011;108(47):19030–5.
79. Rupp C, Friedrich K, Folseraas T, et al. Fut2 genotype is a risk factor for dominant stenosis and biliary candida infections in primary sclerosing cholangitis. Aliment Pharmacol Ther 2014;39(8):873–82.
80. Gaj P, Maryan N, Hennig EE, et al. Pooled sample-based GWAS: a cost-effective alternative for identifying colorectal and prostate cancer risk variants in the polish population. PLoS One 2012;7(4):e35307.
81. Nakagawa H, Hikiba Y, Hirata Y, et al. Loss of liver E-cadherin induces sclerosing cholangitis and promotes carcinogenesis. Proc Natl Acad Sci U S A 2014;111(3):1090–5.
82. Invernizzi P, Miozzo M, Battezzati PM, et al. Frequency of monosomy X in women with primary biliary cirrhosis. Lancet 2004;363(9408):533–5.

83. Miozzo M, Selmi C, Gentilin B, et al. Preferential X chromosome loss but random inactivation characterize primary biliary cirrhosis. Hepatology 2007;46(2):456–62.

84. Lleo A, Oertelt-Prigione S, Bianchi I, et al. Y chromosome loss in male patients with primary biliary cirrhosis. J Autoimmun 2013;41:87–91.

85. Lleo A, Zhang W, Zhao M, et al. DNA methylation profiling of the X chromosome reveals an aberrant demethylation on CXCR3 promoter in primary biliary cirrhosis. Clin Epigenetics 2015;7(1):61.

86. Chuang Y-H, Lian Z-X, Cheng C-M, et al. Increased levels of chemokine receptor CXCR3 and chemokines IP-10 and MIG in patients with primary biliary cirrhosis and their first degree relatives. J Autoimmun 2005;25(2): 126–32.

87. Lleo A, Liao J, Invernizzi P, et al. Immunoglobulin M levels inversely correlate with CD40 ligand promoter methylation in patients with primary biliary cirrhosis. Hepatology 2012;55(1):153–60.

88. Goules A, Tzioufas AG, Manousakis MN, et al. Elevated levels of soluble CD40 ligand (sCD40L) in serum of patients with systemic autoimmune diseases. J Autoimmun 2006;26(3):165–71.

89. Kawamura T, Kanai T, Dohi T, et al. Ectopic CD40 ligand expression on B cells triggers intestinal inflammation. J Immunol 2004;172(10):6388–97.

90. Armstrong MJ, Hegade VS, Robins G. Advances in coeliac disease. Curr Opin Gastroenterol 2012;28(2):104–12.

91. Lee JC, Lyons PA, McKinney EF, et al. Gene expression profiling of CD8+ T cells predicts prognosis in patients with Crohn disease and ulcerative colitis. J Clin Invest 2011;121(10):4170–9.

92. Hirschfield GM, Siminovitch KA. Genetics in PBC: what do the "risk genes" teach us? Clin Rev Allergy Immunol 2014;48(2–3):176–81.

93. Teng MWL, Bowman EP, McElwee JJ, et al. IL-12 and IL-23 cytokines: from discovery to targeted therapies for immune-mediated inflammatory diseases. Nat Med 2015;21(7):719–29.

94. Zhang H, Bernuzzi F, Lleo A, et al. Therapeutic potential of IL-17-mediated signaling pathway in autoimmune liver diseases. Mediators Inflamm 2015; 2015:436450.

95. Heninger A-K, Wentrup S, Al-Saeedi M, et al. Immunomodulation of human intestinal T cells by the synthetic CD80 antagonist RhuDex®. Immun Inflamm Dis 2014;2(3):166–80.

96. Lobatón T, Vermeire S, Van Assche G, et al. Review article: anti-adhesion therapies for inflammatory bowel disease. Aliment Pharmacol Ther 2014;39(6): 579–94.

97. Hart BA, Hintzen RQ, Laman JD. Preclinical assessment of therapeutic antibodies against human CD40 and human interleukin-12/23p40 in a nonhuman primate model of multiple sclerosis. Neurodegener Dis 2008;5(1):38–52.

98. Hassan SB, Sørensen JF, Olsen BN, et al. Anti-CD40-mediated cancer immunotherapy: an update of recent and ongoing clinical trials. Immunopharmacol Immunotoxicol 2014;36(2):96–104.

99. Yellin M, Paliienko I, Balanescu A, et al. A phase II, randomized, double-blind, placebo-controlled study evaluating the efficacy and safety of MDX-1100, a fully human anti-CXCL10 monoclonal antibody, in combination with methotrexate in patients with rheumatoid arthritis. Arthritis Rheum 2012; 64(6):1730–9.

100. Klimatcheva E, Pandina T, Reilly C, et al. CXCL13 antibody for the treatment of autoimmune disorders. BMC Immunol 2015;16:6.

101. Ha SG, Ge XN, Bahaie NS, et al. ORMDL3 promotes eosinophil trafficking and activation via regulation of integrins and CD48. Nat Commun 2013;4:2479.
102. Berce V, Kozmus CEP, Potočnik U. Association among ORMDL3 gene expression, 17q21 polymorphism and response to treatment with inhaled corticosteroids in children with asthma. Pharmacogenomics J 2013;13(6):523–9.
103. Fallarini S, Magliulo L, Paoletti T, et al. Expression of functional GPR35 in human iNKT cells. Biochem Biophys Res Commun 2010;398(3):420–5.
104. Imielinski M, Baldassano RN, Griffiths A, et al. Common variants at five new loci associated with early-onset inflammatory bowel disease. Nat Genet 2009; 41(12):1335–40.
105. Jenkins L, Harries N, Lappin JE, et al. Antagonists of GPR35 display high species ortholog selectivity and varying modes of action. J Pharmacol Exp Ther 2012;343(3):683–95.
106. Harikumar KB, Kunnumakkara AB, Ochi N, et al. A novel small-molecule inhibitor of protein kinase D blocks pancreatic cancer growth in vitro and in vivo. Mol Cancer Ther 2010;9(5):1136–46.

Making Sense of Autoantibodies in Cholestatic Liver Diseases

Simona Marzorati, PhD[a,b], Pietro Invernizzi, MD, PhD[a,c],
Ana Lleo, MD, PhD[a,*]

KEYWORDS

- Autoantibody • Cholestatic diseases • Biliary tree • Mitochondria • Nuclear proteins
- Laboratory tools

KEY POINTS

- Primary biliary cirrhosis (PBC) is a model autoimmune disease; antimitochondrial antibodies against the E2 component of the pyruvate dehydrogenase complex are highly specific, and their presence is a major diagnostic criteria.
- PBC-specific antinuclear antibodies have a prognostic role in PBC because their presence defines a more aggressive phenotype.
- A large number of autoantibodies have been detected in primary sclerosing cholangitis (PSC) patients, but the specificity of these antibodies is generally low, and the frequencies vary largely between different studies.
- The pathogenic role of autoantibodies remains unknown and constitutes a priority for basic and clinical research in both PBC and PSC.

INTRODUCTION

Cholestasis is an impairment of bile formation or bile flow that may affect any age group and presents typical clinical signs: jaundice, pruritus, and fatigue; of note, early biochemical markers are often detected in asymptomatic patients. Most commonly, cholestasis results from obstructive lesions of the extrahepatic biliary tree by gallstones or local malignancies, although hepatocellular cholestasis may be due to impairment in the secretory machinery of hepatocytes and cholangiocytes.[1]

The authors have nothing to disclose.
[a] Liver Unit and Center for Autoimmune Liver Diseases, Humanitas Clinical and Research Center, Via A. Manzoni 113, Rozzano, Milan 20089, Italy; [b] Department of Electronics, Information and Bioengineering, Politecnico di Milano, via Ponzio 34/5, Milan 20133, Italy; [c] Division of Rheumatology, Allergy, and Clinical Immunology, University of California Davis, GBSF, 451 Health Science Drive, Davis, CA 95616, USA
* Corresponding author.
E-mail address: ana.lleo@humanitas.it

Clin Liver Dis 20 (2016) 33–46
http://dx.doi.org/10.1016/j.cld.2015.08.003
1089-3261/16/$ – see front matter © 2016 Elsevier Inc. All rights reserved.
liver.theclinics.com

The signaling of bile major components as well as the digestive function has been gradually unraveled over the last century. Nowadays, bile formation is known as a vital secretory process highly regulated by transcriptional and posttranscriptional mechanisms in hepatocytes, cholangiocytes, and terminal ileum. Moreover, it is widely accepted that accumulation of bile acids within liver cells cause detergent-induced damage of cellular membranes, which ultimately determines the development of necrosis, apoptosis, inflammation, fibrosis, and carcinogenesis.[2] Nevertheless, the molecular mechanisms involved in the development and progression of cholestatic liver diseases (CLD) are still largely unknown.[3]

The most common chronic CLD in adults are associated with immune mechanisms, such as primary biliary cirrhosis (PBC) and primary sclerosing cholangitis (PSC). Antibodies directed against almost all the functional structures of the cell can be detected in these diseases, and its presence plays a central role in the diagnosis and classification of this kind of disorders, although their role in the pathogenesis remains challenging.

PBC is considered a model autoimmune disease on the basis of several features: highly direct and very specific immune response to mitochondrial autoantigens, female predominance, and homogeneity among patients.[4,5] Antimitochondrial antibodies (AMA) against the E2 component of the pyruvate dehydrogenase complex (PDC-E2), the immunodominant mitochondrial autoantigen, are highly specific in PBC and can appear before other histologic or biochemical signs of liver injury.[6] Moreover, specific PBC antinuclear antibodies (ANA) have been shown to have a prognostic significance.[7] PSC is a rare but important cause of CLD and is characterized by chronic inflammation and obliterative fibrosis of the intrahepatic and extrahepatic biliary tree, which leads to bile stasis, hepatic fibrosis, and, ultimately, cirrhosis. The etiopathogenesis of PSC is unknown, although there is growing evidence that (auto) immune-mediated mechanisms play a role.[8] Perinuclear antineutrophil cytoplasmic antibodies (p-ANCA) are the most frequently detected antibodies in PSC but have low specificity for diagnosis.[9]

The clinical care for patients with CLD in recent years has advanced considerably thanks to growing insight into pathophysiological mechanisms and remarkable methodological and technical developments in diagnostic procedures that led to new therapeutic and preventive approaches. This review focuses on the clinical relevance of autoantibodies in CLD with particular attention to recently published data. Moreover, some unanswered questions are discussed, such as the importance of new technologies for autoantibody detection.

AUTOANTIBODIES IN PRIMARY BILIARY CIRRHOSIS

PBC is a chronic cholestatic disease characterized by an orchestrated attack of the biliary epithelial cells (BECs) determining progressive bile duct destruction, and eventually leading to cirrhosis and liver failure.[10] The pathogenesis of the condition involves autoimmune mechanisms that have been largely dissected over the last decade.[11–14]

Antimitochondrial Antibodies

AMAs are the major hallmark of PBC and have mainly a diagnostic rather than prognostic connotation. AMAs were described for the first time in 1965 in a patient affected by PBC[15]; years later Gershwin and colleagues[11] defined, at the molecular level, the targets of AMAs. Subsequently, the autoreactive CD4+ and CD8+ T-cell responses present in human peripheral blood mononuclear cells and liver were dissected.[12,13] These data led to the thesis that a multilineage loss of tolerance to

PDC-E2 is an essential requirement for the 95% of PBC patients that are AMA-positive.[16,17] AMA titer does not correlate with severity or activity of the disease.[18] Despite the controversy reported in literature regarding the importance of its titration among PBC-affected patients,[19,20] AMA titer may differ by more than 200-fold, but in the single patient can remain stable over the years.[21] The measurement of serum AMA is typically based on the immunofluorescent techniques (IIF) (the criteria of positivity, greater than 1:40).[1] Thanks to recent advances in technologies, new assays for AMA detection are now available, such as enzyme-linked immunosorbent assays (ELISA) or Western blotting (**Table 1**). Gershwin and colleagues[11] in 1987 first demonstrated that the target antigen of AMA-M2 is a component of the 2-oxo-acid dehydrogenase complexes (2-OADC), and that AMA are directed against 3 components of this complex family[10]: the E2 subunits of the pyruvate dehydrogenase complex (PDC-E2), the branched chain 2-oxo-acid dehydrogenase complex (BCOADC-E2), and the oxoglutarate dehydrogenase complex (OGDC-E2) as well as the dihydrolipoamide dehydrogenase-binding protein and the E1α subunit of pyruvate dehydrogenase complex (PDC-E1α). Following the nomenclature suggested by this study, it is possible now to classify the majority ($\sim$90%) of patients with antibodies against the major component of 2-oxo-acid dehydrogenase complex family (PDC-E2, BCOADC-E2, OGDC-E2).[10] PDC-E2 has a well-conserved sequence with a high degree of identity across all species[22]; the amino acid motif ExDK in the peptide (the amino acid residues E, D, K are at proteins 170, 172, and 173, respectively) seems to be responsible for its recognition by specific T cells.[23]

Numerous studies suggest a pathogenetic role of AMA in PBC even if it is still not clear how PDC-E2 and other epitopes localized to the inner membrane of mitochondria become targets of autoimmune injury in PBC. Gershwin[24] suggests that a modification of 2-OADC by xenobiotics may alter these self-proteins to cause a breakdown of tolerance facilitating an autoimmune response. It is now known that in PBC patients, PDC-E2 remains immunologically intact in BECs becoming source of the PDC-E2 apotope.[14] Circulating AMA recognizes PDC-E2 in apoptotic bodies, resulting in a complex that stimulates innate immune systems in genetically susceptible individuals.[25]

Anti-nuclear Antibodies

ANA are detected in a wide variety of liver diseases and nonhepatic autoimmune disease.[26] ANAs were first detected in the 1950s by using IIF. Because of the high rate of false positive serum, end point titers are constantly under debate.[26,27] Almost 50% of PBC patients show specific antibodies direct to centromeric proteins, such as DNA, chromatin, or histones.[28] The improvement of laboratory assay (eg, introduction of fixed HEp-2 cells as a source of nuclear antigens) has helped to increase specificity and sensitivity of indirect IIF microscopy assay and allowed the identification of multiple patterns.[29] Generally, on the basis of their different

Table 1 Sensitivity and specificity of antimitochondrial antibodies by different tests			
Methods	Specificity (%)	Sensitivity (%)	References
IIF	98.4	84.6	77,78
Commercially ELISA	95.3	83.2	78–80
MIT3-based ELISA	95	79.7	78,81
WB	91.7	88.3	77,78

intranuclear distributions, IIF-ANA (indirect immunofluorescence antinuclear antibody test) staining patterns recognize homogenous/chromosomal, centromeric, speckled/extrachromosomal, nucleolar, nuclear membrane, nuclear dot, and other disease-defined patterns.[30] Specific patterns for PBC are multiple nuclear dots (MND, detected in 20% of patients) and the rimlike/membranous (RL/M, detected in 20% of patients); by contrast, the anticentromere and the speckled patterns, which are not disease specific, can be found in up to 60% and 30% of patients, respectively.[31–33] The molecular targets of the RL/M pattern are constituents of the nuclear envelope, including gp210, lamin B receptor (LBR), and nucleoporin p62; the MND pattern mainly originates from autoantibodies directed to the Sp100 and the promyelocytic leukemia protein. Anti-gp210 and anti-LBR are extremely specific for PBC (more than 99%), with sensitivity between 10–25% and 1% respectively.[34,35]

Importantly, there is evidence that ANA reactivity correlates with different clinical behavior in PBC[36]; the persistence of anti-gp210 and possibly anti-p62 are strong risk factors for the evolution to end-stage liver disease.[37] The observation that ANA is significantly higher in AMA-negative PBC patients suggests that PBC-specific ANA can be used to confirm diagnosis of PBC in AMA-negative subjects; indeed, in a large series of AMA-negative PBC subjects, 92% of them were found positive for nuclear dots and Sp100 and 99% for nuclear rim and gp210.[38]

AUTOANTIBODIES IN PRIMARY SCLEROSING CHOLANGITIS

PSC is a chronic inflammatory disease of the intrahepatic and extrahepatic biliary tree, leading to progressive bile duct structures and liver cirrhosis.[39] Several mechanisms have been suggested (dysregulation of immune signaling, increase delivery of toxins, damage from toxic bile acids); however, its pathogenesis is still under debate.[40] Immune responses against self-antigens in the bile ducts have been reported to play a role in the etiopathogenesis of PSC[41]; however, whether PSC should be considered an autoimmune or merely immune-mediated disease is still unclear.[8]

The PSC population is heterogeneous, comprising subgroups of regular large-duct PSC, patients with small-duct affection only,[42] and an overlap-syndrome between PSC and autoimmune hepatitis (AIH). The importance of genetic factors in PSC is already demonstrated, such as implication of immune-mediated mechanism[43] and the association with particular human leukocyte antigen haplotypes.[44] Diagnostic signs include cholestatic liver enzyme derangement and typical abnormal cholangiogram.[1]

It has been suggested that the presence of autoantibodies in PSC is the result of a nonspecific dysregulation of the immune system; however, some evidence in PSC highlights the possible presence of specific self-targets in the biliary epithelium and in colon epithelium.[41,45] Indeed, it has been reported that the presence of antibodies against BECs at high frequencies in sera from PSC (63%)[46] and some epitopes have been suggested.[47] Taken together, those data suggest that antigens expressed in the biliary epithelium may determine self-reactive immune responses in PSC; however, the epitope remains to be determined, and the clinical significance of the autoantibodies has never been studied.

The most common and well-studied autoantibodies in PSC are the antineutrophil cytoplasmic antibodies (ANCA) that are detectable in 26% to 94% of PSC patients[48]; however, this antibody has low specificity for diagnosis.[49] ANCA, directed against various subcellular constituents of neutrophil or myeloid cells, are routinely detected by indirect immunofluorescence assays.[50] The IIF ANCA staining pattern has broad, nonhomogeneous enhancement and has been referred to as atypical ANCA, antineutrophil nuclear antibodies, cytoplasmic, and perinuclear (pANCA).

The cytoplasmic antigens targeted by ANCA in PSC are still unknown even though several cytoplasmic proteins have been proposed, including lactoferrin, myeloperoxidase, cathepsin G, proteinase 3 (PR3), and catalase, among others.[51]

Importantly, dissection of the antigenic target of ANCAs would allow prospective studies in order to define their diagnostic potential in PSC. Indeed, the clinical and diagnostic relevance of ANCA is still under debate. ANCA have been proposed to be associated with intestinal affection in PSC; however, a higher prevalence of ANCA in PSC patients with inflammatory bowel disease has not been clearly demonstrated.[52] Furthermore, a few reports associate ANCA with biliary calculi or cholangiocarcinoma but the data need to be consolidated.[53] Finally, the potential prognostic role of pANCA has been investigated, but, even though some studies seem to suggest an association with the presence of end-stage liver disease in pANCA-positive PSC patients,[53] no significant correlation has been clearly demonstrated.[54]

Several other autoantibodies have been detected in the serum of PSC patients, such as ANA (8%–77%)[55] and smooth muscle antibody (0%–83%).[9] However, none of the autoantibodies described in PSC have sufficient specificity or sensitivity to be used for screening or diagnosis.

OTHER AUTOANTIBODIES

Newly available tools allowed identifying other autoantibodies, mostly in conjunction with other autoimmnune diseases, which can be indicators of disease course or outcome. Some of these autoantibodies have been described as having levels and frequencies higher in CLD rather than in other autoimmune diseases: more than 60 autoantibodies have been detected so far in PBC patients, for example.[56]

Of interest, Norman and colleagues[57] recently identified, using high-density human recombinant protein microarrays, 2 potential new biomarkers in PBC: kelch-like 12 (KLHL12) and hexokinase-1 (HK1). Anti-KLHL12 and anti-HK1 antibodies were both highly specific for PBC (≥95%) with a higher sensitivity than anti-gp210 and anti-sp100 antibodies. If validated, this could be of enormous interest, especially in AMA-negative subjects.

An overview of most frequently described autoantibodies (prevalence in CLD >10%) in the literature and their target antigens can be found in **Table 2**.

AUTOANTIBODY DETECTION

The detection of serum autoantibodies has a central role in the diagnosis and classification of CLD. Unfortunately, because of intrinsic limitations of the methodology itself, lack of standardization, and problems concerning interpretation of results, false positive or false negative results are frequently encountered.[49] Many different technologies are widely used, and some of these conventional methods are difficult to manage and time-consuming and present drawbacks and limitations. So far, there is no gold-standard assay (with 100% sensitivity and 100% specificity) for the detection of auto-antibody. Recent technologies have been developed, taking advantage, for example, of antigenic sources (recombinant or native), implementation of accuracy, and reliability of laboratory tools and automation. The possibility of simultaneously testing a high number of analytes overcomes some of the limitations of conventional methods. More recently, functional protein microarrays were also designed to survey thousands of potential antigens in a single experiment and have facilitated rapid and cost-effective identification of biomarkers. Routinely, in clinical practice, IIF is a first-line

Table 2
Autoantibody patterns encountered in cholestatic liver diseases (prevalence >10%) in association with other autoimmune disease with their corresponding target antigens

Autoantibody	Specific Target	Ref.
Anti-CCP	Cyclic citrullinated peptide	82
Anti-HSP	Heat-shock protein	83
Anti-LSP	Liver-specific protein	84
Anti-p97/VCP	p97/valosin-containing protein	85–87
Anti-PS	Phosphatidylserine	88
Anti-β2GPI	β2-glycoprotein I	89,90
Ro52	TRIM21 protein	66
Anti-calreticulina	Calreticulin	91
AGA	Gliadin	92
Anti-LF	Lactoferrin	93
Anti-TG	Thyroglobulin	94
Anti-CA II	Carbonic anhydrase II	95
Anti-a-enolase	α-Enolase	96
Anti-ClpP	Microbial caseinolytic protease P	89
Anti-FH	Fumarate hydratase	97
Anti-tTG	Tissue transglutaminase	88
Anti-TPO	Thyroid peroxidase	94
Anti-EPO	Eosinophil peroxidase	88
Anti-MPO	Myeloperoxidase	9
ARPA (antibody to the β-subunit of bacterial RNA polymerase)	β-Subunit of bacterial RNA polymerase	98
ASCA	*Saccharomyces cerevisiae*	88

screening. If a negative result is obtained, when the clinical evidence of PBC diagnosis is clear, the flowchart recommends using a solid-phase assay such as ELISA.

Indirect Immunofluorescence

IIF staining uses tissue sections or cultured cells as an antigenic source and detects the specific recognition of autoantibodies to native antigens. Most relevant literature in recent years is based on results obtained with the HEp-2 substrate that has largely replaced rodent tissues and has become the standard substrate.[58] However, the International Group of AIH suggested that HEp2 cells should not be used initially as screening because of the high positivity rate in lower dilutions.[59] Despite its widespread use, IIF appears to be a rather insensitive test for some autoantibody detection[32] and still presents numerous disadvantages: (a) is time consuming, (b) cannot be automated, (c) requires substantial experience in interpreting subjective patterns, (d) does not provide information regarding the antigenic specificity, and (e) is not specific in the presence of concurrent antibody reactivity. Moreover, the literature reports that 15% of PBC patients are AMA-negative at routine IIF.[38]

The "International consensus statement on testing and reporting antineutrophil cytoplasmic antibodies (ANCA)" suggests that also for this autoantibody, indirect immunofluorescence is the first method of choice for screening. Then, an enzyme-linked immunoassay should be tested for the major ANCA specificities, PR3, and myeloperoxidase.[50]

Most CLD sera are heterogeneous and present autoantibodies with different specificities. When an overlapping staining pattern is observed and IIF cannot distinguish between various kinds of circulating autoantibodies, complementary methods can help to identify and characterize reactive autoantigens.[60] All the studies suggest that using more than one laboratory assay is mandatory to confirm diagnosis.

Solid Phase Immunoassay

ELISA is a simple, sensitive, inexpensive, and less time-consuming assay widely used to detect autoantibody in sera or plasma of patients affected by cholestatic disease. ELISA produces clear quantitative results and thus is routinely used to overcome all the limitations of IIF assay.

Thanks to the development of a triple-expression hybrid clone coined pMIT3, the current ELISA assay for AMA is able to detect the 3 major immunoglobulin (Ig) classes, with a sensitivity of 90% and specificity of 95%.[61] ELISA is also easily reproducible and reliable in detecting other autoantibodies used for cholestatic disease diagnosis. For gp210 antibody, ELISA conventional assays are 93% sensitive and 96% specific for the detection of gp210 autoantibodies when compared with immunoblotting assay.[62] Also for anti-Sp100 sensitivity and specificity of ELISA, assays are greater than IIF assay (44% and 99%, respectively, for ELISA vs 34% and 98% for IIF). The positive and negative predictive values for anti-Sp100 determined by ELISA were 98%, 60% and 95%, 56% for IIF, respectively.[63] A dual isotype (IgG, IgA) ELISA designed to provide enhanced detection of PBC-specific autoantibodies against both major mitochondrial and nuclear antigens has been developed, validated, and recently became commercially available.[64]

For nonconventional autoantibodies, such as anticardiolipin (aCL), immunologic solid-phase assays (usually ELISA formats) for IgG and IgM aCL antibodies and anti-β2 glycoprotein I antibodies are the widespread method.[65] Further standardization is still required because the methods are limited by poor robustness, reproducibility, and specificity.[65]

Another method used to detect antibodies is the line immunoassay. Using this technique, several antigens are immobilized on strips and are incubated with serum samples obtained from patients.[37] For this reason, line immunoassay is useful to simultaneously measure different autoantibodies especially in all cases where an overlap syndrome is present, as suggested by Saito and colleagues[66] in a recent study. Recently, a new multiplexed line-blot assay (Autoimmune Liver Disease Profile 2 [ALD2]) designed for the diagnosis of autoimmune liver diseases is available. This assay presents a good sensitivity for AMA and also has good diagnostic accuracy for sp100 and gp210 autoantibodies. Combining all the PBC-specific autoantibodies, the overall sensitivity and specificity of the ALD2 assay for PBC is 98.3% and 93.7%, respectively, compared with 96.6% and 96.3% of the conventional IIF assays.[67] Chemiluminescence immunoassay (CIA) is another option to measure autoantibodies. A recent multicentric international study evaluated the frequency of PR3-ANCA in PSC patients measured by both CIA and ELISA and suggested that those 2 methods were more specific than the IIF (83.9%).[68]

Other Immunoassay

Western blot (WB) technique is routinely used to confirm dubious IIF results. Some authors suggest, for example, that WB is the best assay option to detect AMA anti-2OADC.[37] Muratori and colleagues[69] correlated clinical, biochemical, histologic, and immunologic features with AMA patterns defined by WB and were able to dissect the fine details of the AMA reactivity in a large series of PBC patients. Recent advances in proteomics assay were recently used to better dissect pathogenesis of CLD. Using high-content protein microarray, 6 novel PBC-specific autoantigens have been identified.[70] Moreover, combining mass spectrometry with 2D-DIGE (2-dimensional difference in gel electrophoresis), Deng and colleagues[71] investigated differences between AMA-positive and AMA-negative PBC patients opening a new scenario in the pathogenesis of PBC.

Novel Combo Assay

Recent tools, for example, use fluorescence-coded microbeads detected by a multicolor fluorescence image-capture based system with novel pattern recognition algorithms for multiplex testing. Scholz and coauthors[72] applied these tools developing a unique IIF environment for one-step ANA analysis using HEp-2 cells and autoantigen-coated fluorescent beads simultaneously.[72] The assay allows one to overcome drawbacks of the recommended 2-tier ANA testing.[73]

DISCUSSION

Autoantibody presence is an essential element for the diagnosis of CLD, even if not diagnostic on its own. ANA, AMA, and p-ANCA should be determined in all subjects with clinical, biochemical, and histologic features suggestive of CLD. Detection of specific autoantibodies may help the diagnosis in asymptomatic patients, and accurate diagnosis of CLD at early stages is important because early treatment can slow progression, delay liver failure, and improve the survival rate of both PBC and PSC. However, a negative test does not exclude the presence of CLD. Autoantibody titers may vary during the course of the disease, and it is therefore recommended to repeat tests for a correct diagnosis. Sensitive markers to identify these individuals are needed, and new assays may help increase sensitivity. Indeed, advances in serodiagnostics for PBC have resulted in the detection of specific autoantibodies in 95% of patients.[17] Importantly, a significant number of patients, especially PSC patients, do not develop autoantibodies during the whole course of the disease.

Some open questions regarding the clinical significance of autoantibodies in CLD remain to be clarified. First, the pathogenic role of autoantibodies remains unknown and constitutes a priority for basic and clinical research in both PBC and PSC. Indeed, convincing evidence regarding the role of autoantibodies in CLD may be open to the development of specific therapies. Second, autoantibody presence in asymptomatic subjects remains an area for further discussion, especially in the case of highly specific autoantibodies like AMAs. Finally, new biological markers, such as microRNA,[74] genetic polymorphisms,[75] or epigenetics,[76] can help to overcome the current laboratory limitations and help diagnosis and management.

REFERENCES

1. European Association for the Study of the Liver. ASL Clinical Practice Guidelines: management of cholestatic liver diseases. J Hepatol 2009;51(2):237–67.
2. Trauner M, Meier PJ, Boyer JL. Molecular pathogenesis of cholestasis. N Engl J Med 1998;339(17):1217–27.
3. Beuers U, Trauner M, Jansen P, et al. New paradigms in the treatment of hepatic cholestasis: from UDCA to FXR, PXR and beyond. J Hepatol 2015;62(1 Suppl): S25–37.
4. Heathcote J. Update on primary biliary cirrhosis. Can J Gastroenterol 2000;14(1): 43–8.

5. Medina J, Jones EA, Garcia-Monzon C, et al. Immunopathogenesis of cholestatic autoimmune liver diseases. Eur J Clin Invest 2001;31(1):64–71.
6. Kisand KE, Metskula K, Kisand KV, et al. The follow-up of asymptomatic persons with antibodies to pyruvate dehydrogenase in adult population samples. J Gastroenterol 2001;36(4):248–54.
7. Invernizzi P, Podda M, Battezzati PM, et al. Autoantibodies against nuclear pore complexes are associated with more active and severe liver disease in primary biliary cirrhosis. J Hepatol 2001;34(3):366–72.
8. Hirschfield GM, Karlsen TH, Lindor KD, et al. Primary sclerosing cholangitis. Lancet 2013;382(9904):1587–99.
9. Hov JR, Boberg KM, Karlsen TH. Autoantibodies in primary sclerosing cholangitis. World J Gastroenterol 2008;14(24):3781–91.
10. Hirschfield GM, Gershwin ME. The immunobiology and pathophysiology of primary biliary cirrhosis. Annu Rev Pathol 2013;8:303–30.
11. Gershwin ME, Mackay IR, Sturgess A, et al. Identification and specificity of a cDNA encoding the 70 kd mitochondrial antigen recognized in primary biliary cirrhosis. J Immunol 1987;138(10):3525–31.
12. Kita H, Lian ZX, Van de Water J, et al. Identification of HLA-A2-restricted CD8(+) cytotoxic T cell responses in primary biliary cirrhosis: T cell activation is augmented by immune complexes cross-presented by dendritic cells. J Exp Med 2002;195(1):113–23.
13. Shimoda S, Van de Water J, Ansari A, et al. Identification and precursor frequency analysis of a common T cell epitope motif in mitochondrial autoantigens in primary biliary cirrhosis. J Clin Invest 1998;102(10):1831–40.
14. Lleo A, Selmi C, Invernizzi P, et al. Apotopes and the biliary specificity of primary biliary cirrhosis. Hepatology 2009;49(3):871–9.
15. Walker JG, Doniach D, Roitt IM, et al. Serological tests in diagnosis of primary biliary cirrhosis. Lancet 1965;1(7390):827–31.
16. Achenza MI, Meda F, Brunetta E, et al. Serum autoantibodies for the diagnosis and management of autoimmune liver diseases. Expert Rev Gastroenterol Hepatol 2012;6(6):717–29.
17. Oertelt S, Rieger R, Selmi C, et al. A sensitive bead assay for antimitochondrial antibodies: chipping away at AMA-negative primary biliary cirrhosis. Hepatology 2007;45(3):659–65.
18. Invernizzi P, Crosignani A, Battezzati PM, et al. Comparison of the clinical features and clinical course of antimitochondrial antibody-positive and -negative primary biliary cirrhosis. Hepatology 1997;25(5):1090–5.
19. Kim KA, Jeong SH. The diagnosis and treatment of primary biliary cirrhosis. Korean J Hepatol 2011;17(3):173–9.
20. Hohenester S, Oude-Elferink RP, Beuers U. Primary biliary cirrhosis. Semin Immunopathol 2009;31(3):283–307.
21. Van Norstrand MD, Malinchoc M, Lindor KD, et al. Quantitative measurement of autoantibodies to recombinant mitochondrial antigens in patients with primary biliary cirrhosis: relationship of levels of autoantibodies to disease progression. Hepatology 1997;25(1):6–11.
22. Kumagi T, Abe M, Ikeda Y, et al. Infection as a risk factor in the pathogenesis of primary biliary cirrhosis: pros and cons. Dis Markers 2010;29(6): 313–21.
23. Ruvolo G, Pisano C, Candore G, et al. Can the TLR-4-mediated signaling pathway be "a key inflammatory promoter for sporadic TAA"? Mediators Inflamm 2014;2014:349476.

24. Long SA, Quan C, Van de Water J, et al. Immunoreactivity of organic mimeotopes of the E2 component of pyruvate dehydrogenase: connecting xenobiotics with primary biliary cirrhosis. J Immunol 2001;167(5):2956–63.
25. Lleo A, Bowlus CL, Yang GX, et al. Biliary apotopes and anti-mitochondrial antibodies activate innate immune responses in primary biliary cirrhosis. Hepatology 2010;52(3):987–98.
26. Tan EM. Autoantibodies to nuclear antigens (ANA): their immunobiology and medicine. Adv Immunol 1982;33:167–240.
27. Kavanaugh A, Tomar R, Reveille J, et al. Guidelines for clinical use of the antinuclear antibody test and tests for specific autoantibodies to nuclear antigens. American College of Pathologists. Arch Pathol Lab Med 2000;124(1):71–81.
28. Fida S, Myers MA, Whittingham S, et al. Autoantibodies to the transcriptional factor SOX13 in primary biliary cirrhosis compared with other diseases. J Autoimmun 2002;19(4):251–7.
29. Molden DP, Nakamura RM, Tan EM. Standardization of the immunofluorescence test for autoantibody to nuclear antigens (ANA): use of reference sera of defined antibody specificity. Am J Clin Pathol 1984;82(1):57–66.
30. Talwalkar JA, Lindor KD. Primary biliary cirrhosis. Lancet 2003;362(9377):53–61.
31. Rigamonti C, Shand LM, Feudjo M, et al. Clinical features and prognosis of primary biliary cirrhosis associated with systemic sclerosis. Gut 2006;55(3):388–94.
32. Muratori P, Muratori L, Ferrari R, et al. Characterization and clinical impact of antinuclear antibodies in primary biliary cirrhosis. Am J Gastroenterol 2003;98(2): 431–7.
33. Parveen S, Morshed SA, Nishioka M. High prevalence of antibodies to recombinant CENP-B in primary biliary cirrhosis: nuclear immunofluorescence patterns and ELISA reactivities. J Gastroenterol Hepatol 1995;10(4):438–45.
34. Nickowitz RE, Wozniak RW, Schaffner F, et al. Autoantibodies against integral membrane proteins of the nuclear envelope in patients with primary biliary cirrhosis. Gastroenterology 1994;106(1):193–9.
35. Bandin O, Courvalin JC, Poupon R, et al. Specificity and sensitivity of gp210 autoantibodies detected using an enzyme-linked immunosorbent assay and a synthetic polypeptide in the diagnosis of primary biliary cirrhosis. Hepatology 1996;23(5):1020–4.
36. Wesierska-Gadek J, Penner E, Battezzati PM, et al. Correlation of initial autoantibody profile and clinical outcome in primary biliary cirrhosis. Hepatology 2006; 43(5):1135–44.
37. Cancado EL, Abrantes-Lemos CP, Terrabuio DR. The importance of autoantibody detection in autoimmune hepatitis. Front Immunol 2015;6:222.
38. Bizzaro N, Covini G, Rosina F, et al. Overcoming a "probable" diagnosis in antimitochondrial antibody negative primary biliary cirrhosis: study of 100 sera and review of the literature. Clin Rev Allergy Immunol 2012;42(3):288–97.
39. Chapman RW, Arborgh BA, Rhodes JM, et al. Primary sclerosing cholangitis: a review of its clinical features, cholangiography, and hepatic histology. Gut 1980;21(10):870–7.
40. Williamson KD, Chapman RW. Primary sclerosing cholangitis: a clinical update. Br Med Bull 2015;114(1):53–64.
41. Das K, Kar P, Gupta RK, et al. Role of transfusion-transmitted virus in acute viral hepatitis and fulminant hepatic failure of unknown etiology. J Gastroenterol Hepatol 2004;19(4):406–12.
42. Wee A, Ludwig J. Pericholangitis in chronic ulcerative colitis: primary sclerosing cholangitis of the small bile ducts? Ann Intern Med 1985;102(5):581–7.

43. Eksteen B, Grant AJ, Miles A, et al. Hepatic endothelial CCL25 mediates the recruitment of CCR9+ gut-homing lymphocytes to the liver in primary sclerosing cholangitis. J Exp Med 2004;200(11):1511–7.
44. Hov JR, Lleo A, Selmi C, et al. Genetic associations in Italian primary sclerosing cholangitis: heterogeneity across Europe defines a critical role for HLA-C. J Hepatol 2010;52(5):712–7.
45. Mandal A, Dasgupta A, Jeffers L, et al. Autoantibodies in sclerosing cholangitis against a shared peptide in biliary and colon epithelium. Gastroenterology 1994;106(1):185–92.
46. Xu B, Broome U, Ericzon BG, et al. High frequency of autoantibodies in patients with primary sclerosing cholangitis that bind biliary epithelial cells and induce expression of CD44 and production of interleukin 6. Gut 2002;51(1): 120–7.
47. Das KM, Sakamaki S, Vecchi M, et al. The production and characterization of monoclonal antibodies to a human colonic antigen associated with ulcerative colitis: cellular localization of the antigen by using the monoclonal antibody. J Immunol 1987;139(1):77–84.
48. Deniziaut G, Ballot E, Johanet C. Antineutrophil cytoplasmic auto-antibodies (ANCA) in autoimmune hepatitis and primary sclerosing cholangitis. Clin Res Hepatol Gastroenterol 2013;37(1):105–7.
49. Bogdanos DP, Invernizzi P, Mackay IR, et al. Autoimmune liver serology: current diagnostic and clinical challenges. World J Gastroenterol 2008;14(21):3374–87.
50. Savige J, Gillis D, Benson E, et al. International consensus statement on testing and reporting of antineutrophil cytoplasmic antibodies (ANCA). Am J Clin Pathol 1999;111(4):507–13.
51. Roozendaal C, de Jong MA, van den Berg AP, et al. Clinical significance of anti-neutrophil cytoplasmic antibodies (ANCA) in autoimmune liver diseases. J Hepatol 2000;32(5):734–41.
52. Roozendaal C, Van Milligen de Wit AW, Haagsma EB, et al. Antineutrophil cytoplasmic antibodies in primary sclerosing cholangitis: defined specificities may be associated with distinct clinical features. Am J Med 1998;105(5):393–9.
53. Pokorny CS, Norton ID, McCaughan GW, et al. Anti-neutrophil cytoplasmic antibody: a prognostic indicator in primary sclerosing cholangitis. J Gastroenterol Hepatol 1994;9(1):40–4.
54. Lo SK, Fleming KA, Chapman RW. A 2-year follow-up study of anti-neutrophil antibody in primary sclerosing cholangitis: relationship to clinical activity, liver biochemistry and ursodeoxycholic acid treatment. J Hepatol 1994;21(6):974–8.
55. Angulo P, Peter JB, Gershwin ME, et al. Serum autoantibodies in patients with primary sclerosing cholangitis. J Hepatol 2000;32(2):182–7.
56. Hu CJ, Zhang FC, Li YZ, et al. Primary biliary cirrhosis: what do autoantibodies tell us? World J Gastroenterol 2010;16(29):3616–29.
57. Norman GL, Yang CY, Ostendorff HP, et al. Anti-kelch-like 12 and anti-hexokinase 1: novel autoantibodies in primary biliary cirrhosis. Liver Int 2015;35(2):642–51.
58. Forslid J, Heigl Z, Jonsson J, et al. The prevalence of antinuclear antibodies in healthy young persons and adults, comparing rat liver tissue sections with HEp-2 cells as antigen substrate. Clin Exp Rheumatol 1994;12(2):137–41.
59. Vergani D, Alvarez F, Bianchi FB, et al. Liver autoimmune serology: a consensus statement from the committee for autoimmune serology of the International Autoimmune Hepatitis Group. J Hepatol 2004;41(4):677–83.
60. Invernizzi P, Selmi C, Ranftler C, et al. Antinuclear antibodies in primary biliary cirrhosis. Semin Liver Dis 2005;25(3):298–310.

61. Kadokawa Y, Omagari K, Hazama H, et al. Evaluation of newly developed ELISA using "MESACUP-2 test mitochondrial M2" kit for the diagnosis of primary biliary cirrhosis. Clin Biochem 2003;36(3):203–10.

62. Tartakovsky F, Worman HJ. Detection of Gp210 autoantibodies in primary biliary cirrhosis using a recombinant protein containing the predominant autoepitope. Hepatology 1995;21(2):495–500.

63. Bauer A, Habior A, Kraszewska E. Detection of anti-SP100 antibodies in primary biliary cirrhosis. Comparison of ELISA and immunofluorescence. J Immunoassay Immunochem 2013;34(4):346–55.

64. Liu H, Norman GL, Shums Z, et al. PBC screen: an IgG/IgA dual isotype ELISA detecting multiple mitochondrial and nuclear autoantibodies specific for primary biliary cirrhosis. J Autoimmun 2010;35(4):436–42.

65. Raby A, Moffat K, Crowther M. Anticardiolipin antibody and anti-beta 2 glycoprotein I antibody assays. Methods Mol Biol 2013;992:387–405.

66. Saito H, Takahashi A, Abe K, et al. Autoantibodies by line immunoassay in patients with primary biliary cirrhosis. Fukushima J Med Sci 2012;58(2):107–16.

67. Villalta D, Sorrentino MC, Girolami E, et al. Autoantibody profiling of patients with primary biliary cirrhosis using a multiplexed line-blot assay. Clin Chim Acta 2015;438:135–8.

68. Stinton LM, Bentow C, Mahler M, et al. PR3-ANCA: a promising biomarker in primary sclerosing cholangitis (PSC). PLoS One 2014;9(11):e112877.

69. Muratori L, Muratori P, Granito A, et al. The Western immunoblotting pattern of anti-mitochondrial antibodies is independent of the clinical expression of primary biliary cirrhosis. Dig Liver Dis 2005;37(2):108–12.

70. Hu CJ, Song G, Huang W, et al. Identification of new autoantigens for primary biliary cirrhosis using human proteome microarrays. Mol Cell Proteomics 2012;11(9):669–80.

71. Deng C, Hu C, Wang L, et al. Serological comparative proteomics analysis of mitochondrial autoantibody-negative and -positive primary biliary cirrhosis. Electrophoresis 2015;36(14):1588–95.

72. Scholz J, Grossmann K, Knutter I, et al. Second generation analysis of antinuclear antibody (ANA) by combination of screening and confirmatory testing. Clin Chem Lab Med 2015. [Epub ahead of print].

73. Grossmann K, Roggenbuck D, Schroder C, et al. Multiplex assessment of non-organ-specific autoantibodies with a novel microbead-based immunoassay. Cytometry 2011;79(2):118–25.

74. Padgett KA, Lan RY, Leung PC, et al. Primary biliary cirrhosis is associated with altered hepatic microRNA expression. J Autoimmun 2009;32(3–4):246–53.

75. Liu X, Invernizzi P, Lu Y, et al. Genome-wide meta-analyses identify three loci associated with primary biliary cirrhosis. Nat Genet 2010;42(8):658–60.

76. Brooks WH, Le Dantec C, Pers JO, et al. Epigenetics and autoimmunity. J Autoimmun 2010;34(3):J207–19.

77. Muratori P, Muratori L, Gershwin ME, et al. 'True' antimitochondrial antibody-negative primary biliary cirrhosis, low sensitivity of the routine assays, or both? Clin Exp Immunol 2004;135(1):154–8.

78. Hu S, Zhao F, Wang Q, et al. The accuracy of the anti-mitochondrial antibody and the M2 subtype test for diagnosis of primary biliary cirrhosis: a meta-analysis. Clin Chem Lab Med 2014;52(11):1533–42.

79. Hazama H, Omagari K, Masuda J, et al. Automated enzymatic mitochondrial antibody assay for the diagnosis of primary biliary cirrhosis: applications of a routine

diagnostic tool for the detection of antimitochondrial antibodies. J Gastroenterol Hepatol 2002;17(3):316–23.

80. Miyakawa H, Kikuchi K, Jong-Hon K, et al. High sensitivity of a novel ELISA for anti-M2 in primary biliary cirrhosis. J Gastroenterol 2001;36(1):33–8.

81. Gabeta S, Norman GL, Liaskos C, et al. Diagnostic relevance and clinical significance of the new enhanced performance M2 (MIT3) ELISA for the detection of IgA and IgG antimitochondrial antibodies in primary biliary cirrhosis. J Clin Immunol 2007;27(4):378–87.

82. Koga T, Migita K, Miyashita T, et al. Determination of anti-cyclic citrullinated peptide antibodies in the sera of patients with liver diseases. Clin Exp Rheumatol 2008;26(1):121–4.

83. Yamaguchi H, Miura H, Ohsumi K, et al. Detection and characterization of antibodies to bacterial heat-shock protein 60 in sera of patients with primary biliary cirrhosis. Microbiol Immunol 1994;38(6):483–7.

84. Bedlow AJ, Donaldson PT, McFarlane BM, et al. Autoreactivity to hepatocellular antigens in primary biliary cirrhosis and primary sclerosing cholangitis. J Clin Lab Immunol 1989;30(3):103–9.

85. Miyachi K, Matsushima H, Hankins RW, et al. A novel antibody directed against a three-dimensional configuration of a 95-kDa protein in patients with autoimmune hepatic diseases. Scand J Immunol 1998;47(1):63–8.

86. Miyachi K, Hirano Y, Horigome T, et al. Autoantibodies from primary biliary cirrhosis patients with anti-p95c antibodies bind to recombinant p97/VCP and inhibit in vitro nuclear envelope assembly. Clin Exp Immunol 2004;136(3):568–73.

87. Miyachi K, Hosaka H, Nakamura N, et al. Anti-p97/VCP antibodies: an autoantibody marker for a subset of primary biliary cirrhosis patients with milder disease? Scand J Immunol 2006;63(5):376–82.

88. Agmon-Levin N, Shapira Y, Selmi C, et al. A comprehensive evaluation of serum autoantibodies in primary biliary cirrhosis. J Autoimmun 2010;34(1):55–8.

89. Zachou K, Liaskos C, Rigopoulou E, et al. Presence of high avidity anticardiolipin antibodies in patients with autoimmune cholestatic liver diseases. Clin Immunol 2006;119(2):203–12.

90. Gabeta S, Norman GL, Gatselis N, et al. IgA anti-b2GPI antibodies in patients with autoimmune liver diseases. J Clin Immunol 2008;28(5):501–11.

91. Abe K, Ohira H, Kobayashi H, et al. Breakthrough of immune self-tolerance to calreticulin induced by CpG-oligodeoxynucleotides as adjuvant. Fukushima J Med Sci 2007;53(2):95–108.

92. Chatzicostas C, Roussomoustakaki M, Drygiannakis D, et al. Primary biliary cirrhosis and autoimmune cholangitis are not associated with coeliac disease in Crete. BMC Gastroenterol 2002;2:5.

93. Muratori L, Muratori P, Zauli D, et al. Antilactoferrin antibodies in autoimmune liver disease. Clin Exp Immunol 2001;124(3):470–3.

94. Nakamura H, Usa T, Motomura M, et al. Prevalence of interrelated autoantibodies in thyroid diseases and autoimmune disorders. J Endocrinol Invest 2008;31(10):861–5.

95. Ueno Y, Ishii M, Igarashi T, et al. Primary biliary cirrhosis with antibody against carbonic anhydrase II associates with distinct immunological backgrounds. Hepatol Res 2001;20(1):18–27.

96. Akisawa N, Maeda T, Iwasaki S, et al. Identification of an autoantibody against alpha-enolase in primary biliary cirrhosis. J Hepatol 1997;26(4):845–51.

97. Xia Q, Lu F, Yan HP, et al. Autoantibody profiling of Chinese patients with autoimmune hepatitis using immunoproteomic analysis. J Proteome Res 2008;7(5): 1963–70.
98. Roesler KW, Schmider W, Kist M, et al. Identification of beta-subunit of bacterial RNA-polymerase–a non-species-specific bacterial protein–as target of antibodies in primary biliary cirrhosis. Dig Dis Sci 2003;48(3):561–9.

New Thoughts on Immunoglobulin G4– Related Sclerosing Cholangitis

 CrossMark

Wouter L. Smit, MSc[a,c], Emma L. Culver, BSc, MBChB, PhD, MRCP[b,c],
Roger W. Chapman, MD, FRCP[b,c],*

KEYWORDS

- IgG4-related sclerosing cholangitis • IgG4-associated cholangitis
- IgG4-related disease • Autoimmune pancreatitis

KEY POINTS

- Immunoglobulin G4-related sclerosing cholangitis (IgG4-SC) is the biliary manifestation of a multisystem disease known as IgG4-related disease.
- IgG4-SC may present with biliary strictures and/or masses, which makes it extremely difficult to differentiate from primary sclerosing cholangitis or malignancies, such as cholangiocarcinoma and pancreatic cancer.
- Diagnosis of IgG4-SC is based on a combination of clinical, biochemical, radiological, and histologic findings.
- A gold standard diagnostic test for IgG4-SC is still lacking, warranting the identification of more specific disease markers to aid clinicians.

SYNOPSIS

Immunoglobulin G4-related sclerosing cholangitis (IgG4-SC) is a distinct form of chronic cholangitis characterized by infiltration of lymphocytes and abundant IgG4-positive plasma cells in the bile duct wall, elevated IgG4 serum levels in the majority, and a strong response to corticosteroid therapy. It is the biliary manifestation of IgG4-related disease (IRD), a recently recognized fibro-inflammatory multisystem condition.[1] IgG4-SC is most often found in association with autoimmune pancreatitis (AIP), the pancreatic manifestation of IRD. To date, there is no gold standard

The authors have nothing to disclose.
[a] Department of Gastroenterology and Hepatology, Academic Medical Center, University of Amsterdam, Meibergdreef 9, Amsterdam 1105 AZ, The Netherlands; [b] Translational Gastroenterology Unit, John Radcliffe Hospital, Headley Way, Headington, Oxford OX3 9DU, UK; [c] Nuffield Department of Medicine, University of Oxford, Old Road Campus, Oxford OX3 7BN, UK
* Corresponding author. Department of Translational Gastroenterology, John Radcliffe Hospital, Level 5, Headley Way, Headington, Oxford OX3 9DU, UK.
E-mail address: Roger.chapman@ndm.ox.ac.uk

diagnostic test for IgG4-SC; diagnosis is made through a combination of clinical, biochemical, radiological, and histologic features. These features, however, can present similarly to primary sclerosing cholangitis (PSC), cholangiocarcinoma (CCA), or pancreatic cancer (PCa), which complicates and usually delays the diagnostic process. When IgG4-SC is treated during the initial (inflammatory) phase of disease, corticosteroid therapy is very effective. Delayed treatment in a patient with persistent inflammation can eventually lead to irreversible fibrosis and end-stage liver disease. Thus, correctly diagnosing IgG4-SC is critical to avoid unnecessary interventions due to a mistaken diagnosis (for example, surgery or chemotherapy for presumed malignancy) and to prevent fibrotic complications of disease.[2] However, it is essential to exclude malignant disease by adequate imaging and tissue sampling. Evidence suggests that the pathogenesis of IgG4-SC differs from other immune-mediated cholestatic liver diseases like PSC and primary biliary sclerosis (PBC), although fundamental insight into the cause of IgG4-SC is currently lacking. This review provides a comprehensive overview of the current knowledge of the prevalence, clinical features, radiology and histology findings, diagnosis, treatment, natural history, and pathophysiology of IgG4-SC.

Concept of Immunoglobulin G4–Related Disease

IRD is a multisystem disease characterized by unique histopathologic features that include a dense lymphoplasmacytic infiltrate, obliterative phlebitis, and storiform fibrosis, with prominent IgG4-positive plasma cell infiltration in affected organs. Various organs may either simultaneously or consecutively be involved. Almost all organ systems except the brain parenchyma have been reported to be affected.

Brief History

Initial reports of the pancreatobiliary manifestations of IRD date back to 1961, when Sarles and colleagues[3] described an inflammatory disease of the pancreas termed "chronic inflammatory sclerosis of the pancreas." Two years later, Bartholomew and colleagues[4] described cases of sclerosing cholangitis associated with Riedel thyroiditis and "fibrous retroperitonitis". In the 4 decades thereafter, several cases of sclerosing cholangitis were reported in association with inflammation of other organs, such as the pancreas, salivary and lacrimal glands, orbit, mediastinum, and lymph nodes. An association with elevated levels of serum IgG4 was demonstrated in 2001 in patients with AIP.[5] In 2003, after multiple extrapancreatic lesions with similar histologic findings were observed in patients with AIP, the systemic nature of IRD was finally recognized.[6]

Terminology

Several descriptive terms for IRD with concomitant cholangitis have been used through the last decade.[1] The European Association for the Study of the Liver's clinical practice guidelines for cholestatic liver diseases recommended using *IgG4-associated cholangitis*, as clear histologic evidence of sclerosing disease is often absent.[7] However, in 2014 at an international symposium on IRD, the name *IgG4-SC* was agreed on given the fibrotic and potentially irreversible nature of the later stages of the disease, which is the term that is used in this article. With respect to AIP, 2 types have now been recognized (type I and II). Type I AIP is the pancreatic manifestation of IRD and is discussed in this article.[8] Type II AIP has distinct clinical and histologic manifestations (duct-centric sclerosing pancreatitis with granulocytic epithelial lesions) that are unrelated to IRD and are not considered here (**Table 1**).

Table 1	
Hepatopancreatobiliary manifestations of IRD	
Tissue	Condition
Bile ducts (extrahepatic or intrahepatic)	IgG4-SC (with or without pseudotumorous hilar lesions)
Pancreas	AIP (type 1)
Gallbladder	IgG4-related cholecystitis
Liver	IgG4-hepatopathy

Epidemiology and Demographics

Epidemiologic data on the prevalence of IgG4-SC are scarce because of the lack of population-based studies. Most data come from Japanese patients with AIP, whereby the prevalence and incidence is estimated to be 0.8 cases per 100,000 persons and 0.28 to 1.08 per 100,000, respectively.[9] Around 74% of patients with AIP have concomitant IgG4-SC, whereas isolated IgG4-SC is seen only in 8% of cases.[10] It remains to be clarified if the prevalence rates in Western countries are similar. Among patients diagnosed with PSC, the percentage of those with AIP (and likely IgG4-SC) is estimated to be 7%, based on retrospective analysis of patients with PSC who presented with concomitant AIP and responded well to corticosteroid therapy.[11]

CLINICAL FEATURES OF IMMUNOGLOBULIN G4–RELATED SCLEROSING CHOLANGITIS
Clinical Manifestations

The spectrum of clinical manifestations in IgG4-SC is highly variable and depends on the severity of disease activity as well as the presence of associated organ involvement. Most patients present in middle age and are male (male/female ratio 8:1) with symptoms of obstructive jaundice and weight loss related to strictures of the bile ducts.[10] Pancreatic involvement is present in approximately 90% of patients, often causing symptoms of pancreatic exocrine and endocrine insufficiency that include anorexia, weight loss, steatorrhea, and new-onset of diabetes. Mild to moderate abdominal pain, pruritus, malaise, and cholestatic biochemistry are commonly observed. The presence of inflammatory bowel disease is more suggestive of PSC, with colitis reported in about 5% of patients with IRD.

A history of allergy and/or atopy has been described in 40% to 60% of patients with AIP/IgG4-SC, often in association with elevated IgE levels, and may represent a separate disease phenotype.[12] Furthermore, in 2 independent IgG4-SC/AIP cohorts, most patients had a history of blue-collar occupations; the investigators suggested chronic exposure to a variety of chemicals and toxins may be important in disease.[13]

Laboratory Features

The most frequently described laboratory findings are an increased alkaline phosphatase and gamma-glutamyltransferase level, seen in approximately 90% of patients with IgG4-SC. Serum bilirubin levels are often increased, particularly in those with obstructive jaundice, and are usually higher compared with classic PSC.[10] Hypergammaglobulinemia is common and is usually caused by increased IgG4 subclass levels. A cutoff value of 1.4 g/L for serum IgG4 is inadequate for the diagnosis of IgG4-SC because of its limited specificity; moderately increased levels greater than 1.4 to 2.8 g/L can be seen in classic PSC,[14] CCA,[15] PCa,[16] other inflammatory and infective disorders, and 5% of healthy individuals. Markedly increased IgG4 levels of greater than 2.8 g/L (twice the upper limit of normal [2 × ULN]) are more suggestive of IgG4-SC, and levels of greater than 5.6 g/L (4 × ULN) have reported to be 100% specific to distinguish IgG4-SC from CCA.[17] In patients with serum IgG4 between 1.4 and 2.8 g/L, the ratio of serum IgG4/IgG1 greater than 0.24 has additional value for discrimination between IgG4-SC and PSC (**Fig. 1**).[18] The sensitivity of serum IgG4 levels is low, and 20% to 25% of patients present with a normal serum IgG4 at diagnosis.[10,19,20] This subgroup often has a milder clinical phenotype with lower risk of relapse and fewer organs involved. The diagnostic value of biliary IgG4 levels and use of cellular ratios, such as the IgG4-positive plasma cell/mononuclear cell ratio, to differentiate IgG4-SC from PSC have been assessed in small studies and must be further clarified.[21,22]

Eosinophilia and/or elevated IgE levels are seen in approximately 20% to 60% of patients with IgG4-SC, usually in association with a history of allergy and/or atopy. The presence of antinuclear antibodies and other autoantibodies are nonspecific for diagnosis, whereas the presence of perinuclear anti-neutrophil cytoplasmic antibodies (pANCA) is more suggestive of PSC. Elevated carbohydrate antigen 19-9 (Ca 19-9) levels are observed in IgG4-SC (63% in one study) as well as normal or minimally elevated carcinoembryonic antigen (CEA) levels, making these tumor markers not specific enough to distinguish IgG4-SC from malignancies.[23]

Radiographic Features

The spectrum of radiological features in IgG4-SC is variable and nonspecific. The preferred method for assessment of the bile ducts and pancreas is magnetic resonance cholangiopancreatography (MRCP), although computed tomography (CT) abdomen/pelvis with contrast will define other organ manifestations, which may be clinically silent. Cholangiography in IgG4-SC often shows narrowing of the bile ducts and wall thickening, and these abnormalities can be found in all parts of the biliary tract (**Fig. 2**). A common bile duct (CBD) stricture is classic, and involvement of both intrahepatic and extrahepatic bile ducts is evident in approximately 50% of patients.[24] Other imaging modalities, such as abdominal ultrasonography (US),[25] CT,[26] MRCP, endoscopic ultrasound, or intraductal US (IDUS), may show circular and symmetric thickening of the bile duct wall characterized by smooth outer and inner margins and a homogenous internal aspect in IgG4-SC, present in both the stenotic and nonstenotic areas.

Isolated biliary tract disease without evidence of other organ involvement is rare; in most cases, concomitant pancreatic disease is present. Pancreatic imaging typically reveals diffuse sausage-shaped pancreatic enlargement and diffuse irregular narrowing of the pancreatic ducts on CT or MRI (**Fig. 3**). A localized mass lesion, often at the head of the pancreas, with locoregional lymphadenopathy is often seen and is difficult to distinguish from PCa. Changes consistent with acute pancreatitis, atrophic pancreas, and diffuse pancreatic enhancement have been described less commonly. Although the ability of

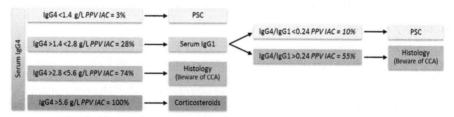

Fig. 1. Proposed diagnostic algorithm for differentiation between IgG4-SC and PSC based on serum IgG4 and IgG1. IAC, Igg4-related associated cholangitis; PPV, positive predictive value. (*From* Boonstra K, Culver EL, de Buy Wenniger LM, et al. Serum immunoglobulin G4 and immunoglobulin G1 for distinguishing immunoglobulin G4-associated cholangitis from primary sclerosing cholangitis. Hepatology 2014;59(5):1961; with permission.)

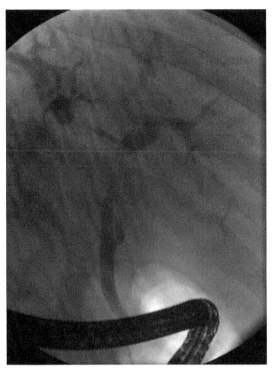

Fig. 2. Endoscopic retrograde cholangiopancreatography: a proximal cystic duct and intra-hepatic duct stricture with distal right and left ductal dilatation. This patient with a normal serum IgG4 had surgery for presumed hilar CCA with the resection specimen demonstrating IgG4-SC.

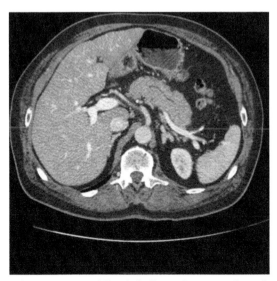

Fig. 3. CT pancreas: The pancreas is diffusely bulky and sausage shaped with enlarged peri-pancreatic and portal lymph nodes. The pancreatic duct is not dilated. Histologically confirmed AIP with the triad of morphologic manifestations and abundant IgG4-positive plasma cells.

MRCP to delineate abnormalities of the main pancreatic duct is limited as compared with endoscopic retrograde cholangiopancreatography in almost half of patients with diffuse-type AIP,[27] it continues to be a valuable noninvasive tool for the detection of pancreatic gland abnormalities as well as for follow-up of patients with IgG4-SC/AIP.

It is challenging to differentiate IgG4-SC from CCA or PSC based on imaging alone. A pancreatic mass or hilar stricture/hepatic mass is highly concerning for PCa, CCA, or hepatocellular carcinoma, respectively, although all can be present in IRD.[23] Segmental strictures, long strictures with prestenotic dilatation, and strictures of the distal CBD are significantly more common in IgG4-SC, whereas bandlike strictures, with a beaded or pruned-tree appearance are more common in classic PSC.[28] A small study showed that irregular inner margin, diverticulumlike out pouching, and disappearance of 3 layers (mucosa, muscularis propria, and subserosa) on IDUS was more specific for PSC than IgG4-SC.[29] However, IDUS findings were insufficient to differentiate between CCA and IgG4-SC.[30]

Histopathology Features

Histopathologic features in IgG4-SC are generally similar to those seen in other organ manifestations of IRD and are characterized by (1) a dense lymphoplasmacytic infiltrate, (2) storiform fibrosis, (3) obliterative phlebitis, and (4) the presence of numerous IgG4-positive plasma cells.[1] Usually the large bile ducts are affected, with diffuse or localized sclerotic and stenotic lesions within the large bile ducts of the hepatic hilus, the extrahepatic bile ducts, and gallbladder. Resected bile ducts appear diffusely thickened, causing a pipe-stem fibrosis–like macroscopic appearance. Biliary epithelium is usually relatively intact, in distinct contrast to the mucosal erosion commonly seen in PSC. Periductal inflammatory mass lesions in the resected hilar and perihilar ducts can be observed.[31] The presence of Ductopenia and periductal fibrosis, typically seen in PSC, argues strongly against IgG4-SC.[32]

The lymphoplasmacytic infiltrates in IgG4-SC consist of evenly distributed lymphocytes that often organize into lymphoid aggregates. There is an abundance of polyclonal T cells (mostly CD4 T-helper cells), and B cells are confined to scattered small cohesive lymphoid aggregates with occasional germinal centers. Polyclonal plasma cells make up an essential component and may predominate the cellular infiltrate. Other immune cells, such as macrophages, eosinophils, and basophils, are also occasionally detectable. More recently, IgE-positive mast cells have been described in the inflammatory infiltrate.[33]

A preponderance of IgG4+ plasma cells in tissue infiltrates is present but is not specific for IgG4-SC, as it can be seen in PSC and CCA too.[34–36] The 2012 Boston histopathologic consensus statement proposed that greater than 50 per high-power field (HPF) in surgical specimens and greater than 10 per HPF in biopsy samples and an IgG4/IgG cell count ratio of greater than 40% are required for the diagnosis of IgG4-SC.[37] However, fewer IgG4+ plasma cells can be seen in patients with longstanding fibrosis, although the IgG4/IgG ratio was found to be particularly helpful in that regard.[37]

The fibro-inflammatory process usually extends to the peribiliary adventitial veins, nerves, and glands. Infiltrating lymphocytes and plasma cells surround and compress the adventitial vein lumen occasionally obliterating it entirely, known as obliterative phlebitis. This obliterative phlebitis is nearly always observed in IgG4-SC and AIP, representing a highly specific diagnostic finding, which is helpful in distinguishing from PSC or CCA.[1]

Fibrosis has a characteristic appearance with deposition of collagen in a swirling or storiform arrangement, seldom observed in other inflammatory and rheumatologic diseases. The cellular makeup depends on the duration of inflammation, with an admixture of fibroblasts and myofibroblasts in the active phase, followed by a pre-dominance of fibroblastic cells in later phases.

Involvement of small intrahepatic bile ducts in IgG4-SC can be observed on liver needle biopsy, which may be especially useful for patients with intrahepatic biliary strictures on cholangiography.[38] The presence of numerous infiltrating IgG4+ plasma cells, small portal inflammatory nodules consisting of spindle-shaped stromal cells and lymphocytes, and central venulitis were specific findings. In AIP, small intrahe-patic ductal changes were reported which included dense periportal fibrosis, marked portal inflammation with numerous plasma cells, lobular inflammation and canalicular cholestasis in perivenular areas.[39] Whether some of these changes are secondary to extrahepatic biliary obstruction of IgG4-SC is uncertain. Tumefactive nodules or in-flammatory pseudotumors of the liver are probably manifestations of intrahepatic IgG4-SC.

DIAGNOSIS

There is no pathognomonic feature of IgG4-SC, and diagnosis is currently based on a combination of clinical, serologic, imaging, and histologic findings. Multiple diagnostic criteria have been proposed to diagnose and distinguish IgG4-SC from disease mimics. The HISORt (histology, imaging, serology, other organ involvement, and response to corticosteroid) criteria, which were originally developed for AIP, were adapted for IgG4-SC, are most widely accepted (**Table 2**). Although these criteria are helpful in clinical practice, every effort should be made to rule out malignant dis-ease (CCA or PCa), which in practice will often require fine-needle aspiration and bi-opsy. Although radiological improvement or resolution of a biliary stricture after 4 weeks of corticosteroid therapy is suggestive of IgG4-SC,[10] it is not diagnostic as the inflammatory infiltrate around malignant strictures in CCA/PCa and in patients with PSC with an elevated serum IgG4 respond to corticosteroids in small series. Recently, a novel qPCR test analyzing the IgG4/IgG RNA-ratio in blood has been shown to achieve excellent diagnostic accuracy (n = 80) and monitoring of treatment response (n = 20) in IgG4-SC and patients with AIP[40] and Doorenspleet, et al. Submit-ted for publication.) (see **Table 2**).

TREATMENT

IgG4-SC, as with AIP and other disease manifestations of IRD, responds dramatically to steroid therapy. The main objectives in the initial phase of treatment are alleviation of symptomatic jaundice and abdominal discomfort, reversal of cholangiographic ap-pearances, and prevention of disease-related fibrotic complications. Some advocate a trial of corticosteroids in those with a high suspicion of disease who do not fulfill the diagnostic criteria of definite IgG4-SC (after best possible exclusion of malignancy) to confirm the diagnosis ex juvantibus; however, this should only be done under close observation and with regular review in centers with experience in managing the disease.

There is no international consensus on an appropriate steroid regimen, duration of treatment, or the management of relapse because of a lack of randomized clinical trials; the most widely applied regimens come from the Mayo Clinic or Japan.[41,42] The first line of treatment typically involves an initial course of 3 to 6 months of corticosteroid therapy beginning at high doses of 40 to 60 mg daily, followed by a slow tapering of 5 mg per week. The response to steroids (through MRCP and biochemical assessment, not symptoms alone) may be assessed at 6 to 8 weeks. Patients with rapid, near-complete resolution can proceed with steroid taper. Patients whose disease improves

Table 2
The HISORt criteria for IgG4-SC

Diagnostic Criterion	Description
1. Histology of bile duct	There is lymphoplasmacytic sclerosing cholangitis on resection specimens (lymphoplasmacytic infiltrate with >10 IgG4-positive cells per HPF within and around bile ducts with associated obliterative phlebitis and storiform fibrosis). Bile duct biopsy specimens often do not provide sufficient tissue for a definitive diagnosis; however, presence of >10 IgG4-positive cells per HPF is suggestive of IgG4-SC.
2. Imaging of bile duct	There are one or more strictures involving intrahepatic, proximal extrahepatic, or intrapancreatic bile ducts. There are fleeting/migrating biliary strictures.
3. Serology	There is an increased serum IgG4 level (normal, 8–140 mg/dL).
4. Other organ involvement	Pancreas: There are classic features of AIP on imaging or histology (diffusely enlarged pancreas with delayed enhancement and capsulelike rim). Suggestive imaging findings include focal pancreatic mass/enlargement without pancreatic duct dilation, multiple pancreatic masses, focal pancreatic duct stricture without upstream dilatation, and pancreatic atrophy. There is retroperitoneal fibrosis. Renal lesions: There are single or multiple parenchymal low-attenuation lesions (round, wedge shaped, or diffuse patchy). There is salivary/lacrimal gland enlargement.
5. Response to steroid therapy	There is normalization of liver enzyme increase or resolution of stricture (although complete resolution of stricture may not be seen early in the course of treatment or in patients with predominantly fibrotic strictures).

From Ohara H, Okazaki K, Tsubouchi H, et al. Clinical diagnostic criteria of IgG4-related sclerosing cholangitis. J Hepatobiliary Pancreat Sci 2012;19(5):538; with permission.

but is slow to resolve or relapse on taper can be treated with further increased doses of corticosteroid and/or initiation of an immunomodulator, typically azathioprine. Other immunomodulators used in the context of extrapancreatic disease and/or intolerance of azathioprine are mycophenolate mofetil and 6-mercaptopurine.[43] Rituximab has shown to be effective in IgG4-SC and has been suggested for patients with incomplete remission, steroid dependency, or steroid/immunomodulator intolerance.[43,44] Biliary stenting may be performed to relieve obstructive jaundice before steroid initiation, being removed once steroid therapy is effective, and in those with a suboptimal clinical response to treatment, particularly in late-stage fibrotic disease.

Complete resolution of strictures and/or normalization of liver tests was reported in approximately two-thirds of patients with IgG4-SC.[10] In AIP, remission rates of almost 100% have been reported.[45] Disease relapse is a common problem in both patients with IgG4-SC and with AIP that may be seen in approximately 50% of patients, occurring after cessation of steroid treatment or during the taper.[10] IgG4-SC is an independent risk factor for relapse, and it is more common in those with proximal biliary strictures and increased IgG4 levels.[10,46]

PROGNOSIS AND NATURAL HISTORY

Because of the short follow-up in most case series, prognosis and natural history of IgG4-SC are not well characterized. Spontaneous remissions are reported in a minority of cases and disease usually recurs. When timely treatment is applied, steroid-responsive IgG4-SC has a favorable prognosis. Without treatment, biliary cirrhosis and its complications can occur, although the rate of progression to advanced fibrosis and prevalence of cirrhosis remains controversial. In cases of extra-biliary organ involvement, severe fibrosis as a result of chronic inflammation may cause permanent organ function loss associated with significant morbidity and mortality.[47] It seems that the risk of any malignancy is increased 2-fold in patients with IgG4-SC/AIP, possibly because of the higher rate of cell proliferation inherent to long-term immune activation.[47]

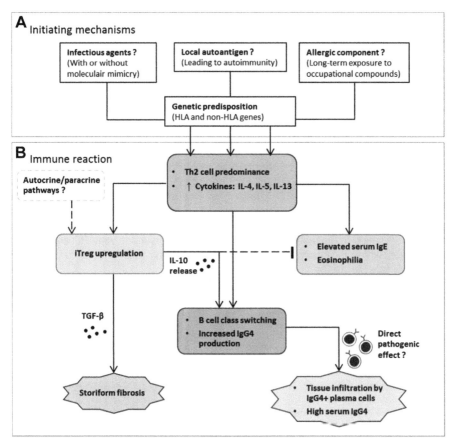

Fig. 4. Disease pathways considered to be involved in the pathogenesis of IRD. Proposed mechanisms involved in disease initiation are infectious agents, local autoantigens, and even allergic components in a genetically predisposed individual (*A*). These initial trigger are thought to activate an immune reaction characterized by increased production of the IL-4, -5, -10, and -13 and tumor growth factor-β (TGF-β) due to Th2 cells that are predominantly activated at affected sites, followed by activation of Treg cells. This immune reaction might cause activated B cells to class switch to IgG4 producing plasma cells (*B*). iTreg, induced regulatory T cell.

PATHOGENESIS OF DISEASE

The etiopathogenetic mechanisms underlying IgG4-SC, as other organ manifestations of IRD, are poorly understood. However, some initial insights into genetic and immunologic aspects of the disease are emerging (**Fig. 4**). Most of these studies have focused on patients with AIP and/or IgG4-sialoadenitis (salivary gland disease), and it is uncertain whether these findings are equally relevant to IgG4-SC. The presence of hypergammaglobulinemia (particularly increased IgG4), frequent detection of nonspecific autoantibodies, infiltration of the affected tissues with immune cells (mostly CD4 T cells, B cells and IgG4-positive plasma cells), and a dramatic response to steroids all strongly indicate an immune-mediated phenomenon. Proposed etiological mechanisms include an autoimmune reaction against a common autoantigen, possibly triggered by a process of molecular mimicry, or chronic exposure to stimulation of one or multiple antigens or allergens.

Role of Genetic Factors

Irrespective of factors that trigger disease, genetic factors may lead to increased disease susceptibility. In AIP, multiple genetic factors have been identified in the Asian population, albeit in small studies (**Table 3**). Associations have been shown with the HLA-II haplotypes (DRB1*0405 and DQB1*0401) as well as single-nucleotide polymorphisms (SNPs) in non-HLA genes, including cytotoxic T-lymphocyte–associated antigen 4 (CTLA-4), tumor necrosis factor-α (TNF- α), and Fc receptor–like (FCR).[48–51] High frequencies of HLA DRB1*0405 and DQB1*0401 were reported in Japanese patients with AIP.[48] This finding was not replicated in Korean patients with AIP, although the nonaspartic acid at DQB1 57 was associated with relapse.[52] The CTLA-4 49A haplotype was reported at higher frequencies in Chinese patients with AIP, whereby the 318C/+49A/CT60G haplotype increased susceptibility to AIP, whereas the TNF-a promoter 863A haplotype was associated with extrapancreatic manifestations.[50] In Japanese patients with AIP, SNPs in CTLA-4 were associated with disease susceptibility, resistance, and risk of relapse,[51] and FCRL3 polymorphisms were linked to disease susceptibility.[49] HLA associations with IRD are different in the West, which is unsurprising given ethnic variation (Culver et al, unpublished data, 2015) (see **Table 3**).

Table 3 Genetic susceptibility factors for patients with AIP			
Proteins	**SNP**	**Association**	**References**
CTLA-4	49A haplotype	Higher frequencies in Chinese patients	Chang et al,[50] 2007
	−318C/+49A/CT60G	AIP susceptibility in Chinese patients	Chang et al,[50] 2007
	+6230 3′, untranslated region	AIP susceptibility in Japanese patients	Umemura et al,[51] 2008
	+6230G/G	AIP susceptibility in Japanese patients	Umemura et al,[51] 2008
	+6230A	AIP resistance in Japanese patients	Umemura et al,[51] 2008
	49A/A and +6230A/A genotypes	AIP relapse in Japanese patients	Umemura et al,[51] 2008
TNF-α	863A haplotype	Extrapancreatic involvement in Chinese patients	Chang et al,[50] 2007
FCR-3	−110A/A genotype	AIP susceptibility in Japanese patients (serum IgG4 correlated to susceptibility alleles)	Umemura et al,[49] 2006

Abbreviation: TNF-α, tumor necrosis factor α.

Role of Autoantibodies and Autoantigens

Based on the theory that IRD is an autoimmune disorder, the specificity of autoantibody responses has been examined in a series of studies in patients with AIP, resulting in the identification of multiple autoantibodies and autoantigens (**Table 4**). Carbonic anhydrase-II (CA-II) is expressed in ductal cells of several exocrine organs (pancreas, salivary gland, biliary duct, and distal renal tubule); lactoferrin can be detected in the lactating breast, bronchial, salivary and gastric glands, as well as pancreatic acinus. These autoantibodies were detected in 54% and 73% of patients with AIP, respectively.[53,54] Other associated autoantibodies in AIP are antipancreatic secretory trypsin inhibitor,[55] antitrypsinogens,[56] antiamylase α-2A,[57] and anti–heat shock protein 10.[58] A proteomics study from Japan identified a 13.1-kDa protein as a candidate autoantigen, although the sequence has not been determined.[59] Loss of tolerance to widely distributed autoantigens may explain the multisystem nature of IRD (see **Table 4**).

Role of Microbial Antigens

After one study reported high prevalence (34.8%) of coexisting gastric ulcers in patients with AIP,[63] a role for Helicobacter pylori (H Pylori) was hypothesized, based on the theory that this organism might trigger disease in a genetically predisposed host via molecular mimicry.[64] Significant homology was shown between human CA-II and α-carbonic anhydrase of Helicobacter pylori in segments containing the binding motif of DRB1*0405, a susceptibility HLA molecule for AIP.[65] Antibodies against H pylori plasminogen-binding protein (PBP) were detected in 94% of patients with AIP in an Italian cohort, and homology was demonstrated between PBP and an enzyme expressed in pancreatic acinar cells.[61] Although these findings are supportive of the aforementioned hypothesis, they have not yet been confirmed elsewhere. A recent study could not detect H pylori DNA in tissue or pancreatic juice from patients with AIP,[66] suggesting no direct infection to be involved. No H pylori infection has been reported in other IgG4-related lesions.

Role of the Immunoglobulin G4 Molecule

IgG4 is normally found in low abundance in serum, accounting for 3% to 6% of total serum IgG in the healthy population. However, under certain situations of chronic or repetitive antigenic exposure, it can represent up to 80%, which is thought to reflect development of humoral tolerance, based on unique antiinflammatory or tolerance-inducing properties related to the IgG4 subclass.[67] IgG4 seems unable to activate complement via the classic pathway as a result of a few amino acid differences to IgG1 in the CH2 domain, which also reduces cellular immune responses due to decreased Fc-gamma receptor binding of effector cells.[68] Amino acid changes in the core hinge also allow the IgG4 molecule to undergo exchange of half-antibodies, generating functionally monovalent half-antibodies that are unable to cross-link antigens or form large immune complexes.[69] Fc-mediated effector function and immune complex formation may be further impaired through Fc tail interaction of IgG4 with other proinflammatory IgG subclasses.[70]

A fundamental question is whether tissue infiltration with IgG4-positive plasma cells and high levels of serum IgG4, seen in most patients, contributes directly to disease pathogenesis. Tolerance-inducing properties of IgG4 might argue for a regulatory function, although pathogenic IgG4 antibodies have been demonstrated in pemphigus vulgaris and myasthenia gravis.[71,72] Furthermore, in patients with AIP, serum IgG4 is able to bind with normal human bile and pancreatic duct epithelia, a reaction that was

Table 4
Main disease-related autoantibody specificities in AIP

Autoantibody/ Autoantigen	Number of Patients with AIP	Origin of Patients	Frequency in AIP (%)	Frequency in Disease and Healthy Controls (%)	References
Anticarbonic anhydrase-II	17	Japanese	59	—	Okazaki et al,[53] 2000
	54	Japanese	28	10.5 chronic alcoholic pancreatitis, 64 Sjögren, 1.9 HCs, 0 HCs	Aparisi et al,[54] 2005
	48	European	12.5	—	Hardt et al,[60] 2008
Antilactoferrin	17	Japanese	76	—	Okazaki et al,[53] 2000
	48	European	20.8	0	Hardt et al,[60] 2008
Plasminogen-binding protein	35	European	94	10 pancreatic cancer, 0 chronic alcoholic pancreatitis, 0 IPMN	Frulloni et al,[61] 2009
Anticarbonic anhydrase-IV	—	Japanese	27	0 HCs, 45 Sjögren	Nishimori et al,[62] 2005
Heat-shock protein 10	—	Japanese	92	81 type I DM, 8 chronic alcoholic pancreatitis, 1.4 HCs	Takizawa et al,[58] 2009
Amylase-2α	15	Japanese	100	88 type 1 DM, 6 type II DM, 0 chronic alcoholic pancreatitis, 0 pancreatic cancer	Endo et al,[57] 2009
Antitrypsinogens	19	German	79	10 non-AIP chronic cholangitis and HCs	Löhr et al,[56] 2010
Antipancreatic secretory trypsin inhibitor	26	Japanese	30.8	0	Asada et al,[55] 2006

Abbreviations: DM, diabetes mellitus; HCs, healthy controls; IPMN, intraductal papillary mucinous neoplasm.
Modified from Smyk DS, Rigopoulou EI, Koutsoumpas AL, et al. Autoantibodies in autoimmune pancreatitis. Int J Rheumatol 2012;2012:940831.

abolished with steroid therapy.[73] In IgG4-SC, the presence of a subset of clonally expanded IgG4-positive B cells in blood and affected tissue was demonstrated, which declined after steroid therapy.[74] In patients with IRD, an oligoclonal IgG4-positive plasmablast expansion was observed during active disease, which declined after B-cell depletion with rituximab.[75] These findings may indicate involvement of specific pathogenic B-cell responses, although alternatively it may reflect an amplified humoral response to an inflammatory environment with polyclonal expansion of preexisting IgG4-switched B cells of multiple specificities.[76]

Role of Immune Cells

T helper 2 (Th2) and T regulatory cells
Inflamed tissue in IRD shows diffuse infiltration of T cells (mostly CD4-positive and to a lesser extent CD8-positive). Histologic examination in patients with IgG4-SC and patients with AIP reveals an increased production of Th2-type cytokines, such as interleukin (IL)-4, IL-5, IL-10, and IL-13.[77] Increased numbers of circulating Th2 cells[78] may be restricted to atopic patients (with a history of rhinitis, bronchial asthma).[12] It is postulated that Th2 responses mediate humoral IgG4 responses, eosinophilia, and elevated serum IgE, supported by in vivo evidence of IL-4– and IL-13–induced switch of naïve B cells to both IgG4 and IgE.[79] IL-10 can potentiate IL-4–mediated class switching to IgG4 while suppressing IgE.[80]

Patients with IgG4-SC and AIP show increased infiltration of inducible-memory T regulatory cells (Tregs) in affected tissue and blood, with upregulation of the regulatory cytokines IL-10 and tumor growth factor-β (TGF-β).[77,81–83] mRNA expression of Tregs-specific Foxp3 (forkhead box P3) was higher in IRD compared with classic autoimmune diseases. Numbers of infiltrating Tregs correlated with IgG4+ plasma cell numbers in a small study in patients with IgG4-SC,[84] whereas, in AIP, circulating Treg cell numbers correlated with serum IgG4 levels.[81] Tregs can exert a regulatory function through IL-10 secretion, inducing IgG4 class switching and promoting the expansion of IgG4-secreting plasma cells.[85,86] Other potential sources of IL-10 include macrophages, dendritic cells, or basophils.[87] TGF-β production from Tregs may stimulate fibroblasts causing fibrogenesis, a prominent feature of advanced-stage disease. Prolonged IL-13 secretion from Tregs (and Th2 cells) could also contribute to this process.[88]

Chemokine signaling
Involvement of chemokine-mediated signaling, which is thought to be involved the pathogenesis of immune-mediated hepatobiliary disorders, such as PBC and PSC, has recently also been implicated in IgG4-SC and AIP.[89] Chemokine (C-C motif) ligand 1 (CCL1) was highly expressed in the pancreatic duct epithelium, peribiliary glands, and vascular endothelial cells of patients with AIP and IgG4-SC, with infiltration of the CCL1-expressing sites by CCR8-positive lymphocytes. The periductal and perivascular cellular infiltrate consisted largely of Tregs and Th2 cells, which was not seen in PSC controls (including patients with PSC with high serum IgG4 levels).[89] These findings may indicate a role for CCL1-CCR8 interaction in lymphocytic recruitment in IgG4-SC/AIP.

The fact that IgG4-SC is associated with AIP, as well as gallbladder and liver involvement, may also suggest locoregional factors play a role in the pathogenesis. Peribiliary glands, physiologically distributed around the extrahepatic and intrahepatic large bile ducts,[90] may be severely damaged in IgG4-SC.[91] These glands are known to contain small amounts of exocrine pancreatic acini.[92]

Innate immune cells
Macrophages, eosinophils, and basophils are often detectable in affected tissue, although their role in pathogenesis is not understood. One study reported the

involvement of IL-10 and TGF-β secreting basophils in tissue of patients with IgG4-related submandibular gland disease.[33] Activation of nucleotide-binding oligomerization domain-containing protein 2 and Toll-like receptor ligands on monocytes or basophils from patients with AIP were shown to enhance IgG4 responses, which was mediated via B-cell activating factor and IL-13, indicating crosstalk between the innate and acquired immune system.[93,94] The relevance of these findings to IgG4-SC remains unclear.

SUMMARY

IgG4-SC is the biliary manifestation of IRD, an increasingly recognized fibro-inflammatory multisystem disease characterized by lymphoplasmacytic infiltration, storiform fibrosis, and obliterative phlebitis with a marked infiltration of IgG4-positive plasma cells in affected tissues. In clinical practice, hepatopancreatobiliary physicians and surgeons must be aware of the possibility of this disease when confronted with patients with unexplained biliary strictures and masses. Diagnosis is established based on a combination of clinical, serologic, radiological, and histologic findings. Correctly differentiating IgG4-SC from disease mimics is crucial, and diagnostic algorithms have been developed to aid disease identification. Steroids are the mainstay of treatment and often successful when initiated in time to prevent fibrotic complications. Disease relapse occurs in half of patients with IRD, with IgG4-SC as an independent risk factor. The early initiation of second-line therapy and/or prolonged corticosteroids in patients with higher-risk IgG4-SC needs to be investigated in prospective controlled trials. Awareness of an increased risk of organ dysfunction and malignancy should encourage close follow-up. Multicenter prospective cohort studies and randomized clinical studies are needed to provide novel biomarkers of disease and to further optimize therapeutic strategies in IgG4-SC. The immunopathogenesis of disease including the role of IgG4 antibodies, Th2 immune response, and genetic factors continues to be unraveled. Identification of a disease-specific autoantigen, autoantibody, pathogen, or allergen remains a focus of research, although it may be that ultimately there is not a single unifying cause.

REFERENCES

1. Björnsson E, Chari ST, Smyrk TC, et al. Immunoglobulin G4 associated cholangitis: description of an emerging clinical entity based on review of the literature. Hepatology 2007;45(6):1547–54.
2. Erdogan D, Kloek JJ, Ten Kate FJW, et al. Immunoglobulin G4-related sclerosing cholangitis in patients resected for presumed malignant bile duct strictures. Br J Surg 2008;95(6):727–34.
3. Sarles H, Sarles JC, Muratore R, et al. Chronic inflammatory sclerosis of the pancreas–an autonomous pancreatic disease? Am J Dig Dis 1961;6:688–98.
4. Bartholomew LG, Cain JC, Woolner LB, et al. Sclerosing cholangitis: its possible association with Riedel's struma and fibrous retroperitonitis. Report of two cases. N Engl J Med 1963;269:8–12.
5. Hamano H, Kawa S, Horiuchi A, et al. High serum IgG4 concentrations in patients with sclerosing pancreatitis. N Engl J Med 2001;344(10):732–8.
6. Kamisawa T, Funata N, Hayashi Y, et al. A new clinicopathological entity of IgG4-related autoimmune disease. J Gastroenterol 2003;38(10):982–4.
7. European Association for the Study of the Liver. EASL clinical practice guidelines: management of cholestatic liver diseases. J Hepatol 2009;51(2):237 67.

8. Kamisawa T, Okamoto A. Autoimmune pancreatitis: proposal of IgG4-related sclerosing disease. J Gastroenterol 2006;41(7):613–25.
9. Umehara H, Okazaki K, Masaki Y, et al. A novel clinical entity, IgG4-related disease (IgG4RD): general concept and details. Mod Rheumatol 2012;22(1): 1–14.
10. Ghazale A, Chari ST, Zhang L, et al. Immunoglobulin G4-associated cholangitis: clinical profile and response to therapy. Gastroenterology 2008;134(3):706–15.
11. Takikawa H, Takamori Y, Tanaka A, et al. Analysis of 388 cases of primary sclerosing cholangitis in Japan. Presence of a subgroup without pancreatic involvement in older patients. Hepatol Res 2004;29(3):153–9.
12. Mattoo H, Della-Torre E, Mahajan VS, et al. Circulating Th2 memory cells in IgG4-related disease are restricted to a defined subset of subjects with atopy. Allergy 2014;69(3):399–402.
13. De Buy Wenniger LJM, Culver EL, Beuers U. Exposure to occupational antigens might predispose to IgG4-related disease. Hepatology 2014;60(4):1453–4.
14. Mendes FD, Jorgensen R, Keach J, et al. Elevated serum IgG4 concentration in patients with primary sclerosing cholangitis. Am J Gastroenterol 2006;101(9): 2070–5.
15. Oseini AM, Chaiteerakij R, Shire AM, et al. Utility of serum immunoglobulin G4 in distinguishing immunoglobulin G4-associated cholangitis from cholangiocarcinoma. Hepatology 2011;54(3):940–8.
16. Ghazale A, Chari ST, Smyrk TC, et al. Value of serum IgG4 in the diagnosis of autoimmune pancreatitis and in distinguishing it from pancreatic cancer. Am J Gastroenterol 2007;102(8):1646–53.
17. Ohara H, Nakazawa T, Kawa S, et al. Establishment of a serum IgG4 cut-off value for the differential diagnosis of IgG4-related sclerosing cholangitis: a Japanese cohort. J Gastroenterol Hepatol 2013;28(7):1247–51.
18. Boonstra K, Culver EL, de Buy Wenniger LM, et al. Serum immunoglobulin G4 and immunoglobulin G1 for distinguishing immunoglobulin G4-associated cholangitis from primary sclerosing cholangitis. Hepatology 2014;59(5):1954–63.
19. Kamisawa T, Takuma K, Tabata T, et al. Serum IgG4-negative autoimmune pancreatitis. J Gastroenterol 2011;46(1):108–16.
20. Sadler R, Chapman RW, Simpson D, et al. The diagnostic significance of serum IgG4 levels in patients with autoimmune pancreatitis: a UK study. Eur J Gastroenterol Hepatol 2011;23(2):139–45.
21. Vosskuhl K, Negm AA, Framke T, et al. Measurement of IgG4 in bile: a new approach for the diagnosis of IgG4-associated cholangiopathy. Endoscopy 2012;44(1):48–52.
22. Uehara T, Hamano H, Kawa S, et al. Distinct clinicopathological entity "autoimmune pancreatitis-associated sclerosing cholangitis". Pathol Int 2005;55(7): 405–11.
23. Hirano K, Shiratori Y, Komatsu Y, et al. Involvement of the biliary system in autoimmune pancreatitis: a follow-up study. Clin Gastroenterol Hepatol 2003;1(6): 453–64.
24. Nishino T, Toki F, Oyama H, et al. Biliary tract involvement in autoimmune pancreatitis. Pancreas 2005;30(1):76–82.
25. Koyama R, Imamura T, Okuda C, et al. Ultrasonographic imaging of bile duct lesions in autoimmune pancreatitis. Pancreas 2008;37(3):259–64.
26. Itoh S, Nagasaka T, Suzuki K, et al. Lymphoplasmacytic sclerosing cholangitis: assessment of clinical, CT, and pathological findings. Clin Radiol 2009;64(11): 1104–14.

27. Kamisawa T, Tu Y, Egawa N, et al. Can MRCP replace ERCP for the diagnosis of autoimmune pancreatitis? Abdom Imaging 2009;34(3):381–4.

28. Nakazawa T, Ohara H, Sano H, et al. Cholangiography can discriminate sclerosing cholangitis with autoimmune pancreatitis from primary sclerosing cholangitis. Gastrointest Endosc 2004;60(6):937–44.

29. Naitoh I, Nakazawa T, Hayashi K, et al. Comparison of intraductal ultrasonography findings between primary sclerosing cholangitis and IgG4-related sclerosing cholangitis. J Gastroenterol Hepatol 2015;30(6):1104–9. Available at: http://doi.wiley.com/10.1111/jgh.12894.

30. Kuwatani M, Kawakami H, Zen Y, et al. Difference from bile duct cancer and relationship between bile duct wall thickness and serum IgG/IgG4 levels in IgG4-related sclerosing cholangitis. Hepatogastroenterology 2014;61(135):1852–6.

31. Zen Y, Fujii T, Sato Y, et al. Pathological classification of hepatic inflammatory pseudotumor with respect to IgG4-related disease. Mod Pathol 2007;20(8):884–94.

32. Deshpande V, Sainani NI, Chung RT, et al. IgG4-associated cholangitis: a comparative histological and immunophenotypic study with primary sclerosing cholangitis on liver biopsy material. Mod Pathol 2009;22(10):1287–95. Nature Publishing Group.

33. Takeuchi M, Sato Y, Ohno K, et al. T helper 2 and regulatory T-cell cytokine production by mast cells: a key factor in the pathogenesis of IgG4-related disease. Mod Pathol 2014;27(8):1126–36.

34. Zhang L, Lewis JT, Abraham SC, et al. IgG4+ plasma cell infiltrates in liver explants with primary sclerosing cholangitis. Am J Surg Pathol 2010;34(1):88–94.

35. Zen Y, Quaglia A, Portmann B. Immunoglobulin G4-positive plasma cell infiltration in explanted livers for primary sclerosing cholangitis. Histopathology 2011;58(3):414–22.

36. Harada K, Shimoda S, Kimura Y, et al. Significance of immunoglobulin G4 (IgG4)-positive cells in extrahepatic cholangiocarcinoma: molecular mechanism of IgG4 reaction in cancer tissue. Hepatology 2012;56(1):157–64.

37. Deshpande V, Zen Y, Chan JK, et al. Consensus statement on the pathology of IgG4-related disease. Mod Pathol 2012;25(9):1181–92.

38. Naitoh I, Zen Y, Nakazawa T, et al. Small bile duct involvement in IgG4-related sclerosing cholangitis: liver biopsy and cholangiography correlation. J Gastroenterol 2011;46(2):269–76.

39. Umemura T, Zen Y, Hamano H, et al. Immunoglobin G4-hepatopathy: association of immunoglobin G4-bearing plasma cells in liver with autoimmune pancreatitis. Hepatology 2007;46(2):463–71.

40. Hubers LM, Doorenspleet ME, Culver EL, et al. IgG4+ B-cell receptor clones in peripheral blood distinguish IgG4-associated cholangitis/autoimmune pancreatitis from primary sclerosing cholangitis. J Hepatol 2015;62(2):S233–4.

41. Ghazale A, Chari ST. Optimising corticosteroid treatment for autoimmune pancreatitis. Gut 2007;56(12):1650–2.

42. Kamisawa T, Okazaki K, Kawa S, et al. Japanese consensus guidelines for management of autoimmune pancreatitis: III. Treatment and prognosis of AIP. J Gastroenterol 2010;45(5):471–7.

43. Hart PA, Topazian MD, Witzig TE, et al. Treatment of relapsing autoimmune pancreatitis with immunomodulators and rituximab: the Mayo Clinic experience. Gut 2013;62(11):1607–15.

44. Topazian M, Witzig TE, Smyrk TC, et al. Rituximab therapy for refractory biliary strictures in immunoglobulin G4-associated cholangitis. Clin Gastroenterol Hepatol 2008;6(3):364–6.

45. Hart PA, Kamisawa T, Brugge WR, et al. Long-term outcomes of autoimmune pancreatitis: a multicentre, international analysis. Gut 2013;62:1771–6.
46. Sandanayake NS, Church NI, Chapman MH, et al. Presentation and management of post-treatment relapse in autoimmune pancreatitis/immunoglobulin G4-associated cholangitis. Clin Gastroenterol Hepatol 2009;7(10):1089–96.
47. Huggett MT, Culver EL, Kumar M, et al. Type 1 autoimmune pancreatitis and IgG4-related sclerosing cholangitis is associated with extrapancreatic organ failure, malignancy, and mortality in a prospective UK cohort. Am J Gastroenterol 2014;109(10):1675–83.
48. Kawa S, Ota M, Yoshizawa K, et al. HLA DRB10405-DQB10401 haplotype is associated with autoimmune pancreatitis in the Japanese population. Gastroenterology 2002;122(5):1264–9.
49. Umemura T, Ota M, Hamano H, et al. Genetic association of Fc receptor-like 3 polymorphisms with autoimmune pancreatitis in Japanese patients. Gut 2006;55(9):1367–8.
50. Chang M-C, Chang Y-T, Tien Y-W, et al. T-cell regulatory gene CTLA-4 polymorphism/haplotype association with autoimmune pancreatitis. Clin Chem 2007;53(9):1700–5.
51. Umemura T, Ota M, Hamano H, et al. Association of autoimmune pancreatitis with cytotoxic T-lymphocyte antigen 4 gene polymorphisms in Japanese patients. Am J Gastroenterol 2008;103(3):588–94.
52. Park DH, Kim M-H, Oh HB, et al. Substitution of aspartic acid at position 57 of the DQbeta1 affects relapse of autoimmune pancreatitis. Gastroenterology 2008;134(2):440–6.
53. Okazaki K, Uchida K, Ohana M, et al. Autoimmune-related pancreatitis is associated with autoantibodies and a Th1/Th2-type cellular immune response. Gastroenterology 2000;118(3):573–81.
54. Aparisi L, Farre A, Gomez-Cambronero L, et al. Antibodies to carbonic anhydrase and IgG4 levels in idiopathic chronic pancreatitis: relevance for diagnosis of autoimmune pancreatitis. Gut 2005;54(5):703–9. Available at: http://www.pubmedcentral.nih.gov/articlerender.fcgi?artid=1774474&tool=pmcentrez&rendertype=abstract. Accessed October 25, 2012.
55. Asada M, Nishio A, Uchida K, et al. Identification of a novel autoantibody against pancreatic secretory trypsin inhibitor in patients with autoimmune pancreatitis. Pancreas 2006;33(1):20–6.
56. Löhr J-M, Faissner R, Koczan D, et al. Autoantibodies against the exocrine pancreas in autoimmune pancreatitis: gene and protein expression profiling and immunoassays identify pancreatic enzymes as a major target of the inflammatory process. Am J Gastroenterol 2010;105(9):2060–71. Available at: http://www.pubmedcentral.nih.gov/articlerender.fcgi?artid=3099227&tool=pmcentrez&rendertype=abstract. Accessed September 27, 2012.
57. Endo T, Takizawa S, Tanaka S, et al. Amylase alpha-2A autoantibodies: novel marker of autoimmune pancreatitis and fulminant type 1 diabetes. Diabetes 2009;58(3):732–7. Available at: http://www.pubmedcentral.nih.gov/articlerender.fcgi?artid=2646073&tool=pmcentrez&rendertype=abstract. Accessed December 2, 2012.
58. Takizawa S, Endo T, Wanjia X, et al. 10 is a new autoantigen in both autoimmune pancreatitis and fulminant type 1 diabetes. Biochem Biophys Res Commun 2009;386(1):192–6.
59. Yamamoto M, Naishiro Y, Suzuki C, et al. Proteomics analysis in 28 patients with systemic IgG4-related plasmacytic syndrome. Rheumatol Int 2010;30(4):565–8.

60. Hardt PD, Ewald N, Bröckling K, et al. Distinct autoantibodies against exocrine pancreatic antigens in European patients with type 1 diabetes mellitus and non-alcoholic chronic pancreatitis. JOP 2008;9(6):683–9.
61. Frulloni L, Lunardi C, Simone R, et al. Identification of a novel antibody associated with autoimmune pancreatitis. N Engl J Med 2009;361(22):2135–42.
62. Nishimori I, Miyaji E, Morimoto K, et al. Serum antibodies to carbonic anhydrase IV in patients with autoimmune pancreatitis. Gut 2005;54(2):274–81.
63. Shinji A, Sano K, Hamano H, et al. Autoimmune pancreatitis is closely associated with gastric ulcer presenting with abundant IgG4-bearing plasma cell infiltration. Gastrointest Endosc 2004;59(4):506–11.
64. Kountouras J, Zavos C, Chatzopoulos D. A concept on the role of Helicobacter pylori infection in autoimmune pancreatitis. J Cell Mol Med 2005;9(1):196–207.
65. Guarneri F, Guarneri C, Benvenga S. Helicobacter pylori and autoimmune pancreatitis: role of carbonic anhydrase via molecular mimicry? J Cell Mol Med 2005;9(3):741–4.
66. Jesnowski R, Isaksson B, Möhrcke C, et al. Helicobacter pylori in autoimmune pancreatitis and pancreatic carcinoma. Pancreatology 2010;10(4):462–6.
67. Aalberse RC, Stapel SO, Schuurman J, et al. Immunoglobulin G4: an odd antibody. Clin Exp Allergy 2009;39(4):469–77.
68. Van der Zee JS, van Swieten P, Aalberse RC. Inhibition of complement activation by IgG4 antibodies. Clin Exp Immunol 1986;64(2):415–22. Available at: http://www.ncbi.nlm.nih.gov/pmc/articles/PMC1542347.
69. Van der Neut Kolfschoten M, Schuurman J, Losen M, et al. Anti-inflammatory activity of human IgG4 antibodies by dynamic Fab arm exchange. Science 2007; 317(5844):1554–7.
70. Kawa S, Kitahara K, Hamano H, et al. A novel immunoglobulin-immunoglobulin interaction in autoimmunity. PLoS One 2008;3(2):e1637.
71. Futei Y, Amagai M, Ishii K, et al. Predominant IgG4 subclass in autoantibodies of pemphigus vulgaris and foliaceus. J Dermatol Sci 2001;26(1):55–61.
72. Huijbers MG, Zhang W, Klooster R, et al. MuSK IgG4 autoantibodies cause myasthenia gravis by inhibiting binding between MuSK and Lrp4. Proc Natl Acad Sci U S A 2013;110(51):20783–8.
73. Aoki S, Nakazawa T, Ohara H, et al. Immunohistochemical study of autoimmune pancreatitis using anti-IgG4 antibody and patients' sera. Histopathology 2005; 47(2):147–58.
74. De Buy Wenniger LJM, Doorenspleet ME, Klarenbeek PL, et al. IgG4+ clones identified by next-generation sequencing dominate the b-cell receptor repertoire in IgG4-associated cholangitis. Hepatology 2013;57(6):2390–8.
75. Mattoo H, Mahajan VS, Della-Torre E, et al. De novo oligoclonal expansions of circulating plasmablasts in active and relapsing IgG4-related disease. J Allergy Clin Immunol 2014;134(3):679–87. Elsevier Ltd. Available at: http://linkinghub. elsevier.com/retrieve/pii/S0091674914005156. Accessed May 11, 2014.
76. Culver EL, Vermeulen E, Makuch M, et al. Increased IgG4 responses to multiple food and animal antigens indicate a polyclonal expansion and differentiation of pre-existing B cells in IgG4-related disease. Ann Rheum Dis 2015;74:994–7.
77. Zen Y, Fujii T, Harada K, et al. Th2 and regulatory immune reactions are increased in immunoglobin G4-related sclerosing pancreatitis and cholangitis. Hepatology 2007;45(6):1538–46.
78. Kanari H, Kagami S, Kashiwakuma D, et al. Role of Th2 cells in IgG4-related lacrimal gland enlargement. Int Arch Allergy Immunol 2010;152(Suppl 1): 47–53.

79. Punnonen J, Aversa G, Cocks BG, et al. Interleukin 4-independent IgG4 and IgE synthesis and CD23 expression by human. Immunology 1993;90(8):3730–4.
80. Jeannin P, Lecoanet S, Delneste Y, et al. IgE versus IgG4 production can be differentially regulated by IL-10. J Immunol 1998;160(7):3555–61.
81. Miyoshi H, Uchida K, Taniguchi T. Circulating Naive and CD4 + CD25high regulatory T cells in patients with autoimmune pancreatitis. Pancreas 2008;36(2): 133–40.
82. Kusuda T, Uchida K, Miyoshi H. Involvement of inducible costimulator - and interleukin 10-positive regulatory T cells in the development of IgG4-related autoimmune pancreatitis. Pancreas 2011;40(7):1120–30.
83. Tsuboi H, Matsuo N, Iizuka M, et al. Analysis of IgG4 class switch-related molecules in IgG4-related disease. Arthritis Res Ther 2012;14(4):R171. BioMed Central Ltd.
84. Koyabu M, Uchida K, Miyoshi H, et al. Analysis of regulatory T cells and IgG4-positive plasma cells among patients of IgG4-related sclerosing cholangitis and autoimmune liver diseases. J Gastroenterol 2010;45(7):732–41.
85. Satoguina JS, Weyand E, Larbi J, et al. T regulatory-1 cells induce IgG4 production by B cells: role of IL-10. J Immunol 2005;174(8):4718–26.
86. Meiler F, Klunker S, Zimmermann M, et al. Distinct regulation of IgE, IgG4 and IgA by T regulatory cells and toll-like receptors. Allergy 2008;63(11):1455–63.
87. Mahajan VS, Mattoo H, Deshpande V, et al. IgG4-related disease. Annu Rev Pathol 2014;9(1):315–47.
88. Wynn TA. Fibrotic disease and the T(H)1/T(H)2 paradigm. Nat Rev Immunol 2004; 4(8):583–94. Available at: http://www.pubmedcentral.nih.gov/articlerender.fcgi? artid=2702150&tool=pmcentrez&rendertype=abstract. Accessed February 21, 2015.
89. Zen Y, Liberal R, Nakanuma Y, et al. Possible involvement of CCL1-CCR8 interaction in lymphocytic recruitment in IgG4-related sclerosing cholangitis. J Hepatol 2013;59(5):1059–64. European Association for the Study of the Liver.
90. Terada T, Nakanuma Y, Ohta G. Glandular elements around the intrahepatic bile ducts in man; their morphology and distribution in normal livers. Liver 1987;7(1): 1–8.
91. Graham RPD, Smyrk TC, Chari ST, et al. Isolated IgG4-related sclerosing cholangitis: a report of 9 cases. Hum Pathol 2014;45(8):1722–9.
92. Terada T, Nakanuma Y, Kakita A. Pathologic observations of intrahepatic peribiliary glands in 1000 consecutive autopsy livers. Heterotopic pancreas in the liver. Gastroenterology 1990;98(5 Pt 1):1333–7.
93. Watanabe T, Yamashita K, Fujikawa S, et al. Involvement of activation of toll-like receptors and nucleotide-binding oligomerization domain-like receptors in enhanced IgG4 responses in autoimmune pancreatitis. Arthritis Rheum 2012; 64(3):914–24.
94. Watanabe T, Yamashita K, Sakurai T, et al. Toll-like receptor activation in basophils contributes to the development of IgG4-related disease. J Gastroenterol 2013; 48(2):247–53.

Primary Sclerosing Cholangitis
Multiple Phenotypes, Multiple Approaches

Souvik Sarkar, MD, Christopher L. Bowlus, MD*

KEYWORDS

- Primary sclerosing cholangitis • Diagnosis • Treatment
- IgG4-related sclerosing cholangitis • Autoimmune hepatitis

KEY POINTS

- Primary sclerosing cholangitis (PSC) presents as a heterogeneous group characterized by segmental strictures of bile ducts, most often in the setting of inflammatory bowel disease (IBD) involving the proximal colon.
- Several phenotypes of PSC have been recognized based on the age of diagnosis, presence or absence of IBD, small duct involvement, immunoglobulin G4 (IgG4) level, dominant strictures, and race.
- Approximately 10% of PSC patients have an elevated serum IgG4 level, which can lead to misdiagnosis of IgG4-related sclerosing cholangitis, which is a separate disease from PSC.
- Future research is needed to develop systems to classify PSC patients into specific phenotypes based on the clinical features that have been described so that the pathogenic mechanisms can be better understood and new targets for drug development identified.

INTRODUCTION

Sclerosing cholangitis refers to a broad array of diseases that cause fibrosis of the bile ducts, usually of medium and large ducts, leading to a segmental pattern of narrowing with proximal dilation. Secondary sclerosing cholangitis may be a complication of several different injuries, inflammatory reactions, or malignancies. In primary sclerosing cholangitis (PSC), in nearly 80% of cases, the underlying insult leading to biliary injury seems to be an extrahepatic manifestation of inflammatory bowel disease (IBD), either ulcerative colitis (UC) or Crohn colitis. Although the typical PSC patient is a young male, 30 to 40 years of age, approximately one-third are women and onset can occur in childhood or late adulthood (**Box 1**).

The authors have nothing to disclose.
Division of Gastroenterology and Hepatology, University of California Davis School of Medicine, 4150 V Street, PSSB 3500, Sacramento, CA 95817, USA
* Corresponding author.
E-mail address: clbowlus@ucdavis.edu

Clin Liver Dis 20 (2016) 67–77
http://dx.doi.org/10.1016/j.cld.2015.08.005
liver.theclinics.com

Box 1
Primary sclerosing cholangitis clinical features

Duct Involvement

- Large duct: classic form
  - Extrahepatic versus intrahepatic versus both
  - Dominant stricture: worse outcomes, especially due to cholangiocarcinoma (CCA)
- Small duct: histologic PSC features but normal cholangiogram, better outcomes

Inflammatory Bowel Disease

- UC: typically mild pancolitis, ileum involvement common
- Crohn disease: more frequent in small duct PSC, better outcome
- Indeterminate colitis
- No IBD: must be confirmed by colonoscopy, better outcome

Serum IgG4

- Normal: typical in 90% of PSC, elevation of total IgG common
- 1 to 2 × upper limit of normal (ULN): ~10% of PSC, may predict poor outcome
- Greater than 2 × ULN: more likely to be IgG4-related sclerosing cholangitis

Autoimmune Overlap

- ALT (alanine aminotransferase) greater than 5 × ULN and IgG greater than 2 × ULN: no diagnostic consensus, consider AIH treatment, may present concurrent with PSC or following AIH treatment

Race or Ethnicity

- European: most data based on those of European descent
- African: more advanced disease at younger age, more Crohn, less male predominance
- Asian, seems rare

Age of Diagnosis

- Pediatric: more overlap with AIH, more responsive to treatment initially
- Young adult: typical presentation, more aggressive
- Older adult: better outcome

DIAGNOSTIC CRITERIA

Unlike primary biliary cholangitis (formerly primary biliary cirrhosis), for which there are agreed-on, validated, diagnostic criteria, there remains a lack of objective criteria on which PSC is diagnosed. Current diagnostics for PSC are limited for several reasons. First, the diagnosis of PSC depends on interpretation of cholangiogram, which is difficult to quantify and limited by technical and interobserver variability. Although magnetic resonance cholangiopancreatography (MRCP) remains the initial diagnostic imaging tool of choice with a sensitivity 86% and specificity 94% for the diagnosis of PSC,[1,2] a negative MRCP does not negate the need for endoscopic retrograde cholangiopancreatography (ERCP) because MRCP lacks sensitivity in early PSC and cholangiocarcinoma and can lack specificity in cirrhosis.[3] Second, in cases of ambiguous cholangiograms, liver biopsy is neither sensitive nor specific for PSC. Even the classic onion-skinning of concentric fibrosis is found in only a minority of PSC cases and may also be present in ischemic cholangitis and other biliary diseases. Third, serum markers, such as perinuclear antineutrophil cytoplasmic antibody (pANCA), are found in up to 95% of PSC patients but are also present in other liver diseases as well as in IBD, particularly UC, without PSC. Finally, excluding secondary causes of sclerosing cholangitis can be difficult, particularly in patients without IBD who may have undergone cholecystectomy during an evaluation of cholestasis or had a history of cholelithiasis. Thus, the diagnostic certainty of PSC ranges from the highest level in a young man with UC and classic intrahepatic and extrahepatic segmental biliary strictures to the lowest level in, for example, an older woman who presents with cholestasis but without any evidence of IBD, a history of cholecystectomy, only minor intrahepatic biliary strictures, and a liver biopsy with nonspecific portal inflammation and biliary fibrosis.

IDENTIFICATION OF PRIMARY SCLEROSING CHOLANGITIS PHENOTYPES

PSC is a rare disease with an incidence rate in North American and Northern Europe of approximately 1 to 1.5 cases per 100,000 person-years and a prevalence rate of 6 to 16 cases per 100,000 inhabitants.[4–6] Estimates of the prevalence of PSC in other parts of the world are very limited but suggested to be substantially lower at 0.95 cases per 1000,000 inhabitants in Japan.[7] This limited the understanding of PSC phenotypes until the recent accumulation of large cohorts at single centers, as well as collaborative efforts such as the International PSC Study Group[8] and the Netherlands EpiPSCPBC (Epidemiology and Natural History of PSC and PBC) Study Group,[9] consisting of several thousand subjects and analysis of transplant databases.[10] These have led to a better understanding of the variety of disease patterns within the larger group of patients diagnosed with PSC. The following are the most notable groups of PSC patients (**Fig. 1**).

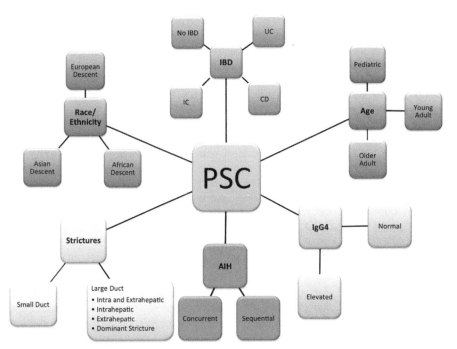

Fig. 1. Multiple clinical features have been identified to describe a variety of PSC phenotypes. In isolation, each has been shown to segregate groups of PSC patients with differences in outcomes or response to treatment. AIH, autoimmune hepatitis; IC, indeterminate colitis.

LARGE DUCT PRIMARY SCLEROSING CHOLANGITIS VARIANTS

The classic form of PSC, which accounts for most PSC cases, as originally described has several characteristic features in addition to the classic cholangiographic features of strictures in the large and medium bile ducts. Namely, large duct PSC occurs predominantly in men (male/female ratio 3:2), is coexistent with IBD in 60% to 80% of cases, and typically presents with cholestasis. The IBD typically is a pancolitis with frequent ileitis and rectal sparing. In addition, the IBD is commonly mild and asymptomatic. The association between PSC and IBD seems to be greater in northern latitudes; although, even there, the frequency of non-IBD PSC is increasing. The natural history of large duct PSC ranges from rapidly progressive to indolent. The mean transplant-free survival has been reported to be from 12 to more than 20 years, with the latter including more recent population-based estimates.[11,12] This group of PSC is the best described and for which there is the best understanding, including the strong association with the human leukocyte antigen (HLA) haplotype defined by HLA-A*01, -B*08, and -DRB1*03.

Special mention should be made regarding the IBD found in PSC, which is commonly asymptomatic. Therefore, all newly diagnosed PSC patients without a diagnosis of IBD must undergo colonoscopy. Interestingly, the IBD typically is a pancolitis, which often shares features of both UC and Crohn colitis with frequent ileitis and rectal sparing.[13] Compared with patients with IBD without PSC, patients with IBD and PSC tend to be younger at presentation, yet have a significantly increased risk of colorectal carcinoma.[14] These patients may also have exacerbation of IBD after liver transplantation for PSC and the risk of pouchitis is significantly increased after proctocolectomy with ileal anal-pouch anastomosis.[14] Of note, PSC does not depend on active intestinal disease and, in fact, can occur after colectomy[13] and immunosuppression. In particular, those that are effective for the treatment of IBD have not been shown to be effective for PSC.[15] Management of IBD remains the same independent of the presence of PSC with the exception that surveillance colonoscopy for dysplasia is recommended to be initiated at the time of PSC diagnosis due to the absence of a lag time in colorectal cancer risk in IBD alone.

With the strong association between PSC and IBD, it is not surprising that they share some common genetic basis. However, only half of the PSC genes that have been identified are also associated with UC, Crohn disease, or both, with the strongest association with UC compared with Crohn disease.[16–21] Notably, most of the genes shared between PSC and IBD are more strongly associated with PSC than with UC or Crohn disease. In addition, network analysis has not identified any common functional pathways to suggest a specific mechanism that predisposes both IBD and PSC. This lack of a more common genetic basis between PSC and UC or Crohn disease supports the clinical notion that PSC-IBD is a unique phenotype.

Stricture Type

Segmental strictures with proximal dilation and sacculation of the bile ducts that create the beaded appearance are the classic finding of PSC on cholangiogram. Typically, these findings are present in the intrahepatic and the extrahepatic bile ducts. Strictures limited to the extrahepatic bile ducts alone are rare, whereas isolated changes of the intrahepatic bile ducts have been reported in 20% to 28% of cases. Dominant strictures, which have been defined as strictures with a diameter of less than 1.5 mm of the common bile duct or less than 1.0 mm of a hepatic duct within 2 cm of the bifurcation, develop in approximately half of PSC patients. The presence of a dominant stricture is of particular concern for cholangiocarcinoma and should be evaluated by brush cytology and/or biopsy. Several studies have shown an association between dominant strictures and poor outcomes even with endoscopic management[22,23] and, recently, this has been suggested to be due to the increased prevalence of cholangiocarcinoma.[24]

Non–Inflammatory Bowel Disease Large Duct Primary Sclerosing Cholangitis

In contrast to PSC in the presence of IBD, PSC in the absence of IBD tends to be equally distributed among men and women, is diagnosed at a much older age,[25] and may have a better prognosis.[26] Although the rarity of PSC without IBD limits the power of genetic analysis, this group of PSC patients seems to share similar HLA risk alleles compared with PSC with IBD.[27]

High–Immunoglobulin G4 Primary Sclerosing Cholangitis

In addition to several autoantibodies, total serum immunoglobulin (Ig) G levels are modestly elevated in approximately 60% of patients and IgM levels can also be elevated. More recently, it has been recognized that IgG4 levels are elevated in approximately 10% of PSC patients but rarely is the level greater than 2.8 g/L or twice the upper limit of normal.[9,28–33] Notably, elevated IgG4 levels have been associated with decreased transplant-free survival in one cohort[28] but not another.[33]

Primary Sclerosing Cholangitis–Autoimmune Hepatitis Overlap

Reports of the frequency of PSC with features that overlap with autoimmune hepatitis (AIH) range between 1% and 53.8%. Likely this is because there remains no agreed-on diagnostic criteria for PSC-AIH overlap.[34] Typically, these patients present with significant elevations of liver transaminases and histologic findings consistent with AIH. However, they may also initially present as a typical case of AIH that becomes cholestatic with the development of sclerosing cholangitis. In some cases, PSC-AIH may respond to immunosuppression. Importantly, autoantibodies, including antinuclear antibodies and antismooth muscle antibodies, are frequent in PSC without evidence of AIH. In addition, 10% or more of patients with AIH may have cholangiographic features on MRCP consistent with PSC.[35,36]

Pediatric Primary Sclerosing Cholangitis

PSC in children seems to have many of the same features as PSC in adults, namely a male predominance and strong association with IBD. However, in children PSC seems much more responsive to therapies and have a higher frequency of overlap with AIH.[37] Autoimmune sclerosing cholangitis is a term used to designate a group of patients with PSC-AIH features with the exceptional reversal of cholangiographic findings with immunosuppression. Recent case series have also reported marked clinical improvement with oral vancomycin in children with PSC. Notably, neither of these therapies has shown similar effects in adults.

Nonwhite Population Large Duct Primary Sclerosing Cholangitis

Most studies of PSC have been performed in northern European populations or populations that descended from northern Europe, leading some clinicians to conclude that PSC is a disease of the white population. However, PSC is a modern disease and, given its association with IBD, it is likely that as the geoepidemiology of IBD changes, the frequency of PSC in nonwhite populations will change with it. To date, there are few data from Asia apart from the IgG4-related sclerosing cholangitis associated with autoimmune pancreatitis (AIP) described in Japan, where PSC seems to be extremely rare.

In contrast, studies of a large health care organization and United States transplant data suggest that the incidence and prevalence rates of PSC among African Americans is at least as great as in white Americans.[10,38] In African Americans there is a less striking male predominance and lower IBD rate. Interestingly, HLA-DR3, which is strongly associated with PSC in European populations, is rare among African Americans and was not associated with PSC in African American subjects. However, the HLA-B8 association is shared between white and African American PSC patients.

SMALL DUCT PRIMARY SCLEROSING CHOLANGITIS

A small group of PSC patients present with clinical and histologic features compatible with PSC, except for the lack of typical cholangiographic findings, and have been defined as small duct PSC.[39] In some series, IBD was required for the diagnosis but not in others. In addition, in the past these patients may have been labeled as antimitochondrial antibody–negative primary biliary cholangitis, formerly known as primary biliary cirrhosis, or autoimmune cholangiopathy. In most cohorts, small duct PSC comprises approximately 10% of the total PSC population, rarely progresses to large duct PSC, and has a generally favorable outcome. Recent analysis of the HLA region shows that small duct PSC without IBD is genetically distinct from large duct PSC.[40]

IMMUNOGLOBULIN G4–RELATED SCLEROSING CHOLANGITIS

The recent description of IgG4-related sclerosing cholangitis often found in association with AIP as one of many diseases associated with elevated IgG4 serum levels and tissue infiltration of IgG4-plasma cell has led to the recognition that some previously diagnosed cases of PSC were, in fact, IgG4-related sclerosing cholangitis.[41] Adding confusion to this issue are findings that serum IgG4 levels are often elevated in PSC and IgG4 plasma cells are frequent in PSC liver explants, but the 2 features do not necessarily correlate.[29,42] In addition, IgG4-related diseases are typically responsive to corticosteroids, which is not seen in PSC. For patients with a serum IgG4 level between 1.4 and 2.8 g/L, a ratio of IgG4 to IgG1 of less than 0.24 suggests a diagnosis of PSC rather than IgG4-sclerosing cholangitis. However, the diagnosis of IgG-4-related sclerosing cholangitis should be based on histology, imaging, serology, and other organ involvement, in addition to response to steroid therapy by the HISORt criteria that were originally developed for the diagnosis of autoimmune pancreatitis.[43]

MULTIPLE APPROACHES
Diagnosis

Understanding the multiple phenotypes of PSC is important for several reasons. First, recognition that PSC may present in an atypical pattern, for example, an older nonwhite woman without IBD, is vital to avoid missed opportunities for diagnosis. Second, proper classification can affect management decisions. For example, a patient with undiagnosed quiescent colitis may not receive the appropriate surveillance for colorectal cancer. Third, patients with IgG4-related sclerosing cholangitis respond well to corticosteroids and some evidence suggest that so do some patients with PSC and elevated serum IgG4 levels, as well as PSC-AIH overlap patients.[30,34] Finally, classification can have a tremendous impact on prognosis. Specifically, those with small duct PSC, normal serum alkaline phosphatase levels, and older age at diagnosis seem to have a more benign course.[39,44–47]

Management

Although there are no therapies other than liver transplantation proven to alter the natural history of PSC, the management of these patients is not simple and includes consideration of ursodeoxycholic acid or other therapies, referral to clinical trials, and monitoring of disease progression to cirrhosis and other outcomes including bacterial cholangitis, cholangiocarcinoma, and colorectal cancer (**Fig. 2**). In addition, PSC patients should be tested for associated autoimmune conditions, nutritional deficiencies, and osteoporosis.

SUMMARY AND DISCUSSION

PSC is a heterogeneous disorder that varies in clinical presentation, natural history, and, potentially, treatment response. Many studies have documented the specific clinical features that may be used to classify a specific phenotype but usually these are analyzed in isolation. A rudimentary calculation suggests that there are more than 3000 potential PSC phenotypes (**Fig. 3**)! The actual number is likely much smaller but,

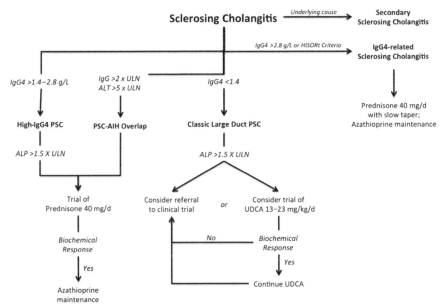

Fig. 2. A proposed management algorithm for PSC patients presenting with sclerosing cholangitis. Data are limited to case series for PSC patients with elevated IgG4 levels or PSC-AIH overlap and response-guided treatment with ursodeoxycholic acid (UDCA) has not been prospectively validated.[30,48,49] A biochemical response is defined by a reduction in alkaline phosphatase to lower than 1.5 × ULN. In addition to treatment, monitoring and surveillance studies should include those to investigate liver disease progression (laboratories, transient elastography, MR elastography), malignancy (annual colonoscopy if IBD is present, annual abdominal imaging and serum CA19-9), and comorbid conditions (bone density scan, fat soluble vitamins, celiac disease serologies). ALP, alkaline phosphatase; HISORt, Histology, Imaging, Serology, other Organ involvement, Response to Therapy; ULN, upper limit of normal.

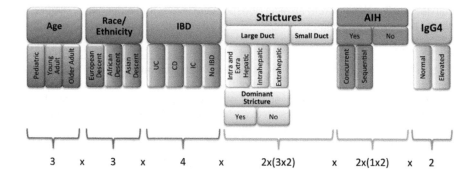

>3,000 Possible PSC Phenotypes

Fig. 3. Possible combinations of clinical features associated with PSC phenotypes. Not included is gender.

for a rare disease, fully appreciating the variability in clinical phenotypes and their significance requires the ongoing collaboration of international consortia as well as larger participation from patient advocacy groups and large health care systems. In addition, as larger numbers of subjects are studied in more detail, a systems-based approach to classifying subphenotypes will need to be considered to unravel the complexity and heterogeneous nature of PSC. Correlating genetic data with these phenotypes will begin to reveal the mechanisms responsible for this heterogeneity. Ultimately, the goal is to develop a better understanding of the pathogenic mechanisms underlying each PSC phenotype so that therapies may be individualized for each patient.

REFERENCES

1. Dave M, Elmunzer BJ, Dwamena BA, et al. Primary sclerosing cholangitis: meta-analysis of diagnostic performance of MR cholangiopancreatography. Radiology 2010;256(2):387–96.
2. Hekimoglu K, Ustundag Y, Dusak A, et al. MRCP vs. ERCP in the evaluation of biliary pathologies: review of current literature. J Dig Dis 2008;9(3):162–9.
3. Weber C, Kuhlencordt R, Grotelueschen R, et al. Magnetic resonance cholangiopancreatography in the diagnosis of primary sclerosing cholangitis. Endoscopy 2008;40(9):739–45.
4. Bambha K, Kim WR, Talwalkar J, et al. Incidence, clinical spectrum, and outcomes of primary sclerosing cholangitis in a united states community. Gastroenterology 2003;125(5):1364–9.
5. Eaton JE, Talwalkar JA, Lazaridis KN, et al. Pathogenesis of primary sclerosing cholangitis and advances in diagnosis and management. Gastroenterology 2013;145(3):521–36.
6. Lindkvist B, Benito de Valle M, Gullberg B, et al. Incidence and prevalence of primary sclerosing cholangitis in a defined adult population in Sweden. Hepatology 2010;52(2):571–7.

7. Tanaka A, Takikawa H. Geoepidemiology of primary sclerosing cholangitis: a critical review. J Autoimmun 2013;46:35–40.
8. Weismüller TJ, Talwalkar JA, Ponsioen CY, et al. Primary sclerosing cholangitis from a global perspective—a multicenter, retrospective, observational study of the International PSC Study Group. J Hepatol 2014;60(1):S3.
9. Boonstra K, Culver EL, de Buy Wenniger LM, et al. Serum immunoglobulin G4 and immunoglobulin G1 for distinguishing immunoglobulin G4-associated cholangitis from primary sclerosing cholangitis. Hepatology 2014;59(5): 1954–63.
10. Bowlus CL, Li CS, Karlsen TH, et al. Primary sclerosing cholangitis in genetically diverse populations listed for liver transplantation: unique clinical and human leukocyte antigen associations. Liver Transpl 2010;16(11):1324–30.
11. Yanai H, Matalon S, Rosenblatt A, et al. Prognosis of primary sclerosing cholangitis in Israel is independent of coexisting inflammatory bowel disease. J Crohns Colitis 2015;9(2):177–84.
12. Boonstra K, Weersma RK, van Erpecum KJ, et al. Population-based epidemiology, malignancy risk, and outcome of primary sclerosing cholangitis. Hepatology 2013; 58(6):2045–55.
13. Loftus EV Jr, Harewood GC, Loftus CG, et al. PSC-IBD: a unique form of inflammatory bowel disease associated with primary sclerosing cholangitis. Gut 2005; 54(1):91–6.
14. de Vries AB, Janse M, Blokzijl H, et al. Distinctive inflammatory bowel disease phenotype in primary sclerosing cholangitis. World J Gastroenterol 2015;21(6): 1956–71.
15. Bowlus CL. Cutting edge issues in primary sclerosing cholangitis. Clin Rev Allergy Immunol 2011;41(2):139–50.
16. Karlsen TH, Franke A, Melum E, et al. Genome-wide association analysis in primary sclerosing cholangitis. Gastroenterology 2010;138(3):1102–11.
17. Eike MC, Nordang GB, Karlsen TH, et al. The FCRL3 -169T>C polymorphism is associated with rheumatoid arthritis and shows suggestive evidence of involvement with juvenile idiopathic arthritis in a Scandinavian panel of autoimmune diseases. Ann Rheum Dis 2008;67(9):1287–91.
18. Karlsen TH, Hampe J, Wiencke K, et al. Genetic polymorphisms associated with inflammatory bowel disease do not confer risk for primary sclerosing cholangitis. Am J Gastroenterol 2007;102(1):115–21.
19. Gaj P, Habior A, Mikula M, et al. Lack of evidence for association of primary sclerosing cholangitis and primary biliary cirrhosis with risk alleles for Crohn's disease in Polish patients. BMC Med Genet 2008;9:81.
20. Mitchell SA, Grove J, Spurkland A, et al. Association of the tumour necrosis factor alpha -308 but not the interleukin 10 -627 promoter polymorphism with genetic susceptibility to primary sclerosing cholangitis. Gut 2001;49(2): 288–94.
21. Liu JZ, Hov JR, Folseraas T, et al. Dense genotyping of immune-related disease regions identifies nine new risk loci for primary sclerosing cholangitis. Nat Genet 2013;45(6):670–5.
22. Bjornsson E, Lindqvist-Ottosson J, Asztely M, et al. Dominant strictures in patients with primary sclerosing cholangitis. Am J Gastroenterol 2004;99(3): 502–8.
23. Rudolph G, Gotthardt D, Kloters-Plachky P, et al. Influence of dominant bile duct stenoses and biliary infections on outcome in primary sclerosing cholangitis. J Hepatol 2009;51(1):149–55.

24. Chapman MH, Webster GJ, Bannoo S, et al. Cholangiocarcinoma and dominant strictures in patients with primary sclerosing cholangitis: a 25-year single-centre experience. Eur J Gastroenterol Hepatol 2012;24(9):1051–8.
25. Eaton JE, Juran BD, Atkinson EJ, et al. A comprehensive assessment of environmental exposures among 1000 North American patients with primary sclerosing cholangitis, with and without inflammatory bowel disease. Aliment Pharmacol Ther 2015;41(10):980–90.
26. Ngu JH, Gearry RB, Wright AJ, et al. Inflammatory bowel disease is associated with poor outcomes of patients with primary sclerosing cholangitis. Clin Gastroenterol Hepatol 2011;9(12):1092–7 [quiz: e135].
27. Karlsen TH, Boberg KM, Vatn M, et al. Different HLA class II associations in ulcerative colitis patients with and without primary sclerosing cholangitis. Genes Immun 2007;8(3):275–8.
28. Mendes FD, Jorgensen R, Keach J, et al. Elevated serum IgG4 concentration in patients with primary sclerosing cholangitis. Am J Gastroenterol 2006;101(9): 2070–5.
29. Zhang L, Lewis JT, Abraham SC, et al. IgG4+ plasma cell infiltrates in liver explants with primary sclerosing cholangitis. Am J Surg Pathol 2010;34(1): 88–94.
30. Bjornsson E, Chari S, Silveira M, et al. Primary sclerosing cholangitis associated with elevated immunoglobulin G4: clinical characteristics and response to therapy. Am J Ther 2011;18(3):198–205.
31. Vosskuhl K, Negm AA, Framke T, et al. Measurement of IgG4 in bile: a new approach for the diagnosis of IgG4-associated cholangiopathy. Endoscopy 2012;44(1):48–52.
32. Parhizkar B, Mohammad Alizadeh AH, Asadzadeh Aghdaee H, et al. Primary sclerosing cholangitis associated with elevated immunoglobulin-G4: a preliminary study. ISRN Gastroenterol 2012;2012:325743.
33. Benito de Valle M, Muller T, Bjornsson E, et al. The impact of elevated serum IgG4 levels in patients with primary sclerosing cholangitis. Dig Liver Dis 2014;46(10): 903–8.
34. Boberg KM, Chapman RW, Hirschfield GM, et al. Overlap syndromes: the International Autoimmune Hepatitis Group (IAIHG) position statement on a controversial issue. J Hepatol 2011;54(2):374–85.
35. Abdalian R, Dhar P, Jhaveri K, et al. Prevalence of sclerosing cholangitis in adults with autoimmune hepatitis: evaluating the role of routine magnetic resonance imaging. Hepatology 2008;47(3):949–57.
36. Lewin M, Vilgrain V, Ozenne V, et al. Prevalence of sclerosing cholangitis in adults with autoimmune hepatitis: a prospective magnetic resonance imaging and histological study. Hepatology 2009;50(2):528–37.
37. Miloh T, Arnon R, Shneider B, et al. A retrospective single-center review of primary sclerosing cholangitis in children. Clin Gastroenterol Hepatol 2009;7(2): 239–45.
38. Toy E, Balasubramanian S, Selmi C, et al. The prevalence, incidence and natural history of primary sclerosing cholangitis in an ethnically diverse population. BMC Gastroenterol 2011;11:83.
39. Bjornsson E, Olsson R, Bergquist A, et al. The natural history of small-duct primary sclerosing cholangitis. Gastroenterology 2008;134(4):975–80.
40. Naess S, Bjornsson E, Anmarkrud JA, et al. Small duct primary sclerosing cholangitis without inflammatory bowel disease is genetically different from large duct disease. Liver Int 2014;34(10):1488–95.

41. Nakazawa T, Ohara H, Sano H, et al. Clinical differences between primary sclerosing cholangitis and sclerosing cholangitis with autoimmune pancreatitis. Pancreas 2005;30(1):20–5.
42. Fischer S, Trivedi PJ, Ward S, et al. Frequency and significance of igg4 immunohistochemical staining in liver explants from patients with primary sclerosing cholangitis. Int J Exp Pathol 2014;95(3):209–15.
43. Chari ST. Diagnosis of autoimmune pancreatitis using its five cardinal features: introducing the Mayo clinic's HISORt criteria. J Gastroenterol 2007;42(Suppl 18): 39–41.
44. Stanich PP, Bjornsson E, Gossard AA, et al. Alkaline phosphatase normalization is associated with better prognosis in primary sclerosing cholangitis. Dig Liver Dis 2011;43(4):309–13.
45. Al Mamari S, Djordjevic J, Halliday JS, et al. Improvement of serum alkaline phosphatase to <1.5 upper limit of normal predicts better outcome and reduced risk of cholangiocarcinoma in primary sclerosing cholangitis. J Hepatol 2013;58(2): 329–34.
46. Lindstrom L, Hultcrantz R, Boberg KM, et al. Association between reduced levels of alkaline phosphatase and survival times of patients with primary sclerosing cholangitis. Clin Gastroenterol Hepatol 2013;11(7):841–6.
47. Rupp C, Rossler A, Halibasic E, et al. Reduction in alkaline phosphatase is associated with longer survival in primary sclerosing cholangitis, independent of dominant stenosis. Aliment Pharmacol Ther 2014;40(11–12):1292–301.
48. Tabibian JH, Lindor KD. Ursodeoxycholic acid in primary sclerosing cholangitis: if withdrawal is bad, then administration is good (right?). Hepatology 2014;60(3): 785–8.
49. Wunsch E, Trottier J, Milkiewicz M, et al. Prospective evaluation of ursodeoxycholic acid withdrawal in patients with primary sclerosing cholangitis. Hepatology 2014;60(3):931–40.

Cancer Risk and Surveillance in Primary Sclerosing Cholangitis

Trine Folseraas, MD, PhD[a,b,c], Kirsten Muri Boberg, MD, PhD[a,b,c],*

KEYWORDS

- Primary sclerosing cholangitis • Carcinoma • Dysplasia • Cholangiocarcinoma
- Inflammatory bowel disease • Surveillance • Brush cytology

KEY POINTS

- Primary sclerosing cholangitis (PSC) is associated with a major lifetime risk of gastrointestinal cancers, including cholangiocarcinoma, gallbladder carcinoma, and colorectal cancer.
- There is no evidence-based algorithm for surveillance of PSC patients with respect to cancer development.
- Cancer surveillance with interval ultrasound of the gallbladder in all adult PSC patients and colonoscopies in PSC patients with inflammatory bowel disease have been recommended in the guidelines for management of PSC.
- Interval imaging with magnetic resonance imaging or ultrasound and measurements of serum carbohydrate antigen 19-9, aiming at early detection of cholangiocarcinoma in PSC, has also been advocated.

A BRIEF INTRODUCTION TO PRIMARY SCLEROSING CHOLANGITIS AND PRIMARY SCLEROSING CHOLANGITIS–ASSOCIATED CANCER RISK

Primary sclerosing cholangitis (PSC) is a chronic, progressive, inflammatory, and cholestatic condition characterized by fibrotic strictures and intervening dilatations of the bile ducts.[1–3] The cause of PSC is largely unknown but identified genetic risk factors indicate the relevance of immune-mediated mechanisms to pathogenesis.[4]

The authors have nothing to disclose.
[a] Section of Gastroenterology, Department of Transplantation Medicine, Division of Cancer Medicine, Surgery and Transplantation, Oslo University Hospital, Rikshospitalet, Oslo, Norway;
[b] Norwegian PSC Research Center, Department of Transplantation Medicine, Division of Cancer Medicine, Surgery and Transplantation, Oslo University Hospital, Rikshospitalet, Oslo, Norway;
[c] Institute of Clinical Medicine, University of Oslo, Rikshospitalet, Oslo, Norway
* Corresponding author. Section of Gastroenterology, Department of Transplantation Medicine, Division of Cancer Medicine, Surgery and Transplantation, Rikshospitalet, Oslo University Hospital, 4950 Nydalen, Oslo N-0424, Norway.
E-mail address: kboberg@ous-hf.no

Clin Liver Dis 20 (2016) 79–98
http://dx.doi.org/10.1016/j.cld.2015.08.014
1089-3261/16/$ – see front matter © 2016 Elsevier Inc. All rights reserved.

In the absence of any pharmacologic treatment regimens with unequivocal evidence for efficacy on disease progression, most patients will gradually develop liver cirrhosis and end-stage liver disease. Orthotopic liver transplantation (OLT) represents the only curative option.[5–7]

The reported prevalence and annual incidence of PSC in the population ranges from 3.9 to 16.2 per 100,000 and 0.41 to 1.3 per 100,000, respectively. Across the populations studied, PSC most commonly affects adults with a median age at onset of 30 to 40 years. The disease is also diagnosed in children and elderly individuals, although less frequently. A male preponderance is observed with a male to female ratio of approximately 2 to 1.[8]

Inflammatory bowel disease (IBD) is present in 62% to 83% of PSC patients of Northern European decent, whereas lower frequencies of 20% to 50% are observed in PSC patients in southern Europe and Asia.[8] According to commonly accepted criteria, the IBD diagnosis in PSC is compatible with ulcerative colitis (UC) in 80% to 90% of the patients, whereas the remaining 10% to 20% is compatible with Crohn disease (CD) or unclassified IBD.[9] However, several clinical reports indicate that the IBD phenotype in PSC may represent a third IBD entity (PSC-IBD), characterized by clinical features distinct from both classic UC and CD.

PSC is associated with a major lifetime risk of gastrointestinal cancers (**Tables 1–3**). The risk of cholangiocarcinoma (CCA) predominates; however, an increased frequency of gallbladder carcinoma (GBC), hepatocellular carcinoma (HCC) and colorectal carcinoma (CRC) is also observed.[10–15] In a large national-based Swedish study comprising 604 PSC subjects, a 161-times increased risk for hepatobiliary malignancies and a 10-times increased risk for CRC in PSC subjects compared with the general population was reported.[12] The overall frequency of hepatobiliary malignancies was 13%. This study also reported a 10- to 14-times increased risk of pancreatic carcinoma in the presence of PSC. A limitation of the study, however, was the potential diagnostic misclassification of carcinomas originating from the distal common bile duct and the caput of the pancreas. Thus, strong evidence for an association between PSC and cancer development in the pancreas is lacking.[15]

Cancer development is a major determinant for poor prognosis in PSC. More than 40% of the mortality in PSC patients is caused by associated cancers. Cancer-related death far exceeds death caused by end-stage liver disease and other nonmalignant complications of the disease.[12,13,16] Early-stage detection and treatment of PSC-associated cancers are crucial for a favorable prognosis. Lack of accurate diagnostic methods for early detection of CCA and the limited therapeutic options for advanced stage of this malignancy are among the main challenges in current handling of PSC patients.

This article reviews the epidemiology of cancer risk in PSC based on reports in published literature and discusses current recommendations and strategies for cancer surveillance in PSC.

PRINCIPLES OF CANCER SURVEILLANCE

In general, cancer surveillance is a strategy aiming at early detection of cancer in a targeted asymptomatic population preidentified as at risk for cancer development.[15] Several guiding principles have been outlined for accurate and cost-effective cancer surveillance (**Box 1**).

In the published guidelines on PSC from the European Association for the Study of the Liver (EASL) and the American Association for the Study of Liver Diseases (AASLD), strategies for surveillance of PSC-associated cancers are discussed and a

Table 1
Reported frequencies of cholangiocarcinoma in primary sclerosing cholangitis

Geographic Population	Period of Data Registration	PSC Patients Included n	PSC-CCA Detected n (%)	Number of CCA Diagnosed Coincident with Diagnosis of PSC n (% of Total CCA)	Number of CCA Detected ≤1 y after PSC Diagnosis n (% of Total CCA)	Median Follow-up (y)	Reference
US	1989–1998	1009	43 (4.3)	15 (35)	NA	NA	Kaya et al,[89] 2001
Sweden	1970–1998	604	81 (13.3)[b]	NA	30 (37)	5.7	Bergquist et al,[12] 2002
Netherlands	2000–2011	590	41 (6.9)	5 (12)	6 (15)	7.7	Boonstra et al,[16] 2013
Norway, Sweden, Italy, Spain, UK[a]	NA–1998	394	48 (12.2)	NA	24 (50)	4.7	Boberg et al,[26] 2002
UK	1981–2004	370	48 (13.0)	NA	NA	4.9	Morris-Stiff et al,[90] 2008
Sweden	NA–1992	305	24 (7.9)	NA	9 (38)	5.3	Broome et al,[7] 1996
Netherlands	1980–2000	211	15 (7.1)	NA	NA	9	Claessen et al,[13] 2009
Belgium	NA–2005	200	13 (6.5)	4 (31)[d]	NA	12.4	Fevery et al,[91] 2012
Netherlands	1970–1999	174	18 (10.3)	6 (33)	NA	6.3	Ponsioen et al,[92] 2002
US	1970–1997	161	11 (6.8)[c]	NA	NA	11.5	Burak et al,[27] 2004
US	1984–1997	139	25 (19.9)	12 (48)	NA	13	Ahrendt et al,[21] 1999
UK	1972–1989	126	8 (6.3)	NA	NA	5.8	Farrant et al,[6] 1991
Belgium	1975–2001	125	8 (6.4)	NA	4 (50)	9	Fevery et al,[28] 2007
Sweden	1964–1991	125	14 (11.2)	NA	7 (50)	10	Kornfeld et al,[23] 1997
Italy	1973–1993	117	3 (2.8)	NA	NA	4	Okolicsanyi et al,[24] 1996

Abbreviations: CCA, cholangiocarcinoma; n, size of sample; NA, not applicable; UK, United Kingdom; US, United States.
[a] Includes patients from Norway, Sweden, Italy, Spain, and the United Kingdom.
[b] Includes cholangiocarcinoma, gallbladder carcinoma, and hepatocellular carcinoma.
[c] Additional 13 subjects excluded from study because CCA was present at time of PSC diagnosis.
[d] Coincident or shortly after diagnosis of CCA.

Table 2
Reported frequencies of gallbladder carcinoma in primary sclerosing cholangitis

Geographic Population	Period of Data Registration	PSC Patients Included n	PSC-GBC Detected n (%)	Reference
US	1996–2005	72	10 (13.8)	Lewis et al,[54] 2007
US	NA	121	3 (2.5)	Brandt et al,[52] 1988
Sweden	1970–2005	286	10 (3.5)	Said et al,[11] 2008
US	1977–1999	102[a]	7 (6.9)	Buckles et al,[53] 2002
US	1995–2008	57[a]	12 (21.1)	Eaton et al,[55] 2012

Abbreviations: GBC, gallbladder carcinoma; n, size of sample; US, United States.
[a] Includes only PSC patients who underwent cholecystectomy.

limited set of recommendations presented, based on relevant published information.[17,18] However, strict evidence for performing cancer surveillance in PSC meeting the criteria for effective surveillance described above is, at present, not established. Specifically, ambiguity exists about which diagnostic modalities should be applied for surveillance and, in the case of positive findings, which treatment approaches should be followed for improved prognosis for PSC patients.

CHOLANGIOCARCINOMA IN PATIENTS WITH PRIMARY SCLEROSING CHOLANGITIS
Epidemiology of Cholangiocarcinoma in Primary Sclerosing Cholangitis

The reported lifetime risk for CCA in patients with PSC ranges from 8% to 36%,[7,12,19,20] and the 10-year cumulative incidence from 11% to 31%.[12,21–23] Population-based studies show lower frequencies of PSC-CCA (6.3%–13%) than transplant center series, the latter presumably overestimating the true prevalence of CCA in the overall PSC-population. In addition, population differences are known to be present. Frequencies of CCA are lower in patients from southern Europe and Asia (3%–4%) than in other parts of the world.[24,25] Up to 50% of CCAs are diagnosed concurrently with PSC or within the first year of diagnosis of PSC.[12,26] Thereafter, the estimated yearly incidence is 0.5% to 1.5%.[12,27,28] The CCAs in PSC may develop from the intrahepatic, the perihilar (so-called Klatskin tumor), or distal extrahepatic

Table 3
Reported frequencies of colorectal carcinoma in primary sclerosing cholangitis

Geographic Population	Period of Data Registration	PSC Patients Included n	PSC-CRC Detected n (%)	Median Follow-up (y)	Reference
Netherlands	2000–2011	590	20 (3.4)	7.7	Boonstra et al,[16] 2013
Netherlands	1980–2000	211	16 (7.6)	9	Claessen et al,[13] 2009
Belgium	NA–2005	200	10 (5.0)	12.4	Fevery et al,[91] 2012
Sweden	1992–2008	199	2 (1.0)	6.5	de Valle et al,[14] 2012
UK	NA	166	2 (1.2)	11	Braden et al,[70] 2012
Germany	1987–2007	171	7 (4.1)	6.9	Rudolph et al,[75] 2010
Sweden	1978–2006	28	3 (1.1)	15	Lindstrom et al,[69] 2011[a]

The overview excludes PSC patients with colonic dysplasia.
Abbreviations: CRC, colorectal carcinoma; n, size of sample; UK, United Kingdom.
[a] Includes only PSC patients with CD.

Box 1
Principles of disease surveillance
1. Presence of a clearly defined at-risk surveillance population
2. High diagnostic accuracy of surveillance modality
3. Available, accessible, and acceptable surveillance modality
4. Available, effective, and evidence-based treatment approaches for the disease considered for surveillance
5. Process from surveillance to treatment should be cost-effective and increase the survival of the surveillance population.

bile ducts; hilar origin of carcinoma is the most common (approximately two-thirds of cases).[29] For an overview of the main epidemiologic studies performed in PSC-associated CCA, see **Table 1**.

The pathogenesis of PSC-associated CCA is poorly understood but several studies support the view that CCA development involves an inflammation-induced hyperplasia-dysplasia-carcinoma sequence.[29,30] Several studies have focused on detecting risk factors or predictors associated with CCA development in PSC. The primary aim was to identify a subset of PSC subjects at higher risk for CCA development that would have increased benefit from dedicated surveillance. Alcohol consumption, smoking, and genetic variants in the *NKG2D-*, *hMYH-*, and *NEIL1* genes have been suggested to increase risk for CCA in PSC.[17,27,31] Old age at PSC diagnosis, elevated serum bilirubin, Mayo risk score greater than 4, variceal bleeding, presence of colorectal neoplasia (CRN) coexisting with UC, and long duration of IBD in PSC have been identified as potential predictors of CCA development.[14,24,26] These risk factors and predictors only infer small to modest increments to risk and are not helpful in the clinical setting to identify a subgroup of PSC patients at a high risk for developing CCA. In the absence of any useful clinical markers for patients at high risk, current CCA surveillance strategies should include all PSC patients regardless of phenotype characteristics. However, awareness and diagnostic awareness of potential CCA should be particularly directed at patients that have received their PSC diagnosis within the last 1 to 2 years, based on the close proximity of diagnosis of PSC and CCA in most patients.

Surveillance Strategies in Primary Sclerosing Cholangitis–Associated Cholangiocarcinoma

At present, no unifying, evidence-based guidelines for CCA surveillance in PSC exist. Current proposals attempt to incorporate a surveillance strategy that adequately meets the guiding principles for accurate and effective cancer surveillance (see **Box 1**).[15,17,18,32–34] Fundamentally, a defined at-risk population for which surveillance would be extremely meaningful is present because PSC patients have a markedly increased risk of CCA development. On the other hand, accurate diagnostic modalities to detect CCA in PSC patients and effective treatment alternatives are, to a large extent, lacking. The main clinical challenges relate to the problems of identifying early, potentially asymptomatic stages of cancers and distinguishing benign bile duct strictures from malignant changes. Current diagnostic approaches include a combination of imaging modalities, results from biliary brush cytology, and analysis of the serum tumor marker carbohydrate antigen 19-9 (CA19-9).[17,18,31]

Diagnostic Modalities Relevant for Surveillance of Primary Sclerosing Cholangitis–Cholangiocarcinoma

Noninvasive imaging

Based on reports of the performance of different diagnostic modalities for CCA in PSC (**Table 4**), a rational approach for CCA surveillance includes radiologic imaging of the biliary tree at regular intervals.[15,32–34] Both MRI with magnetic resonance cholangio-pancreatography (MRCP) and ultrasound are noninvasive modalities that may visualize a mass lesion, polyp, or thickening of the bile duct wall with proximal biliary dilatation consistent with a potential CCA lesion. MRI may be superior to ultrasound at identifying small lesions and at providing additional information, including typical signal intensity and enhancement of lesion.[15] MRI combined with MRCP (MRI/MRCP) is associated with a sensitivity of 89% and specificity of 75%.[35] Ultrasound, in most cases a less expensive, more available, and acceptable modality than MRI/MRCP, has demonstrated a sensitivity and specificity of 57% and 94%, respectively.[35] Computerized tomography has sensitivity and specificity comparable to MRI/MRCP (see **Table 4**) but is a less agreeable modality to be used in surveillance because of inherent contrast and radiation exposure. PET scan does not contribute to higher diagnostic accuracy in detection of premalignant or early-stage CCA in PSC but can be of value in staging of PSC-CCA once diagnosed by another modality.[36]

Serum carbohydrate antigen 19-9

The use of serum biomarkers for CCA could potentially provide an alternative or complement to imaging in screening. The only validated and available serum biomarker at present is CA19-9. The diagnostic accuracy of elevated CA19-9 for unmasking CCA in PSC is, however, suboptimal. Low levels of CA19-9 may be observed in presence of CCA and elevated levels are also observed in cholangitis resulting from benign PSC

Table 4
Diagnostic performance of different modalities used in diagnosis of cholangiocarcinoma in primary sclerosing cholangitis

Modality	Sensitivity %	Specificity %	Accuracy %	Reference
Ultrasound	57	94	90	[35]
MRI	63	79	76	[35]
MRCP	78	76	76	[35]
CT	75	80	79	[35]
ERCP	91	66	69	[35]
MRI/MCRP	89	75	76	[35]
CA19-9 (cutoff ≥20 IU/mL)	78	67	68	[35]
CA 19-9 (cutoff ≥130 IU/mL)	13	100	90	[35]
CA 19-9 + ultrasound[a]	91	62	65	[35]
CA 19-9 + MRI/MRCP[a]	100	38	47	[35]
CA 19-9 + CT[a]	100	38	47	[35]
CA 19-9 + ERCP[a]	100	43	49	[35]
Biliary brush cytology	43	97	NA	[39]
FISH	51	93	NA	[43]

Abbreviations: CT, computerized tomography; ERCP, endoscopic retrograde cholangiopancreatography; FISH, fluorescence in situ hybridization; MRCP, magnetic resonance cholangiopancreatography.
[a] CA19-9 cutoff greater than or equal to 20 IU/mL.

bile duct changes, secondary bacterial cholangitis, and other malignancies. CA19-9 values greater than or equal to 20 IU/mL may enable detection of early-stage CCA; however, diagnostic performance is low with a sensitivity of 78% and specificity of 67% for presence of CCA.[35] CA19-9 values greater than or equal to 20 IU/mL and CCA-suspicious findings using MRI/MRCP increases sensitivity to 100% but decreases specificity to 38% and, in total, reduces diagnostic accuracy compared with CA19-9 or MRI/MRCP alone.[35] Setting a higher cut-off value for CA19-9 increases specificity but reduces the sensitivity of the test (see **Table 4**). One should be aware that approximately 7% of PSC patients will be CA19-9–negative as a result of specific inactivating polymorphisms in the *FUT3* gene leading to lack of expression of the CA19-9 epitope.[37] In this subgroup of patients, CA19-9 screening will not be informative. It has not been common in clinical practice to determine *FUT3* genotypes in PSC patients to predetermine CA19-9 test utility.[37]

Endoscopic retrograde cholangiopancreatography
Endoscopic retrograde cholangiopancreatography (ERCP) with brush cytology sampling from the biliary ducts has been considered an alternative surveillance strategy for CCA in PSC. The sensitivity and specificity of ERCP findings indicative for CCA have been reported to be 91% and 66%, respectively, if ERCP is used alone.[35] Including only definite findings of biliary stenosis with a polypoid bile duct lesion decreases sensitivity of the test to 13%. Combining ERCP indicative findings of CCA with elevated CA19-9 levels, in general, increases sensitivity of CCA detection at the cost of specificity (see **Table 4**).

Biliary brush cytology
Because there is evidence that development of CCA occurs in a multistep sequence from hyperplasia via dysplasia to carcinoma, a combination of ERCP with cytologic examination of brush samples taken from stenotic parts of the bile ducts or randomly throughout the biliary tree may provide additional information of CCA risk.[30]

Challenges associated with brush cytology sampling relate to obtaining adequate cellular material for excluding malignancy because CCA is frequently surrounded by depositions of fibrotic and connective tissue (desmoplastic response).[38] Thus, in general, conventional brush cytology has low sensitivity for definite diagnosis of CCA in PSC, although specificity is acceptable. A meta-analysis comprising 747 PSC subjects showed a sensitivity and specificity for positive brush cytology of 43% and 93%, respectively.[39] Repeated brush sampling may increase sensitivity.[40] Equivocal cytology, that is, findings of atypical cells or other features suspicious for but not definitive for malignancy, is a challenge frequently met in clinical practice for which there are no established guidelines for management. DNA methylation analyses using biliary brush samples could potentially serve as a supplement to conventional brush cytology in this setting.[41] Testing for specific methylation patterns in 4 genes (*CDO1*, *CNRIP1*, *SEPT9*, and *VIM*) has demonstrated a sensitivity of 85% and a specificity of 98% for CCA detection.[41] Methylation profiling of this gene panel outperforms the diagnostic accuracy of conventional brush cytology but has not yet been put into routine clinical practice.[41]

Fluorescence in situ hybridization
Fluorescence in situ hybridization (FISH), which uses labeled DNA probes to detect aneusomy (abnormal loss or gain of chromosomes or chromosomal loci) in individual cells, may add value to the diagnostic performance of conventional brush cytology in detecting CCA.[42] In a meta-analysis including 828 subjects, the pooled sensitivity and specificity for positive FISH (trisomy, tetrasomy, and polysomy) for detection of CCA

were 68% and 70%, respectively.[43] In another study assessing biliary brush samples from 30 PSC subjects without definitive radiological or histologic signs of malignancy, polysomy at time of first FISH assessment was associated with a diagnosis of CCA in 75% of the subjects during 3 years follow-up.[44] Subjects with serial polysomy FISH results were at higher risk of developing CCA than those with subsequent nonpolysomy results, 69% and 18% developing CCA in these 2 groups, respectively.[44] PSC subjects with polysomy detected in 2 or more areas of the biliary tree when brushings had been performed in more than 1 location during a single procedure (multifocal polysomy) have recently been reported to be more likely to be diagnosed with CCA compared with subjects with polysomy detected in a single location.[45] Results from the same study also indicated that findings of multifocal polysomy are a stronger predictor for CCA development than serial polysomy.[45] FISH testing overall increases the diagnostic yield of brush cytology and should be used as a complement to conventional brush cytology, if available. FISH polysomy assessments are of special value in patients with equivocal cytology results or other cases of suspicious but not verified CCA.

Based on the imperfect diagnostic performance of different ERCP-based test combinations in detecting CCA, it is difficult to justify use of this invasive procedure in regular surveillance of PSC-CCA. The risk of complications associated with the procedure, such as bleeding, perforation, pancreatitis, and cholangitis, also makes ERCP a less favorable option to be used in initial surveillance.[46] Therefore, current practice in most centers of using ERCP with brushing, with or without FISH, as a second-line procedure in patients with suspicious CCA and/or dominant stenosis on noninvasive imaging, new or worsening symptoms, change in serum cholestatic parameters, or rapidly increasing or continuously elevated CA19-9, seems rational.

Treatment Options Relevant for Primary Sclerosing Cholangitis–Cholangiocarcinoma Surveillance

Once CCA has been diagnosed, therapeutic options are limited. Curative treatment possibilities include surgical resection of the tumor in the absence of liver cirrhosis. However, in most cases, the frequent advanced infiltrative growth and wide-spread dysplasia at time of diagnosis of CCA in PSC limit the potential for radical resection.[17,21] When surgical treatment is performed with negative tumor margins, it is still associated with a dismal prognosis with 3-year survival around 20%.[47] Following neoadjuvant therapy, liver transplantation can be considered in highly selected cases of limited-stage, unresectable, perihilar CCA with a 5-year survival rate of 65%.[48] Liver transplantation following neoadjuvant therapy has been advocated in patients of limited-stage CCA, including patients with unicentric mass lesion less than or equal to 3 cm in radial diameter and no intrahepatic or extrahepatic metastases or TNM stage less than or equal to 2, and CA19-9 less than or equal to 100 IU/mL.[49,50] Palliative treatment of patients not eligible for surgery includes endoscopic stenting, photodynamic therapy, and chemotherapy.[51] There is currently no randomized study showing a clear survival benefit for a specific chemotherapeutic regimen in PSC-CCA.[51] Overall, the prognosis of PSC-CCA is dismal with median survival of around 5 months in patients who are not available for curative treatment.[21]

The management of findings of isolated low-grade dysplasia (LGD) or high-grade dysplasia (HGD) from brush cytology sampling is notoriously difficult because dysplasia is a strong predictor for CCA development but the absolute fraction of patients that progresses from dysplasia to carcinoma and the time factor involved are not well-established.[30] The EASL guidelines state that liver transplantation could be considered in patients with dysplasia.[18] However, because around one-third of patients with biliary dysplasia have been reported not to have CCA on follow-up and the time interval for progression from dysplasia to carcinoma has not been established, both the indication and timing of transplantation in this patient group remains controversial.[30]

Suggested Surveillance Strategy for Primary Sclerosing Cholangitis–Cholangiocarcinoma

The EASL and AASLD guidelines for management of PSC do not recommend regular evaluation for PSC-CCA but do advocate for evaluation if deterioration of constitutional performance status or alterations in liver biochemical parameters occur.[17,18] In absence of high-quality evidence and lack of clear support in the guidelines, more recent PSC management proposals advise an interval surveillance strategy with annual MRI/MRCP or ultrasound in combination with serum CA19-9, proceeding to second-line evaluation with ERCP with biliary brush sampling and FISH in cases of suspicious CCA findings on imaging and/or continuously elevated CA 19.9.[15,32–34] In **Fig. 1** the authors suggest a procedure for surveillance taking both the EASL and AASLD guidelines, and more recent publications assessing surveillance strategies in PSC-CCA, into account.[15,17,18,32–34] Cost-effectiveness studies are, however, required to evaluate when to ideally initiate surveillance for PSC-CCA, with which diagnostic tools, and for which treatment purpose.

GALLBLADDER CARCINOMA IN PATIENTS WITH PRIMARY SCLEROSING CHOLANGITIS
Epidemiology of Gallbladder Carcinoma in Primary Sclerosing Cholangitis

PSC patients have increased frequency of multiple gallbladder abnormalities, including gallstones, cholecystitis, and benign and malignant gall bladder lesions.[11,52–55] In a study from Sweden investigating the presence of gallbladder abnormalities in 286 PSC subjects followed between 1970 and 2005, 41% had 1 or more abnormal gallbladder findings, with gallstones identified in 25%, cholecystitis in 25%, and gallbladder mass lesions in 6%. In 56% of cases, the mass lesion constituted a GBC. Overall, GBC was present in 3.5% of the total subject population.[11] Another study including 121 PSC subjects estimated a prevalence of 4% of mass lesions in the PSC population and, among these, 75% represented malignant neoplasms.[52] In other series reporting only on PSC subjects who have undergone cholecystectomy, that is, introducing a selection bias likely to overestimate the true prevalence of GBC in PSC, the frequencies of GBC range from 5.5% to 21.1%.[53,55] In comparison, incidental GBCs were identified in 0.35% of subjects in the general population undergoing laparoscopic cholecystectomies for gallstone.[56] For an overview of the main epidemiologic studies performed in PSC-associated GBC, see **Table 2**.

Predictors for presence of malignancy in gallbladder mass lesions and polyps in PSC are not thoroughly studied; however, for GBC in the general population, the size of the gallbladder lesion seems to be an important factor.[55,57] In 57 subjects that had undergone cholecystectomy, 9 out of 11 (82%) subjects with a gallbladder mass and 2 out of 14 (14%) subjects with a polyp had GBC.[55] Using receiver operating characteristics estimates, the best cutoff size for detection of neoplasia was 0.80 cm with a sensitivity and specificity of 100% and 70% for gallbladder neoplasia, respectively.[55] No cases of dysplasia were detected in lesions less than 0.80 cm. In non-PSC subjects, other risk factors for presence of GBC within mass lesions or polyps include rapid and sessile growth, imaging features of vascularity and local invasion, chronic inflammation secondary to gallstones, or infections and old age at time of identification

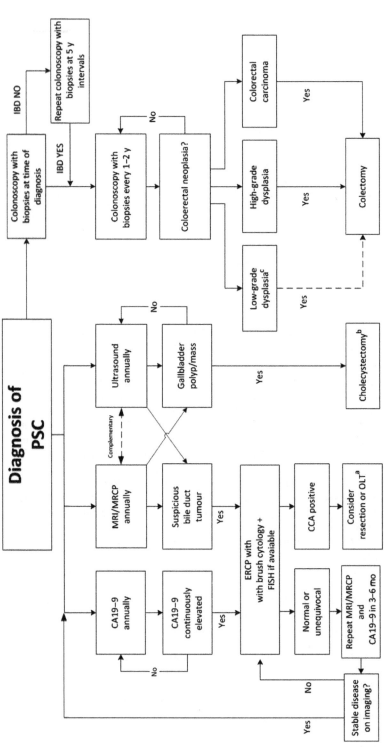

Fig. 1. Suggested procedure for cancer surveillance in PSC. [a] See main text for treatment alternatives of confirmed CCA in PSC. [b] A more individualized approach with close observation with interval imaging every 3 to 6 months in patients with high postoperative risk for complications, for example, assessed by preoperative Child-Pugh score, in gallbladder lesions less than 0.80 cm without other malignant risk features has been suggested.[33,55] [c] Endoscopic treatment of polypoid (polyp) LGD lesions followed by colonoscopy within 6 months has been suggested.[15] Chromoendoscopy with endoscopic treatment followed by colonoscopy control within 6 months has also been suggested in flat LGD lesions in patients with high postoperative risk for complications or compromised liver function.[15] (*Adapted from* Refs.[15,17,18,32–34])

of the lesion.[57–59] These risk factors may also apply to PSC patients. Chronic inflammation resulting from primary PSC-affection, gallstone formation, and recurrent episodes of bacterial cholecystitis, presumably plays an important role in malignant transformation of the gallbladder epithelium in PSC through an inflammation-dysplasia-carcinoma sequence.[15] An association between gallbladder dysplasia and adenocarcinoma on 1 side, and bile duct dysplasia and CCA on the other, has been reported, supporting the concept of a neoplastic field effect along the entire biliary tree.[54]

SURVEILLANCE STRATEGIES IN PRIMARY SCLEROSING CHOLANGITIS–ASSOCIATED GALLBLADDER CARCINOMA
Diagnostic Modalities Relevant for Surveillance of Primary Sclerosing Cholangitis–Gallbladder Carcinoma

Based on the increased frequency of mass lesions in PSC and the high risk that these lesions harbor malignancy, both the AASLD and the EASL guidelines recommend annual abdominal ultrasound for the detection of gallbladder mass lesions in PSC patients.[17,18] Ultrasound is a reasonable modality for surveillance for this purpose, demonstrating superior diagnostic accuracy compared with most other imaging modalities because it is available and acceptable to most patients, and it is cost-effective.[60] Although ultrasound is the most common modality of choice in daily practice, adequate monitoring of the gallbladder may also be performed with MRI/MRCP if these modalities are used for other follow-up purposes, such as surveillance of CCA or HCC.[15] Robust evidence supporting the practice of annual ultrasound screening for gallbladder abnormalities in PSC is, however, lacking. Also, the potential benefits and risks of instituting a widespread screening program for gallbladder malignancy in this population have not been well defined.[55]

Treatment Options Relevant for Primary Sclerosing Cholangitis–Gallbladder Carcinoma Surveillance

The AASLD and the EASL guidelines recommend cholecystectomy for all PSC gallbladder lesions regardless of size.[17,18] In early-stage GBC, cholecystectomy represents a curative option but early-stage disease only comprises about 10% of GBC patients.[61,62] Cholecystectomy is also an independent predictor for increased survival time in more advanced stages of GBC.[61] Median survival for localized, regional, and distant stages of GBC is, however, dismal, with median survival for these stages of 20, 5, and 2 months, respectively.[61]

Knowledge is limited about the natural history and malignant potential of small gallbladder lesions (<1.0 cm) in PSC. The cholecystectomy strategy for any size lesion is based on the potential of curative resection in early-stage disease and reports of a limited number of cases of dysplasia and adenocarcinomas in lesions less than 1.0 cm.[57,63] In addition, reports of a spectrum of metaplasia-dysplasia alterations in the background gallbladder epithelium in the presence of GBC, call for for an aggressive treatment strategy of any size lesion.[11,54] It is, however, uncertain if small lesions should preferably be closely observed instead of being subjected directly to resection. PSC patients, both with and without cirrhosis, show an increased morbidity rate following cholecystectomy compared with patients without liver disease.[55] Therefore, it has been suggested to consider a more individualized approach with close observation of patients with high postoperative risk for complications; for example, assessment by preoperative Child-Pugh score in lesions less than 0.80 cm without other malignant risk features.[33,55]

Recommended Surveillance Strategy for Primary Sclerosing Cholangitis–Gallbladder Carcinoma

Current recommendations for surveillance of PSC patients with regard to GBC are summarized in **Fig. 1**.

HEPATOCELLULAR CARCINOMA IN PATIENTS WITH PRIMARY SCLEROSING CHOLANGITIS

In 2 studies assessing prevalence of HCC in transplanted PSC subjects, HCC was found in 2% and 4% of the subjects, respectively.[12,64] Incidence rates of HCC in PSC have not been well studied and it is not established whether the increased occurrence of HCC in PSC patients depends on concurrent cirrhosis or if PSC is an independent risk factor for HCC regardless of cirrhotic stage. A cost-benefit analysis of HCC in general suggests that an HCC incidence of 1.5% per year or above in a cirrhotic-stage liver disease legitimizes regular HCC screening.[65] Based on this threshold, it is doubtful that HCC-screening should be initiated in cirrhotic PSC patients because incidence rates are likely to be lower. Surveillance conducted for CCA or GBC with ultrasound or MRI/MRCP may, however, serve the dual purpose of identifying HCC and may also provide more data about incidence and prevalence rates of HCC in cirrhotic and non-cirrhotic PSC patients.

COLORECTAL CARCINOMA IN PATIENTS WITH PRIMARY SCLEROSING CHOLANGITIS
Epidemiology of Colorectal Carcinoma in Primary Sclerosing Cholangitis

IBD is a widely accepted risk factor for CRC development and CRN has been reported to account for more than 30% of the mortality in UC.[66] In PSC patients with UC, the risk of colorectal malignancies is even higher than the risk in UC patients without hepatobiliary disease. A large meta-analysis comprising 16,844 subjects (564 PSC and 16,280 UC) indicated a 4-fold increased risk of CRC in PSC subjects with concurrent UC compared with subjects with UC alone. Therefore, it provided strong support to the contention that PSC serves as an independent risk factor for colonic dysplasia in UC.[10] The cumulative incidence of CRC and dysplasia in coexisting PSC and UC compared with UC alone is reported to be 9% versus 2% after 10 years and 20% to 31% versus 5% after 20 years from diagnosis.[13,67,68] PSC may also be a risk factor for CRN development in CD, although this association seems less clear.[69,70] The subset of PSC patients without IBD has not independently been demonstrated to have an increased risk of CRC.

The risk of colonic neoplasms is present early in the course of coexisting IBD in PSC.[71] Neoplasia in PSC patients with colitis has a predilection for the right side of the colon with more than 60% of the neoplastic lesions being located proximal to the splenic flexure.[71,72] PSC-IBD patients with CRC are younger at onset of IBD symptoms (19 vs 29 years) and at diagnosis of CRC (38 vs 48 years) compared with patients who develop CRC based on IBD without PSC. The colitis-CRC interval (17 vs 20 years) is, however, similar in the 2 groups.[73] For a summary of the main epidemiologic studies performed in PSC-associated CRC, see **Table 3**.

Risk factors for malignant transformation in IBD, in general, include duration and anatomic extent of disease, family history of CRC, and the presence of PSC.[66] Long duration of IBD is also a risk factor for malignancy in PSC.[66] Importantly, IBD in PSC patients often runs a quiescent, subclinical course and the IBD is, in many cases, first diagnosed on active screening with colonoscopy and biopsies. IBD disease duration in PSC is, therefore, often underestimated.[67] The higher frequency of total colitis in PSC-IBD patients than in patients with UC alone could also in part explain the increased risk of neoplasia in PSC-UC.[74] Differences in genetic susceptibility risk factors in IBD in PSC compared with ordinary IBD could also explain differences in cancer risk between the 2 entities. Potentially, PSC-IBD harbors a genetic profile with increased risk of neoplasia.[4] Presence of dominant biliary strictures in PSC has been suggested to increase the risk for both colorectal and hepatobiliary malignancies.[75] The increased risk of CRC in the proximal part of the colon where concentration of bile acids is high could suggest a role for bile acids in CRC carcinogenesis in PSC.[66,72] Also, IBD remains a risk factor for CRC development in PSC following OLT. Firm evidence for OLT conferring an additional CRC risk in PSC is still lacking but some reports have indicated a higher CRC risk after OLT.[66,76]

SURVEILLANCE STRATEGIES IN PRIMARY SCLEROSING CHOLANGITIS–ASSOCIATED COLORECTAL CARCINOMA

Diagnostic Modalities Relevant to Surveillance of Primary Sclerosing Cholangitis–Colorectal Carcinoma

Given the increased risk of CRC in PSC patients, the EASL and AASLD guidelines recommend full colonoscopy with biopsies at the time of diagnosis of PSC. In cases of concurrent PSC and IBD, colonoscopy with biopsies should be performed at annual (EASL) or annual to biannual basis (AASLD).[17,18] The IBD in PSC is often asymptomatic with only mild colonic inflammation; however, it already harbors a high risk of CRC soon after the diagnosis of coexistent of PSC and IBD. This is the rationale for recommending a full colonoscopy with biopsies at the time of initial diagnosis of PSC and, subsequently, every 5 years thereafter in those who have not received a diagnosis of IBD, regardless of the presence of symptoms.[17,18]

Colonoscopic surveillance should include all PSC patients with IBD, regardless of subtype.[17,18] Because CRN risk even may increase after OLT, annual or biannual colonoscopy screening should be continued in PSC patients posttransplant.[76] The ideal procedure for sampling of colonic screening biopsies in PSC has not been clearly outlined in the guidelines but principles from CRC screening in IBD in general should also guide screening for PSC-IBD.[77] Because colitis in PSC is frequently not macroscopically visible, sampling of random 4-quadrant biopsies at least every 10 cm throughout the colon is also advisable in PSC patients with macroscopically normal-appearing mucosa.[77] In addition, thorough biopsy sampling from any suspicious lesion should be performed. For the initial diagnosis of IBD in PSC, biopsies should also include normal-appearing mucosa because evidence of microscopic colitis may not be macroscopically apparent. The role of confocal endomicroscopy, narrow band-imaging, and chromoendoscopy to enhance diagnostic accuracy for CRN in PSC-IBD remains to be determined; however, chromoendoscopy may serve as a tool to identify flat lesions in LGD that could potentially be removed by endoscopic therapy.

Treatment Options Relevant to Surveillance of Primary Sclerosing Cholangitis–Colorectal Carcinoma

Optimal treatment options following surveillance colonoscopy findings in PSC-IBD are not clearly delineated based on available outcome studies and not discussed in depth in the guidelines. The AASLD guidelines underscore that patients with IBD and PSC should be treated according to guidelines for IBD.[17] Screening, not only with the purpose of detecting neoplastic lesions but also for defining intensity and extent of intestinal inflammation, to enable adequate decision-making with regard IBD treatment, is essential to reduce risk of inflammation-induced neoplastic development in PSC-IBD patients.

CRN complicating PSC-IBD represents a range of neoplastic disease stages from LGD to HGD and carcinoma. When HGD or carcinoma is present and agreed on by 2 independent pathologists, proctocolectomy is recommended.[33] Proctocolectomy is, in principle, usually also performed for LGD lesions. However, additional outcome studies are warranted to assess this practice. Reports indicating that risk of progression of LGD to HGD and cancer may be increased in PSC-IBD also support a colectomy strategy in this group of patients.[78] However, proctocolectomy may negatively affect the natural course of the hepatobiliary disease and lead to worsened prognosis, especially in PSC patients with cirrhosis or compromised hepatic function.[15,79] Furthermore, high rates of pouchitis and remaining risk for carcinoma development in the pouch in PSC-IBD after ileal pouch-anal anastomosis (IPAA) and difficult-to-treat peristomal varices after ileostomy following colectomy have been reported.[15] These factors require an individualized approach in LGD cases. Targeted local endoscopic therapy for polypoid and, potentially, flat dysplastic lesions, followed by close observation with colonoscopies at 6 month intervals in LGD cases, has been suggested as a reasonable strategy in this group.[15] The optimal pouch surveillance strategy in PSC-IBD patients with IPAA remains undefined.

The role of ursodeoxycholic acid (UCDA) as a chemopreventive agent against CRC development in PSC is debated. Retrospective studies of relatively small numbers of subjects have shown that treatment with UCDA is associated to decreased prevalence of CRN and decreased development of CRC.[80] Other studies have not been able to verify this effect and high-dose UCDA has been reported to increase risk of CRN and CRC.[81–83] The EASL recommendation suggests the use of UCDA in prevention of CRC, in particular in high-risk patients, including patients with long-duration or extensive IBD or family history of CRC.[18] The AASLD guidelines do not recommend routine use of UCDA as a chemopreventive agent based on the conflicting information available and potential negative side-effects of UCDA.[17]

Recommended surveillance strategy for primary sclerosing cholangitis–colorectal carcinoma

Current recommendations for follow-up of PSC patients with regard to CRC are summarized in **Fig. 1**.

CANCER SURVEILLANCE IN SPECIFIC PRIMARY SCLEROSING CHOLANGITIS SUBPOPULATIONS
Cancer Surveillance in Pediatric Primary Sclerosing Cholangitis

PSC is relatively rare in children with a reported incidence less than 20% that of the adult PSC population.[84] CCA is uncommonly observed in pediatric PSC and, similarly, mass lesions of the gallbladder are rarely seen.[85] Routine screening for detecting biliary tract cancer in children with PSC is, therefore, not recommended.[17] IBD is identified in approximately 60% of cases of pediatric PSC.[86] Thus, it is reasonable to consider full colonoscopy in children with a new diagnosis of PSC and, subsequently, in children with symptoms of active IBD.[17] Risk of CRC development is, however, low in PSC-IBD children and interval colonoscopy as part of CRC screening before 16 years of age is advised against.[17]

Cancer Surveillance in Primary Sclerosing Cholangitis Patients Posttransplant

Recurrence of PSC occurs in 20% to 25% of patients within the first 10 years after OLT.[87] De novo CCA in recurrent PSC has been described but whether recurrent PSC patients harbor an increased risk of hepatobiliary cancer is not known.[88] Longstanding inflammation is potentially essential for inducing a hyperplasia-dysplasia-carcinoma sequence in recurrent disease, thus long-term follow-up of patients with recurrent PSC is needed to establish evidence for a potentially increased hepatobiliary cancer risk and to determine a rationale for interval cancer surveillance in this patient group.

As discussed above, CRC risk does not dissipate after OLT. Annual or biannual colonoscopy screening should, therefore, be continued in PSC patients posttransplant.

SUMMARY

With the associated high time risk of hepatobiliary and colorectal cancers, PSC should be considered a premalignant condition. Cancer has, during the last decade, become the dominant cause of mortality in PSC patients. Implementation of surveillance is warranted to provide early detection and treatment of PSC-associated cancers to improve overall survival in this patient group. For CCA, in particular, accurate diagnostic modalities and efficient treatment options governing establishment of efficient screening are lacking. In the absence of evidence-based, accurate, and cost-effective strategies, more pragmatic approaches to cancer surveillance in PSC have been suggested in the AASLD and EASL PSC management guidelines and in more recent reviews on the topic.[15,17,18,32–34] In view of the strict principles for initiating efficient surveillance, screening based on pragmatic assessments is suboptimal but may, despite lack of evidence, provide better care for the patients than a more conservative approach. Moreover, continuous evaluation of surveillance programs initiated based on pragmatic assessments may ultimately provide future evidence about the level of benefit of such strategies.

Better general understanding of the natural history of PSC and, specifically, of PSC-associated cancers is required to drive the development of more efficient surveillance strategies. Herein, dedicated investigation of the genetic, epigenetic, and molecular profiles in PSC-associated cancers that could further guide the establishment of accurate biomarkers for detection of preneoplastic and early stages of cancer, and potentially of targeted therapy, is warranted.

REFERENCES

1. Chapman RW, Arborgh BA, Rhodes JM, et al. Primary sclerosing cholangitis: a review of its clinical features, cholangiography, and hepatic histology. Gut 1980;21(10):870–7.
2. Wiesner RH, Grambsch PM, Dickson ER, et al. Primary sclerosing cholangitis: natural history, prognostic factors and survival analysis. Hepatology 1989;10(4): 430–6.
3. Schrumpf E, Elgjo K, Fausa O, et al. Sclerosing cholangitis in ulcerative colitis. Scand J Gastroenterol 1980;15(6):689–97.
4. Folseraas T, Liaskou E, Anderson CA, et al. Genetics in PSC: what do the "risk genes" teach us? Clin Rev Allergy Immunol 2015;48(2–3):154–64.
5. Aadland E, Schrumpf E, Fausa O, et al. Primary sclerosing cholangitis: a long-term follow-up study. Scand J Gastroenterol 1987;22(6):655–64.
6. Farrant JM, Hayllar KM, Wilkinson ML, et al. Natural history and prognostic variables in primary sclerosing cholangitis. Gastroenterology 1991;100(6):1710–7.
7. Broome U, Olsson R, Loof L, et al. Natural history and prognostic factors in 305 Swedish patients with primary sclerosing cholangitis. Gut 1996;38(4):610–5.
8. Karlsen TH, Schrumpf E, Boberg KM. Update on primary sclerosing cholangitis. Dig Liver Dis 2010;42(6):390–400.
9. Fausa O, Schrumpf E, Elgjo K. Relationship of inflammatory bowel disease and primary sclerosing cholangitis. Semin Liver Dis 1991;11(1):31–9.

10. Soetikno RM, Lin OS, Heidenreich PA, et al. Increased risk of colorectal neoplasia in patients with primary sclerosing cholangitis and ulcerative colitis: a meta-analysis. Gastrointest Endosc 2002;56(1):48–54.
11. Said K, Glaumann H, Bergquist A. Gallbladder disease in patients with primary sclerosing cholangitis. J Hepatol 2008;48(4):598–605.
12. Bergquist A, Ekbom A, Olsson R, et al. Hepatic and extrahepatic malignancies in primary sclerosing cholangitis. J Hepatol 2002;36(3):321–7.
13. Claessen MM, Vleggaar FP, Tytgat KM, et al. High lifetime risk of cancer in primary sclerosing cholangitis. J Hepatol 2009;50(1):158–64.
14. de Valle MB, Bjornsson E, Lindkvist B. Mortality and cancer risk related to primary sclerosing cholangitis in a Swedish population-based cohort. Liver Int 2012; 32(3):441–8.
15. Razumilava N, Gores GJ, Lindor KD. Cancer surveillance in patients with primary sclerosing cholangitis. Hepatology 2011;54(5):1842–52.
16. Boonstra K, Weersma RK, van Erpecum KJ, et al. Population-based epidemiology, malignancy risk, and outcome of primary sclerosing cholangitis. Hepatology 2013;58(6):2045–55.
17. Chapman R, Fevery J, Kalloo A, et al. Diagnosis and management of primary sclerosing cholangitis. Hepatology 2010;51(2):660–78.
18. European Association for the Study of the Liver. EASL clinical practice guidelines: management of cholestatic liver diseases. J Hepatol 2009;51(2):237–67.
19. Miros M, Kerlin P, Walker N, et al. Predicting cholangiocarcinoma in patients with primary sclerosing cholangitis before transplantation. Gut 1991;32(11):1369–73.
20. Nashan B, Schlitt HJ, Tusch G, et al. Biliary malignancies in primary sclerosing cholangitis: timing for liver transplantation. Hepatology 1996;23(5):1105–11.
21. Ahrendt SA, Pitt HA, Nakeeb A, et al. Diagnosis and management of cholangiocarcinoma in primary sclerosing cholangitis. J Gastrointest Surg 1999;3(4): 357–67.
22. Farges O, Malassagne B, Sebagh M, et al. Primary sclerosing cholangitis: liver transplantation or biliary surgery. Surgery 1995;117(2):146–55.
23. Kornfeld D, Ekbom A, Ihre T. Survival and risk of cholangiocarcinoma in patients with primary sclerosing cholangitis. A population-based study. Scand J Gastroenterol 1997;32(10):1042–5.
24. Okolicsanyi L, Fabris L, Viaggi S, et al. Primary sclerosing cholangitis: clinical presentation, natural history and prognostic variables: an Italian multicentre study. The Italian PSC Study Group. Eur J Gastroenterol Hepatol 1996;8(7):685–91.
25. Takikawa H, Manabe T. Primary sclerosing cholangitis in Japan–analysis of 192 cases. J Gastroenterol 1997;32(1):134–7.
26. Boberg KM, Bergquist A, Mitchell S, et al. Cholangiocarcinoma in primary sclerosing cholangitis: risk factors and clinical presentation. Scand J Gastroenterol 2002;37(10):1205–11.
27. Burak K, Angulo P, Pasha TM, et al. Incidence and risk factors for cholangiocarcinoma in primary sclerosing cholangitis. Am J Gastroenterol 2004;99(3):523–6.
28. Fevery J, Verslype C, Lai G, et al. Incidence, diagnosis, and therapy of cholangiocarcinoma in patients with primary sclerosing cholangitis. Dig Dis Sci 2007; 52(11):3123–35.
29. Fevery J, Verslype C. An update on cholangiocarcinoma associated with primary sclerosing cholangitis. Curr Opin Gastroenterol 2010;26(3):236–45.
30. Lewis JT, Talwalkar JA, Rosen CB, et al. Precancerous bile duct pathology in end-stage primary sclerosing cholangitis, with and without cholangiocarcinoma. Am J Surg Pathol 2010;34(1):27–34.

31. Boberg KM, Lind GE. Primary sclerosing cholangitis and malignancy. Best Pract Res Clin Gastroenterol 2011;25(6):753–64.
32. Eaton JE, Talwalkar JA. Primary sclerosing cholangitis: current and future management strategies. Curr Hepat Rep 2013;12(1):28–36.
33. Trauner M, Halilbasic E, Baghdasaryan A, et al. Primary sclerosing cholangitis: new approaches to diagnosis, surveillance and treatment. Dig Dis 2012; 30(Suppl 1):39–47.
34. Bergquist A, von Seth E. Epidemiology of cholangiocarcinoma. Best Pract Res Clin Gastroenterol 2015;29(2):221–32.
35. Charatcharoenwitthaya P, Enders FB, Halling KC, et al. Utility of serum tumor markers, imaging, and biliary cytology for detecting cholangiocarcinoma in primary sclerosing cholangitis. Hepatology 2008;48(4):1106–17.
36. Sangfelt P, Sundin A, Wanders A, et al. Monitoring dominant strictures in primary sclerosing cholangitis with brush cytology and FDG-PET. J Hepatol 2014;61(6): 1352–7.
37. Wannhoff A, Hov JR, Folseraas T, et al. FUT2 and FUT3 genotype determines CA19-9 cut-off values for detection of cholangiocarcinoma in patients with primary sclerosing cholangitis. J Hepatol 2013;59(6):1278–84.
38. Boberg KM, Jebsen P, Clausen OP, et al. Diagnostic benefit of biliary brush cytology in cholangiocarcinoma in primary sclerosing cholangitis. J Hepatol 2006;45(4):568–74.
39. Trikudanathan G, Navaneethan U, Njei B, et al. Diagnostic yield of bile duct brushings for cholangiocarcinoma in primary sclerosing cholangitis: a systematic review and meta-analysis. Gastrointest Endosc 2014;79(5):783–9.
40. Rabinovitz M, Zajko AB, Hassanein T, et al. Diagnostic value of brush cytology in the diagnosis of bile duct carcinoma: a study in 65 patients with bile duct strictures. Hepatology 1990;12(4 Pt 1):747–52.
41. Andresen K, Boberg KM, Vedeld HM, et al. Four DNA methylation biomarkers in biliary brush samples accurately identify the presence of cholangiocarcinoma. Hepatology 2015;61(5):1651–9.
42. Bangarulingam SY, Bjornsson E, Enders F, et al. Long-term outcomes of positive fluorescence in situ hybridization tests in primary sclerosing cholangitis. Hepatology 2010;51(1):174–80.
43. Navaneethan U, Njei B, Venkatesh PG, et al. Fluorescence in situ hybridization for diagnosis of cholangiocarcinoma in primary sclerosing cholangitis: a systematic review and meta-analysis. Gastrointest Endosc 2014;79(6): 943–50.e3.
44. Barr Fritcher EG, Kipp BR, Voss JS, et al. Primary sclerosing cholangitis patients with serial polysomy fluorescence in situ hybridization results are at increased risk of cholangiocarcinoma. Am J Gastroenterol 2011;106(11):2023–8.
45. Eaton JE, Barr Fritcher EG, Gores GJ, et al. Biliary multifocal chromosomal polysomy and cholangiocarcinoma in primary sclerosing cholangitis. Am J Gastroenterol 2015;110(2):299–309.
46. Bangarulingam SY, Gossard AA, Petersen BT, et al. Complications of endoscopic retrograde cholangiopancreatography in primary sclerosing cholangitis. Am J Gastroenterol 2009;104(4):855–60.
47. Rosen CB, Heimbach JK, Gores GJ. Liver transplantation for cholangiocarcinoma. Transpl Int 2010;23(7):692–7.
48. Darwish Murad S, Kim WR, Harnois DM, et al. Efficacy of neoadjuvant chemoradiation, followed by liver transplantation, for perihilar cholangiocarcinoma at 12 US centers. Gastroenterology 2012;143(1):88–98.e3.

49. Friman S, Foss A, Isoniemi H, et al. Liver transplantation for cholangiocarcinoma: selection is essential for acceptable results. Scand J Gastroenterol 2011;46(3): 370–5.

50. Gores GJ, Nagorney DM, Rosen CB. Cholangiocarcinoma: is transplantation an option? For whom? J Hepatol 2007;47(4):455–9.

51. Blechacz B, Gores GJ. Cholangiocarcinoma: advances in pathogenesis, diagnosis, and treatment. Hepatology 2008;48(1):308–21.

52. Brandt DJ, MacCarty RL, Charboneau JW, et al. Gallbladder disease in patients with primary sclerosing cholangitis. AJR Am J Roentgenol 1988;150(3):571–4.

53. Buckles DC, Lindor KD, Larusso NF, et al. In primary sclerosing cholangitis, gallbladder polyps are frequently malignant. Am J Gastroenterol 2002;97(5): 1138–42.

54. Lewis JT, Talwalkar JA, Rosen CB, et al. Prevalence and risk factors for gallbladder neoplasia in patients with primary sclerosing cholangitis: evidence for a metaplasia-dysplasia-carcinoma sequence. Am J Surg Pathol 2007;31(6): 907–13.

55. Eaton JE, Thackeray EW, Lindor KD. Likelihood of malignancy in gallbladder polyps and outcomes following cholecystectomy in primary sclerosing cholangitis. Am J Gastroenterol 2012;107(3):431–9.

56. Paolucci V, Schaeff B, Schneider M, et al. Tumor seeding following laparoscopy: international survey. World J Surg 1999;23(10):989–95.

57. Zielinski MD, Atwell TD, Davis PW, et al. Comparison of surgically resected polypoid lesions of the gallbladder to their pre-operative ultrasound characteristics. J Gastrointest Surg 2009;13(1):19–25.

58. Mainprize KS, Gould SW, Gilbert JM. Surgical management of polypoid lesions of the gallbladder. Br J Surg 2000;87(4):414–7.

59. Lee JS, Lee KT, Jung JH, et al. Factors associated with malignancy in gallbladder polyps without gallbladder stone. Korean J Gastroenterol 2008;52(2):97–105.

60. Inui K, Yoshino J, Miyoshi H. Diagnosis of gallbladder tumors. Intern Med 2011; 50(11):1133–6.

61. Kiran RP, Pokala N, Dudrick SJ. Incidence pattern and survival for gallbladder cancer over three decades–an analysis of 10301 patients. Ann Surg Oncol 2007;14(2):827–32.

62. Fong Y, Wagman L, Gonen M, et al. Evidence-based gallbladder cancer staging: changing cancer staging by analysis of data from the National Cancer Database. Ann Surg 2006;243(6):767–71.

63. Leung UC, Wong PY, Roberts RH, et al. Gall bladder polyps in sclerosing cholangitis: does the 1-cm rule apply? ANZ J Surg 2007;77(5):355–7.

64. Harnois DM, Gores GJ, Ludwig J, et al. Are patients with cirrhotic stage primary sclerosing cholangitis at risk for the development of hepatocellular cancer? J Hepatol 1997;27(3):512–6.

65. Bruix J, Sherman M, American Association for the Study of Liver D. Management of hepatocellular carcinoma: an update. Hepatology 2011;53(3):1020–2.

66. Wang R, Leong RW. Primary sclerosing cholangitis as an independent risk factor for colorectal cancer in the context of inflammatory bowel disease: a review of the literature. World J Gastroenterol 2014;20(27):8783–9.

67. Broome U, Bergquist A. Primary sclerosing cholangitis, inflammatory bowel disease, and colon cancer. Semin Liver Dis 2006;26(1):31–41.

68. Leidenius MH, Farkkila MA, Karkkainen P, et al. Colorectal dysplasia and carcinoma in patients with ulcerative colitis and primary sclerosing cholangitis. Scand J Gastroenterol 1997;32(7):706–11.

69. Lindstrom L, Lapidus A, Ost A, et al. Increased risk of colorectal cancer and dysplasia in patients with Crohn's colitis and primary sclerosing cholangitis. Dis Colon Rectum 2011;54(11):1392–7.
70. Braden B, Halliday J, Aryasingha S, et al. Risk for colorectal neoplasia in patients with colonic Crohn's disease and concomitant primary sclerosing cholangitis. Clin Gastroenterol Hepatol 2012;10(3):303–8.
71. Thackeray EW, Charatcharoenwitthaya P, Elfaki D, et al. Colon neoplasms develop early in the course of inflammatory bowel disease and primary sclerosing cholangitis. Clin Gastroenterol Hepatol 2011;9(1):52–6.
72. Claessen MM, Lutgens MW, van Buuren HR, et al. More right-sided IBD-associated colorectal cancer in patients with primary sclerosing cholangitis. Inflamm Bowel Dis 2009;15(9):1331–6.
73. Brackmann S, Andersen SN, Aamodt G, et al. Relationship between clinical parameters and the colitis-colorectal cancer interval in a cohort of patients with colorectal cancer in inflammatory bowel disease. Scand J Gastroenterol 2009;44(1): 46–55.
74. Loftus EV Jr, Harewood GC, Loftus CG, et al. PSC-IBD: a unique form of inflammatory bowel disease associated with primary sclerosing cholangitis. Gut 2005; 54(1):91–6.
75. Rudolph G, Gotthardt D, Kloeters-Plachky P, et al. In PSC with dominant bile duct stenosis, IBD is associated with an increase of carcinomas and reduced survival. J Hepatol 2010;53(2):313–7.
76. Jorgensen KK, Lindstrom L, Cvancarova M, et al. Colorectal neoplasia in patients with primary sclerosing cholangitis undergoing liver transplantation: a Nordic multicenter study. Scand J Gastroenterol 2012;47(8–9):1021–9.
77. Itzkowitz SH, Present DH, Crohn's and Colitis Foundation of America Colon Cancer in IBD Study Group. Consensus conference: colorectal cancer screening and surveillance in inflammatory bowel disease. Inflamm Bowel Dis 2005;11(3): 314–21.
78. Eaton JE, Smyrk TC, Imam M, et al. The fate of indefinite and low-grade dysplasia in ulcerative colitis and primary sclerosing cholangitis colitis before and after liver transplantation. Aliment Pharmacol Ther 2013;38(8):977–87.
79. Treeprasertsuk S, Bjornsson E, Sinakos E, et al. Outcome of patients with primary sclerosing cholangitis and ulcerative colitis undergoing colectomy. World J Gastrointest Pharmacol Ther 2013;4(3):61–8.
80. Pardi DS, Loftus EV Jr, Kremers WK, et al. Ursodeoxycholic acid as a chemopreventive agent in patients with ulcerative colitis and primary sclerosing cholangitis. Gastroenterology 2003;124(4):889–93.
81. Wolf JM, Rybicki LA, Lashner BA. The impact of ursodeoxycholic acid on cancer, dysplasia and mortality in ulcerative colitis patients with primary sclerosing cholangitis. Aliment Pharmacol Ther 2005;22(9):783–8.
82. Eaton JE, Silveira MG, Pardi DS, et al. High-dose ursodeoxycholic acid is associated with the development of colorectal neoplasia in patients with ulcerative colitis and primary sclerosing cholangitis. Am J Gastroenterol 2011;106(9):1638–45.
83. Lindor KD, Kowdley KV, Luketic VA, et al. High-dose ursodeoxycholic acid for the treatment of primary sclerosing cholangitis. Hepatology 2009;50(3):808–14.
84. Card TR, Solaymani-Dodaran M, West J. Incidence and mortality of primary sclerosing cholangitis in the UK: a population-based cohort study. J Hepatol 2008; 48(6):939–44.
85. Bjornsson E, Angulo P. Cholangiocarcinoma in young individuals with and without primary sclerosing cholangitis. Am J Gastroenterol 2007;102(8):1677–82.

86. Miloh T, Arnon R, Shneider B, et al. A retrospective single-center review of primary sclerosing cholangitis in children. Clin Gastroenterol Hepatol 2009;7(2): 239–45.

87. Campsen J, Zimmerman MA, Trotter JF, et al. Clinically recurrent primary sclerosing cholangitis following liver transplantation: a time course. Liver Transpl 2008;14(2):181–5.

88. Heneghan MA, Tuttle-Newhall JE, Suhocki PV, et al. De-novo cholangiocarcinoma in the setting of recurrent primary sclerosing cholangitis following liver transplant. Am J Transplant 2003;3(5):634–8.

89. Kaya M, de Groen PC, Angulo P, et al. Treatment of cholangiocarcinoma complicating primary sclerosing cholangitis: the Mayo clinic experience. Am J Gastroenterol 2001;96(4):1164–9.

90. Morris-Stiff G, Bhati C, Olliff S, et al. Cholangiocarcinoma complicating primary sclerosing cholangitis: a 24-year experience. Dig Surg 2008;25(2):126–32.

91. Fevery J, Henckaerts L, Van Oirbeek R, et al. Malignancies and mortality in 200 patients with primary sclerosering cholangitis: a long-term single-centre study. Liver Int 2012;32(2):214–22.

92. Ponsioen CY, Vrouenraets SM, Prawirodirdjo W, et al. Natural history of primary sclerosing cholangitis and prognostic value of cholangiography in a Dutch population. Gut 2002;51(4):562–6.

Sclerosing Cholangitis in Children and Adolescents

Giorgina Mieli-Vergani, MD, PhD, FRCP, FRCPCH[a],*, Diego Vergani, MD, PhD, FRCPath, FRCP[b]

KEYWORDS

- Juvenile sclerosing cholangitis • Primary sclerosing cholangitis
- Autoimmune sclerosing cholangitis • Autoimmune hepatitis
- Inflammatory bowel disease • Liver transplant • Children • Adolescents

KEY POINTS

- Sclerosing cholangitis in pediatric age recognizes different etiologies, management, and prognosis depending on the underlying cause.
- Sclerosing cholangitis is frequently associated with inflammatory bowel disease (ulcerative colitis, Crohn disease, indeterminate colitis).
- A high proportion of patients with sclerosing cholangitis have autoimmune features similar to those of autoimmune hepatitis type 1 and respond biochemically to immunosuppressive treatment, but the bile duct disease progresses in half of them leading to liver transplant.
- Sclerosing cholangitis can recur after liver transplant, particularly in patients with strong autoimmune features.
- Severity of liver disease and risk of recurrence after transplant are linked to the severity of the inflammatory bowel disease.

DEFINITION

Sclerosing cholangitis is a chronic disorder characterized by inflammation and progressive obliterative fibrosis of the intrahepatic and/or extrahepatic bile ducts. It has long been considered a disease confined to adulthood, but it is now clear that it occurs in all age groups, with some features being unique to children. Sclerosing cholangitis progresses slowly to biliary cirrhosis, liver failure, and, particularly in adults, cholangiocarcinoma (CC).

HISTORIC BACKGROUND

Sclerosing cholangitis was first described in adult patients in 1924 by the Parisian surgeon Delbet,[1] who reported a patient with "irregular fibrosis and stenosis of the biliary

The authors have nothing to disclose.
[a] Paediatric Liver, GI and Nutrition Centre, King's College Hospital, Denmark Hill, London SE5 9RS, UK; [b] Institute of Liver Studies, King's College Hospital, Denmark Hill, London SE5 9RS, UK
* Corresponding author.
E-mail address: giorgina.vergani@kcl.ac.uk

tree." In 1927, Miller[2] referred to a similar condition as "benign stricture of common bile duct." In 1964,[3] the term "primary sclerosing cholangitis" (PSC) was used for the first time to distinguish sclerosing cholangitis without an obvious etiology from sclerosing cholangitis secondary to lesions of the bile ducts or systemic disease, such as primary or secondary immunodeficiencies. Until the advent of endoscopic retrograde cholangiopancreatography (ERCP) and percutaneous transhepatic cholangiography, recognition was rare, being made at laparotomy in patients with persistent jaundice. With the availability of ERCP and more recently magnetic resonance cholangiopancreatography (MRCP) the reported prevalence of sclerosing cholangitis in adults and children is increasing. The association of sclerosing cholangitis with inflammatory bowel disease (IBD) was first clearly established in 1966,[4] although inflammatory involvement of the liver parenchyma in IBD had been described in 1899 by Lister.[5]

SCLEROSING CHOLANGITIS IN CHILDREN AND ADOLESCENTS

With the growing use of biliary imaging in the form of ERCP and, more recently, noninvasive MRCP, sclerosing cholangitis is diagnosed with increasing frequency also in pediatric age. It is an important cause of morbidity and mortality, accounting for some 2% of pediatric liver transplants in the United States between 1988 and 2008 (United Network for Organ Sharing Data Report - October 2009. http://www.unos.org/data/).

The term PSC, universally used in adult patients, is not accurate to describe pediatric SC: "primary" denotes ignorance about etiology and pathogenesis, whereas in pediatrics[6–10] there are well-defined forms of sclerosing cholangitis. In the neonatal period, pathologic features of severe sclerosing cholangitis characterize biliary atresia and neonatal sclerosing cholangitis, a condition inherited in an autosomal-recessive manner.[11] Other inherited diseases, systemic malignancies, and immunologic defects may produce a clinical picture similar to adult PSC. For example, mild to moderate defects in the ABCB4 (MDR3) gene are a likely cause of several cases of small duct sclerosing cholangitis in children and adults.[12,13] Sclerosing cholangitis may also complicate a wide variety of disorders, including primary and secondary immunodeficiencies, Langerhans cell histiocytosis (LCH), psoriasis, cystic fibrosis, reticulum cell sarcoma, and sickle cell anemia. Moreover, an overlap syndrome between autoimmune hepatitis (AIH) and sclerosing cholangitis (autoimmune sclerosing cholangitis [ASC]) is significantly more common in children than in adults. Only in those pediatric patients in whom SC occurs without any of the previously mentioned defining features should the name of "primary" be used.

DIAGNOSIS

The diagnosis of sclerosing cholangitis is usually based on the demonstration of radiologic evidence of bile duct disease, with or without biliary features on liver histology. More recently, a condition called small-duct PSC has been described, whereby chronic cholestasis and hepatic histology compatible with sclerosing cholangitis are associated with normal cholangiography.[14] In pediatrics, all disorders described previously that can be associated with sclerosing cholangitis should be excluded.

Several papers have compared the accuracy of MRCP with that of ERCP in the diagnosis of sclerosing cholangitis in adults and children. With the availability of more advanced magnetic resonance instrumentation and matching software, coupled with increased radiologic expertise, the sensitivity and specificity of MRCP ranks in the high 80s and is comparable with that of ERCP,[15,16] although ERCP may still be more accurate in the diagnosis of early changes[17] and allows therapeutic interventions in the case of strictures.[18] MRCP is reported to be 84% sensitive and accurate in the diagnosis of pediatric sclerosing cholangitis.[8,19]

The classic histologic feature of adult PSC, periductular onion skin fibrosis, is rare, a high proportion of pediatric patients having variable degrees of interface hepatitis at diagnosis.[6,20] In view of the presence of interface hepatitis on liver biopsy and the frequent positivity for circulating autoantibodies,[6,10,20] the differential diagnosis between AIH and ASC relies on the demonstration of bile duct damage at presentation. Neither the original nor the simplified International Autoimmune Hepatitis Group scoring systems devised for the diagnosis of AIH[21–23] are suitable to discriminate between AIH and ASC[6,9,10,24,25] because they do not include cholangiographic studies at disease onset.

EPIDEMIOLOGY

The reported incidence and prevalence of PSC in adults range from 0 to 1.3 and from 0 to 16.2 per 100,000, respectively.[26] Little is known about the epidemiology of pediatric sclerosing cholangitis, probably because of its rarity and heterogeneous etiology. The incidence of PSC was estimated to be 0.23 per 100,000 children in Calgary[27] and 0.2 per 100,000 children in Utah.[28] In the latter study, the prevalence of pediatric PSC was 1.5 per 100,000,[28] whereas the incidence and prevalence of ASC per 100,000 were 0.1 and 0.6, respectively.[28]

GENETIC FEATURES

ASC and adult-type PSC are complex trait diseases (ie, conditions not inherited in a mendelian autosomal-dominant, autosomal-recessive, or sex-linked fashion). The mode of inheritance of a complex trait disorder is unknown and involves one or more genes operating alone or in concert to increase or reduce the risk of the trait, and interacting with environmental factors.

Susceptibility to juvenile ASC is associated with possession of the HLA haplotype DRB1*13 (DR13).[1,29] Susceptibility to PSC in adults is associated with two main HLA haplotypes, DRB1*0301-DQA1*0501-DQB1*0201 (referred to as DR3) and HLA-DRB1*1301-DQA1*0103-DQB1*0603 (referred to as DR6).[30] The role of additional genes encoded within or without the HLA region has been investigated in patient cohorts mainly comprising adults, but also including children. The main contribution of genetic susceptibility to PSC comes from the Oslo group,[30–34] which follows a particularly well-characterized patient population. Through the use of seven microsatellite markers, Wiencke and colleagues[30] have shown that a gene in linkage disequilibrium with microsatellite D6S265 contributes to PSC susceptibility in individuals carrying the DR6 haplotype. They also show that the PSC-associated DR3 haplotype extends more telomerically than previously reported and that DR11 may have a protective effect on the development of PSC. Karlsen and colleagues[33] have reported that the frequency of HLA-Bw4 and-C2, ligands for the inhibitory receptors on natural killer cells KIRs 3DL1 and 2DL1, is significantly reduced in patients with PSC exerting a protective role. In two further papers Karlsen and colleagues[32] dissociate susceptibility to PSC from that to IBD. In the first report they show that associations with HLA class II genes are different in the two conditions; similarly, in the second paper[31] they show that IBD-associated polymorphisms do not play a major predisposing role to PSC. The same group has reported that polymorphisms in the steroid and xenobiotic receptor gene influence survival in PSC, with median survival being significantly reduced in patients homozygous for an allele in this region.[22,34]

Henckaerts and colleagues[35] hypothesize that CC-type chemokine receptor 5 (CCR5) would be an interesting candidate gene for susceptibility to PSC because of its chromosomal location within the IBD susceptibility region. They found that the frequency of the CCR5-D32 mutation in PSC is significantly lower than in patients with IBD and healthy control subjects, suggesting a protective effect of this mutation for PSC.

Bergquist and colleagues[36] have shown that first-degree relatives of patients with PSC have an increased risk of PSC, indicating the importance of genetic factors in the cause of this condition. Moreover, first-degree relatives of patients with PSC without IBD have an increased risk of developing ulcerative colitis (UC), suggesting a shared genetic susceptibility between UC and PSC.

Two studies have focused on cystic fibrosis transmembrane conductance regulator in PSC. Pall and colleagues[37] found that the chloride channel function is markedly decreased in patients with PSC, whereas Henckaerts and colleagues[38] reported that cystic fibrosis transmembrane conductance regulator variants affecting the functional properties of the cystic fibrosis transmembrane conductance regulator protein offer protection against the development of PSC.

PEDIATRIC SERIES

There is a limited number of published series of pediatric sclerosing cholangitis.[6–10,28] In these reports the incidence of the various clinical forms of sclerosing cholangitis differs depending on the year of publication and the center where the study was conducted, reflecting different study designs, pattern of referral, and diagnostic protocols. Most of these series are retrospective and cholangiographic studies, performed by ERCP, percutaneous cholangiography, or more recently MRCP, were prompted by biochemical and/or histologic features of cholestatic disease.[7–10,28] Only one study, published in 2001, differs from all the other series, because it was prospective and aimed at establishing the relative incidence of AIH and ASC among children presenting with liver disease and positive autoimmune serology (autoantibodies; increased levels of IgG), by performing cholangiograms at disease onset, irrespective of biochemical or histologic evidence of cholestatic disease.[6] Other forms of sclerosing cholangitis seen over the same period of observation were excluded from this prospective study.

In all published series, boys are more affected than girls; 20% to 40% of patients have intrahepatic cholangiopathy with normal extrahepatic bile ducts; and IBD is strongly associated with the diagnosis of sclerosing cholangitis, being found in 60% to 90% of cases according to study design.[6–10,28] More than two-thirds of the cases have UC, and the others have Crohn disease or indeterminate colitis. IBD can precede the diagnosis of liver disease by many years, be diagnosed at the same time, or develop during follow-up. The prevalence of IBD is higher in those centers where surveillance enteroscopy is performed even in the absence of clinical symptoms of IBD.[6] It is advisable to consider surveillance colonoscopy in all children who are newly diagnosed with sclerosing cholangitis and to have a low threshold for performing this procedure in those who have symptoms consistent with IBD (eg, diarrhea, growth failure, anemia).

Retrospective Studies

The first relatively large retrospective series of children with sclerosing cholangitis was published in 1994.[7] It comprised 56 children with a variety of underlying pathologies, including immunodeficiencies, LCH, neonatal sclerosing cholangitis, and psoriasis.

Eight children had associated autoimmune features, including six with IBD, and two with AIH/sclerosing cholangitis overlap syndrome, one of whom had IBD. Ten children had no associated disease. Patients with autoimmune features received immunosuppressive treatment of IBD and had an overall better outcome than the other disease groups, with an estimated 10-year survival rate of 86%. The 10 with no associated conditions had a particularly poor prognosis, three dying and four requiring liver transplantation during a mean of 7 ± 4.3 years of follow-up.

In 1995 Wilschanski and colleagues[8] described 32 children with sclerosing cholangitis. Excluding two with associated immunodeficiencies, 30 children were diagnosed as having PSC. Interestingly, at presentation half of the children had normal levels of alkaline phosphatase (γ-glutamyl transpeptidase [GGT] levels were not measured). Prognosis at a mean follow-up of 3.8 years was poor for nine patients with evidence of overlap between AIH and sclerosing cholangitis (six with IBD), five requiring liver transplantation, and for four patients with incidental finding of abdominal organomegly (one with IBD), two needing transplant. Prognosis in 17 further patients (one with IBD) presenting with chronic liver disease and prominent features of cholestasis, similar to adult PSC, was better, with only three developing end-stage liver disease requiring grafting. In this series the prognosis of AIH/PSC overlap syndrome was particularly severe and not ameliorated by immunosuppressive treatment, although no information is provided regarding the timing of treatment implementation during the course of the disease or the immunosuppressive drugs used.

A report by Feldstein and colleagues[9] describes 55 patients with sclerosing cholangitis. Seventy-two percent were positive for antineutrophil cytoplasmic antibody, 68% for antinuclear (ANA) and/or anti-smooth muscle (SMA) antibodies, and 70% had high levels of IgG. IBD was present in 81%. Based on the presence of interface hepatitis on liver biopsy, 14 patients were labeled as AIH/PSC overlap, whereas 38 children were diagnosed as PSC. Forty-one of the 55 children were treated either with ursodeoxycholic acid (UDCA) alone, with immunosuppressive drugs (corticosteroids with or without azathioprine) alone, or a combination of UDCA and immunosuppression, with variable response. The overall outcome was poor, with 11 patients requiring liver transplantation over a mean of 6.6 ± 4.4 years of follow-up, the median (50%) survival free of liver transplantation being 12.7 years. The prognosis of children with PSC or AIH/PSC was similar and was not ultimately affected by treatment. Three of 11 (27%) transplanted children had recurrence of PSC in the graft within 6 years from surgery.

Miloh and colleagues[10] describe 47 patients with sclerosing cholangitis. Based on absence or presence of interface hepatitis on liver biopsy, 35 were diagnosed as having PSC and 12 as having AIH/PSC overlap syndrome. All patients with overlap syndrome had positive ANA and/or SMA and/or increased IgG levels. Autoantibodies were present also in 32% of patients with PSC. In this series, where cholangiographic studies were mainly performed by MRCP, no radiologic biliary involvement was detected despite histologic evidence of sclerosing cholangitis in an unusually high proportion (36%) of patients. These patients were diagnosed as having small-duct PSC.[14] Whether this is caused by the lower sensitivity of the MRCP compared with the ERCP in detecting biliary changes remains to be verified. Patients with AIH/PSC overlap syndrome were treated with UDCA and immunosuppression, whereas those with PSC with UDCA alone, with amelioration of biochemical parameters in both groups. After a median of 6.5 years, however, nine children required liver transplantation, one experiencing disease recurrence 10 years later. Transplant-free survival was marginally better in patients with small-duct PSC than in the others.

Deneau and colleagues[28] performed a large pediatric population–based study in Utah between 1986 and 2011. They identified 29 children with PSC (96.6% with IBD) and 12 with overlap syndrome (ASC, 75% with IBD). After a mean follow-up of 5.9 years, their outcome was compared with that of 44 children diagnosed with AIH over the same time period. Although no information is provided regarding treatment, it is interesting that survival with native liver was marginally better in ASC and AIH compared with PSC, the probability of developing complicated liver disease within 5 years from diagnosis being 37% for PSC, 25% for ASC, and 15% for AIH. Also of interest is that this is the only study reporting the development of CC in 2 of 29 patients with PSC, both with UC, one of whom died, whereas the other was alive 3 years after chemotherapy, radiation, and liver transplant.

Prospective Study

Progression from AIH to sclerosing cholangitis has been reported in children and adults.[40–43] However, in these reports no cholangiographic studies were performed at disease presentation, challenging the concept of progression from one disease to the other. To establish the relative prevalence, the response to treatment, and the outcome of AIH versus ASC, a prospective study was initiated at the King's College Hospital tertiary referral center in 1984 and patients were recruited over a period of 16 years.[6] Interim results were published in 2001,[6] and the patient cohort is being followed up to date. In this study, all children with serologic (ie, positive autoantibodies, high IgG levels) and histologic (ie, interface hepatitis; **Fig. 1**) features of autoimmune liver disease underwent a cholangiogram at the time of presentation, independently of the presence of biochemical or histologic evidence of cholestasis. Surveillance enteroscopy to investigate for possible IBD was performed in all cases, independently of symptoms. Approximately 50% of the patients enrolled in this prospective study had alterations of the bile ducts characteristic of sclerosing cholangitis, although they were generally less advanced than those observed in adult-type PSC (**Fig. 2**) and were diagnosed as having ASC. A quarter of the children with ASC, despite abnormal cholangiograms, had no histologic features that suggested bile duct involvement, and the diagnosis of sclerosing cholangitis was only possible because

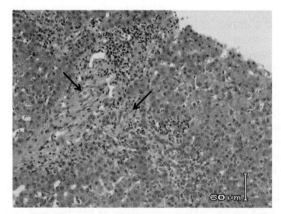

Fig. 1. Dense portal tract inflammatory infiltrate comprising lymphocyte and plasma cells and invading the surrounding parenchyma (interface hepatitis) in a child with autoimmune sclerosing cholangitis. The arrows show bile duct damage (hematoxylin-eosin, original magnification × 40).

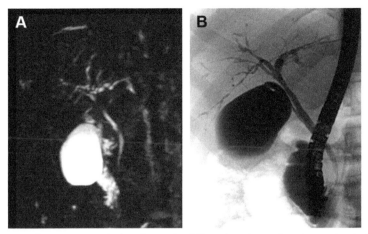

Fig. 2. Magnetic resonance cholangiography (*A*) and endoscopic retrograde cholangiography (*B*) of a child with autoimmune sclerosing cholangitis showing a diffuse cholangiopathy with ductal changes in both lobes. The extrahepatic bile ducts have normal appearance.

of the cholangiographic studies. Virtually all patients with ASC were seropositive for ANA and/or SMA, antibodies typical of AIH type 1, only one patient being positive for anti–liver kidney microsomal type 1 (anti-LKM1), the antibody characterizing AIH type 2. In contrast to AIH, which had a clear female preponderance, ASC was diagnosed in a similar proportion of boys and girls. The mode of presentation of ASC was similar to that of AIH type 1 (**Table 1**). IBD was present in 45% of children with ASC compared with 20% of those with typical AIH type 1, and 90% of children with ASC had greatly increased serum IgG levels. At the time of presentation, standard liver function tests, including alkaline phosphatase and GGT levels, did not help in discriminating between AIH and ASC, although the alkaline phosphatase/aspartate amino transferase ratio was significantly higher in ASC (**Table 2**). Atypical perinuclear antineutrophil cytoplasmic antibodies, whose target is located within the nuclear membrane leading to the name of perinuclear antineutrophil nuclear antibody (pANNA), were present in 74% of patients with ASC compared with 45% of patients with AIH type 1 and 11% of those with AIH type 2. Antisoluble liver antigen antibodies were found in some 50% of patients with ASC, defining a more severe disease course.[44] Evolution from AIH to ASC was documented in one patient during the published prospective series[6] and has been observed in two further patients during follow-up,[45] suggesting that AIH and ASC may be part of the same pathogenic process. During the same observation period of the prospective study, nine children with cholangiographic evidence of bile duct disease, but no positivity for ANA, SMA, or anti-LKM1 at the time of presentation, were diagnosed as having PSC. Three had UC treated with immunosuppressive drugs at the time of referral, one had thyroiditis, three a family history of autoimmune disorders, and four were pANNA positive. After an observation period of 6 years, six of the nine children were alive and stable, four on treatment with UDCA alone and two on UDCA plus immunosuppressive drugs for IBD, one had died of ischemic hepatitis, and two were lost to follow-up.

Currently, in our center imaging of the biliary system by MRCP, followed by ERCP if MRCP is not informative, and colonoscopy is part of the evaluation of all children with liver disease associated with autoimmune features.

Table 1
Comparison between the clinical presentation of childhood autoimmune hepatitis and autoimmune sclerosing cholangitis

Parameter	AIH Type 1	AIH Type 2	ASC
Median age in years	11	7	12
Mode of presentation (%)			
Acute hepatitis	47	40	37
Acute liver failure	3	25	0
Insidious onset	38	25	37
Complication of chronic liver disease	12	10	26
Associated immune diseases (%)	22	20	48
Inflammatory bowel disease (%)	20	12	45
Abnormal cholangiogram (%)	0	0	100
ANA/SMA (%)	100	25	96
Anti-LKM-1 (%)	0	100	4
pANNA (%)	45	11	74
Anti-SLA (%)	58	58	41
Interface hepatitis (%)	92	94	60
Biliary features (%)	28	6	31
Cirrhosis (%)	69	38	15

Abbreviations: AIH, autoimmune hepatitis; ANA, antinuclear antibodies; anti-LKM-1, anti–liver kidney microsomal type 1 antibody; ASC, autoimmune sclerosing cholangitis; pANNA, peripheral antinuclear neutrophil antibodies; SLA, soluble liver antigen; SMA, anti–smooth muscle antibodies.

Data from Gregorio GV, Portmann B, Karani, et al. Autoimmune hepatitis/sclerosing cholangitis overlap syndrome in childhood: a 16-year prospective study. Hepatology 2001;33(3):544–53.

TREATMENT AND PROGNOSIS

Treatment and prognosis of sclerosing cholangitis depend on the underlying pathology. Management of sclerosing cholangitis associated with immunodeficiency syndromes, LCH, or metabolic/genetic disorders is closely related to the ability of

Table 2
Comparison between the biochemical parameters at presentation of childhood autoimmune hepatitis and autoimmune sclerosing cholangitis

	AIH	ASC
Bilirubin (nv <20 mmol/L)	35 (4–306)	20 (4–179)
Albumin (nv >35 g/L)	35 (25–47)	39 (27–54)
AST (nv <50 IU/L)	333 (24–4830)	102 (18–1215)
INR (nv <1.2)	1.2 (0.96–2.5)	1.1 (0.9–1.6)
GGT (nv <50 IU/L)	76 (29–383)	129 (13–948)
AP (nv <350 IU/L)	356 (131–878)	303 (104–1710)
AP/AST ratio	1.14 (0.05–14.75)	3.96 (0.20–14.20)

Abbreviations: AIH, autoimmune hepatitis; AP, alkaline phosphatase; ASC, autoimmune sclerosing cholangitis; AST, aspartate aminotransferase; GGT, γ-glutamyl transpeptidase; INR, international normalized ratio; nv, normal values.

Data from Gregorio GV, Portmann B, Karani, et al. Autoimmune hepatitis/sclerosing cholangitis overlap syndrome in childhood: a 16-year prospective study. Hepatology 2001;33(3):544–53.

controlling the primary disease. For sclerosing cholangitis without associated pathologies, no standard mode of treatment is presently advocated.[46] Based on a reported beneficial effect in adult PSC, UDCA is used also for the treatment of childhood sclerosing cholangitis, but whether it is helpful in arresting the progression of the bile duct disease remains to be established. In adults with PSC high-dose UDCA was initially reported as more beneficial than standard doses,[47] but a randomized double-blind controlled study from the Mayo Clinic shows that high-dose UDCA has a negative effect.[48] It is prudent, therefore, to use doses not higher than 15 to 20 mg/kg/day.

A beneficial effect of oral vancomycin (50 mg/kg per day) has been reported in 14 patients with sclerosing cholangitis and IBD, 12 positive for autoantibodies.[49] All showed a marked improvement in transaminase and GGT levels, erythrocyte sedimentation rate, and clinical symptoms on prolonged oral vancomycin treatment, the best improvement being observed in patients who were not cirrhotic at treatment start. Four patients positive for ANA, SMA, and/or perinuclear antineutrophil cytoplasmic antibodies became negative after an average of 3 months of vancomycin treatment. Suspension of treatment was associated with relapse of biochemical abnormalities in four patients, who improved again after retreatment. Despite severe cholangitic changes before treatment, the liver histology of three children rebiopsied while on vancomycin is reported as normal. Whether these children represent a subgroup of PSC in whom infectious causes play a major pathogenic role remains to be clarified. These results await confirmation in a larger number of patients. Whether vancomycin acts through its antibiotic, immunomodulatory,[50] or choleretic[51] properties remains to be elucidated.

The King's prospective study shows that in ASC treatment with steroids and azathioprine, using the same schedule as in AIH, in association with UDCA, is beneficial in abating the parenchymal inflammatory lesions, but is less effective in controlling bile duct damage. Although resolution of liver test abnormalities is seen within a few months in most patients, the medium- to long-term prognosis of ASC is worse than that of AIH because of progression of cholangiopathy despite treatment in some 50% of patients, with 20% of them eventually requiring liver transplantation.[6,45] Similarly, in the series by Miloh and colleagues,[10] although all patients with overlap AIH/sclerosing cholangitis syndrome were reported to have a favorable biochemical response to immunosuppression and UDCA treatment, 25% required liver transplantation during the 12-year observation period. Response to immunosuppressive drugs was less satisfactory in sclerosing cholangitis patients with autoimmune features described by Wilschanski and colleagues[8] and Feldstein and colleagues,[9] possibly because of long-standing liver disease before starting treatment.

It is our experience that reactivation of the liver disease often follows flares of the intestinal disease in sclerosing cholangitis patients with IBD. In this context, it is of note that none of the published series of sclerosing cholangitis in pediatric patients gives details of the severity of the IBD or of the effectiveness of its treatment, information that would be important to verify whether ability to control efficiently IBD has a major role in preventing liver disease progression.

CHOLANGIOCARCINOMA

In adult patients with PSC the incidence and prevalence of CC are reportedly between 5% and 36% and 0.6% per year, respectively.[52] In pediatrics, there are only three cases of CC described in patients with PSC, two by Deneau and colleagues[28] and one by Ross and colleagues.[39] The three patients were 17.9, 18, and 14 years of age at the time of CC diagnosis; all had UC and developed CC 6 years, 4.2 years, and 14 months after the diagnosis of PSC, respectively. None of the patients with ASC enrolled in the King's prospective study has developed CC over an observation period of 30 years. Long-term follow-up of cases identified in pediatric age is needed to establish the incidence and prevalence of CC in this group of patients.

LIVER TRANSPLANTATION

Liver transplantation is indicated in patients with sclerosing cholangitis who develop end-stage liver disease. Approximately 20% to 30% of children with sclerosing cholangitis require liver transplantation in the medium term. After transplantation, recurrence of disease is reported in 27%[9] to 67%[45] of patients, the highest risk of relapse being observed in patients with florid autoimmune features and poorly controlled IBD.[10,45] In these patients it is prudent to continue steroid-based immunosuppression at a higher dose than that used for patients not transplanted for autoimmune liver disease, because recurrence may occur years after transplantation. Recurrence of sclerosing cholangitis, which leads to retransplantation in a high proportion of patients, seems to be associated with poorly controlled IBD. In this context it is of interest that PSC recurrence in adults with IBD can be prevented by pre–liver transplant colectomy.[53–55] A paper focusing on risk factors for recurrence of PSC after living donor liver transplantation describes disease recurrence in 11 of 20 (55%) patients.[56] Risk factors for recurrence were cytomegalovirus disease within 3 months posttransplant and grafts from related donors. Multivariate analysis showed that younger age (<30 years of age, including children and adolescents) was an independent risk factor for recurrence.

SUMMARY

In pediatrics, sclerosing cholangitis is the result of several different pathologies. A high proportion of patients have associated IBD and autoimmune features. Prospective studies on large cohorts of children with sclerosing cholangitis are needed for a better understanding of diagnostic pathways and pathogenic mechanisms, including the role of intestinal inflammation, with the aim of devising more effective treatment to improve the outcome of this devastating disease.

REFERENCES

1. Delbet P. Retrecissement du choledoque: cholecystoduodenostomie. Bull Mem Soc Nat Chir 1924;50:1144–6.
2. Miller R. Benign stricture of common bile duct. Ann Surg 1927;86:296–303.
3. Holubitsky IB, McKenzie AD. Primary sclerosing cholangitis of the extrahepatic bile ducts. Can J Surg 1964;7:277–83.
4. Warren KW, Athanassiades S, Monge JI. Primary sclerosing cholangitis. A study of forty-two cases. Am J Surg 1966;111(1):23–38.
5. Lister JD. A specimen of diffuse ulcerative colitis with secondary diffuse hepatitis. Trans Pathol Soc Lon 1899;50:130–4.
6. Gregorio GV, Portmann B, Karani J, et al. Autoimmune hepatitis/sclerosing cholangitis overlap syndrome in childhood: a 16-year prospective study. Hepatology 2001;33(3):544–53.
7. Debray D, Pariente D, Urvoas E, et al. Sclerosing cholangitis in children. J Pediatr 1994;124(1):49–56.

8. Wilschanski M, Chait P, Wade JA, et al. Primary sclerosing cholangitis in 32 children: clinical, laboratory, and radiographic features, with survival analysis. Hepatology 1995;22(5):1415–22.
9. Feldstein AE, Perrault J, El-Youssif M, et al. Primary sclerosing cholangitis in children: a long-term follow-up study. Hepatology 2003;38(1):210–7.
10. Miloh T, Arnon R, Shneider B, et al. A retrospective single-center review of primary sclerosing cholangitis in children. Clin Gastroenterol Hepatol 2009;7(2): 239–45.
11. Baker AJ, Portmann B, Westaby D, et al. Neonatal sclerosing cholangitis in two siblings: a category of progressive intrahepatic cholestasis. J Pediatr Gastroenterol Nutr 1993;17(3):317–22.
12. Jacquemin E, De Vree JM, Cresteil D, et al. The wide spectrum of multidrug resistance 3 deficiency: from neonatal cholestasis to cirrhosis of adulthood. Gastroenterology 2001;120(6):1448–58.
13. Ziol M, Barbu V, Rosmorduc O, et al. ABCB4 heterozygous gene mutations associated with fibrosing cholestatic liver disease in adults. Gastroenterology 2008; 135(1):131–41.
14. Wee A, Ludwig J. Pericholangitis in chronic ulcerative colitis: primary sclerosing cholangitis of the small bile ducts? Ann Intern Med 1985;102(5):581–7.
15. Berstad AE, Aabakken L, Smith HJ, et al. Diagnostic accuracy of magnetic resonance and endoscopic retrograde cholangiography in primary sclerosing cholangitis. Clin Gastroenterol Hepatol 2006;4(4):514–20.
16. Moff SL, Kamel IR, Eustace J, et al. Diagnosis of primary sclerosing cholangitis: a blinded comparative study using magnetic resonance cholangiography and endoscopic retrograde cholangiography. Gastrointest Endosc 2006;64(2): 219–23.
17. Weber C, Kuhlencordt R, Grotelueschen R, et al. Magnetic resonance cholangiopancreatography in the diagnosis of primary sclerosing cholangitis. Endoscopy 2008;40(9):739–45.
18. Rocca R, Castellino F, Daperno M, et al. Therapeutic ERCP in paediatric patients. Dig Liver Dis 2005;37(5):357–62.
19. Chavhan GB, Roberts E, Moineddin R, et al. Primary sclerosing cholangitis in children: utility of magnetic resonance cholangiopancreatography. Pediatr Radiol 2008;38(8):868–73.
20. Batres LA, Russo P, Mathews M, et al. Primary sclerosing cholangitis in children: a histologic follow-up study. Pediatr Dev Pathol 2005;8(5):568–76.
21. Johnson PJ, McFarlane IG. Meeting report: International Autoimmune Hepatitis Group. Hepatology 1993;18(4):998–1005.
22. Alvarez F, Berg PA, Bianchi FB, et al. International Autoimmune Hepatitis Group report: review of criteria for diagnosis of autoimmune hepatitis. J Hepatol 1999; 31:929–38.
23. Hennes EM, Zeniya M, Czaja AJ, et al. Simplified criteria for the diagnosis of autoimmune hepatitis. Hepatology 2008;48(1):169–76.
24. Hiejima E, Komatsu H, Sogo T, et al. Utility of simplified criteria for the diagnosis of autoimmune hepatitis in children. J Pediatr Gastroenterol Nutr 2011;52(4):470–3.
25. Ebbeson RL, Schreiber RA. Diagnosing autoimmune hepatitis in children: is the International Autoimmune Hepatitis Group scoring system useful? Clin Gastroenterol Hepatol 2004;2(10):935–40.
26. Boonstra K, Beuers U, Ponsioen CY. Epidemiology of primary sclerosing cholangitis and primary biliary cirrhosis: a systematic review. J Hepatol 2012;56(5): 1181–8.

27. Kaplan GG, Laupland KB, Butzner D, et al. The burden of large and small duct primary sclerosing cholangitis in adults and children: a population-based analysis. Am J Gastroenterol 2007;102(5):1042–9.
28. Deneau M, Jensen MK, Holmen J, et al. Primary sclerosing cholangitis, autoimmune hepatitis, and overlap in Utah children: epidemiology and natural history. Hepatology 2013;58(4):1392–400.
29. Vergani D, Mieli-Vergani G. Autoimmune hepatitis and PSC connection. Clin Liver Dis 2008;12(1):187–202.
30. Wiencke K, Karlsen TH, Boberg KM, et al. Primary sclerosing cholangitis is associated with extended HLA-DR3 and HLA-DR6 haplotypes. Tissue Antigens 2007; 69(2):161–9.
31. Karlsen TH, Hampe J, Wiencke K, et al. Genetic polymorphisms associated with inflammatory bowel disease do not confer risk for primary sclerosing cholangitis. Am J Gastroenterol 2007;102(1):115–21.
32. Karlsen TH, Boberg KM, Vatn M, et al. Different HLA class II associations in ulcerative colitis patients with and without primary sclerosing cholangitis. Genes Immun 2007;8(3):275–8.
33. Karlsen TH, Boberg KM, Olsson M, et al. Particular genetic variants of ligands for natural killer cell receptors may contribute to the HLA associated risk of primary sclerosing cholangitis. J Hepatol 2007;46(5):899–906.
34. Karlsen TH, Lie BA, Frey Froslie K, et al. Polymorphisms in the steroid and xenobiotic receptor gene influence survival in primary sclerosing cholangitis. Gastroenterology 2006;131(3):781–7.
35. Henckaerts L, Fevery J, Van Steenbergen W, et al. CC-type chemokine receptor 5-Delta32 mutation protects against primary sclerosing cholangitis. Inflamm Bowel Dis 2006;12(4):272–7.
36. Bergquist A, Montgomery SM, Bahmanyar S, et al. Increased risk of primary sclerosing cholangitis and ulcerative colitis in first-degree relatives of patients with primary sclerosing cholangitis. Clin Gastroenterol Hepatol 2008;6(8):939–43.
37. Pall H, Zielenski J, Jonas MM, et al. Primary sclerosing cholangitis in childhood is associated with abnormalities in cystic fibrosis-mediated chloride channel function. J Pediatr 2007;151(3):255–9.
38. Henckaerts L, Jaspers M, Van Steenbergen W, et al. Cystic fibrosis transmembrane conductance regulator gene polymorphisms in patients with primary sclerosing cholangitis. J Hepatol 2009;50(1):150–7.
39. Ross AM 4th, Anupindi SA, Balis UJ. Case records of the Massachusetts General Hospital. Weekly clinicopathological exercises. Case 11-2003. A 14-year-old boy with ulcerative colitis, primary sclerosing cholangitis, and partial duodenal obstruction. N Engl J Med 2003;348(15):1464–76.
40. el-Shabrawi M, Wilkinson ML, Portmann B, et al. Primary sclerosing cholangitis in childhood. Gastroenterology 1987;92(5 Pt 1):1226–35.
41. McNair AN, Moloney M, Portmann BC, et al. Autoimmune hepatitis overlapping with primary sclerosing cholangitis in five cases. Am J Gastroenterol 1998; 93(5):777–84.
42. Gohlke F, Lohse AW, Dienes HP, et al. Evidence for an overlap syndrome of autoimmune hepatitis and primary sclerosing cholangitis. J Hepatol 1996;24(6):699–705.
43. Wurbs D, Klein R, Terracciano LM, et al. 28-year-old woman with a combined hepatitis/cholestatic syndrome. Hepatology 1995;22(5):1598–605.
44. Ma Y, Okamoto M, Thomas MG, et al. Antibodies to conformational epitopes of soluble liver antigen define a severe form of autoimmune liver disease. Hepatology 2002;35(3):658–64.

45. Scalori A, Heneghan M, Hadzic N, et al. Outcome and survival in childhood onset autoimmune sclerosing cholangitis and autoimmune hepatitis: a 13-year follow up study. Hepatology 2007;46S:555A.
46. Ibrahim SH, Lindor KD. Current management of primary sclerosing cholangitis in pediatric patients. Paediatr Drugs 2011;13(2):87–95.
47. Mitchell SA, Bansi DS, Hunt N, et al. A preliminary trial of high-dose ursodeoxycholic acid in primary sclerosing cholangitis. Gastroenterology 2001;121(4): 900–7.
48. Lindor KD, Kowdley KV, Luketic VA, et al. High-dose ursodeoxycholic acid for the treatment of primary sclerosing cholangitis. Hepatology 2009;50(3):808–14.
49. Davies YK, Cox KM, Abdullah BA, et al. Long-term treatment of primary sclerosing cholangitis in children with oral vancomycin: an immunomodulating antibiotic. J Pediatr Gastroenterol Nutr 2008;47(1):61–7.
50. Abarbanel DN, Seki SM, Davies Y, et al. Immunomodulatory effect of vancomycin on Treg in pediatric inflammatory bowel disease and primary sclerosing cholangitis. J Clin Immunol 2013;33(2):397–406.
51. Vrieze A, Out C, Fuentes S, et al. Impact of oral vancomycin on gut microbiota, bile acid metabolism, and insulin sensitivity. J Hepatol 2014;60(4):824–31.
52. Burak K, Angulo P, Pasha TM, et al. Incidence and risk factors for cholangiocarcinoma in primary sclerosing cholangitis. Am J Gastroenterol 2004;99(3):523–6.
53. Alabraba E, Nightingale P, Gunson B, et al. A re-evaluation of the risk factors for the recurrence of primary sclerosing cholangitis in liver allografts. Liver Transpl 2009;15(3):330–40.
54. Vera A, Moledina S, Gunson B, et al. Risk factors for recurrence of primary sclerosing cholangitis of liver allograft. Lancet 2002;360(9349):1943–4.
55. Cholongitas E, Shusang V, Papatheodoridis GV, et al. Risk factors for recurrence of primary sclerosing cholangitis after liver transplantation. Liver Transpl 2008; 14(2):138–43.
56. Egawa H, Taira K, Teramukai S, et al. Risk factors for recurrence of primary sclerosing cholangitis after living donor liver transplantation: a single center experience. Dig Dis Sci 2009;54(6):1347–54.

Novel Therapies on Primary Biliary Cirrhosis

Frank Czul, MD[a], Cynthia Levy, MD[b],*

KEYWORDS

- Primary biliary cirrhosis • Ursodeoxycholic acid • Novel therapies • Treatment
- Immunomodulation • Biochemical response • Biomarkers

KEY POINTS

- Increased serum alkaline phosphatase and bilirubin levels are strongly associated with reduced transplant-free survival in patients with primary biliary cirrhosis (PBC).
- Biochemical response to ursodeoxycholic acid (UDCA) in PBC is a strong predictor of long-term outcome with failure to respond in approximately 40% of patients.
- Obeticholic acid, a farnesoid X receptor agonist, demonstrated biochemical efficacy when given to patients with PBC with an inadequate response to UDCA therapy.
- Treatment with fibrates may be beneficial for patients with PBC and incomplete response to UDCA, in particular in cases with early-stage disease.
- Novel immunologic and molecular therapies, including anti-CD20, anti–interleukin-12, anti–C-X-C motif ligand 10, cytotoxic T-lymphocyte antigen 4 immunoglobulin, mesenchymal stem cells, and antiretroviral therapies are currently under investigation.

BACKGROUND

Primary biliary cirrhosis (PBC) is a chronic cholestatic disease of presumed autoimmune etiology, characterized by inflammation and progressive destruction of the small intrahepatic bile ducts, which can eventually progress to cirrhosis.[1]

The annual incidence rate for PBC ranges between 0.7 and 49 cases per million and the prevalence rate ranges between 6.7 and 402 cases per million,[2] predominantly affecting women, who are usually diagnosed in their 50s and mainly in an asymptomatic stage. The precise pathogenesis of PBC remains unclear; however, the disease is thought to develop due to a combination of genetic predisposition and environmental triggers.[3]

The authors have nothing to disclose.
[a] University of Miami Miller School of Medicine, 1500 Northwest, 12th Avenue, Suite 1101, Miami, FL 33136, USA; [b] Division of Hepatology, University of Miami Miller School of Medicine, University of Miami, 1500 Northwest, 12th Avenue, Suite 1101, Miami, FL 33136, USA
* Corresponding author.
E-mail address: clevy@med.miami.edu

Clin Liver Dis 20 (2016) 113–130
http://dx.doi.org/10.1016/j.cld.2015.08.006
liver.theclinics.com

The diagnosis of PBC is generally confirmed in the presence of serum liver biochemistries showing a cholestatic pattern, a positive antimitochondrial antibody (AMA), exclusion of drug-induced liver injury, and lack of biliary ductal abnormalities on cross-sectional abdominal imaging.[4,5] Liver biopsy is helpful when overlap syndrome with autoimmune hepatitis is suspected or when an alternative diagnosis is considered. In addition, liver biopsy can be used for staging in patients with an otherwise uncomplicated presentation.[6]

Management of patients with PBC embraces disease-specific therapy. The goals of treatment are to[7]

- Slow down the disease progression
- Alleviate symptoms
- Improve quality of life by preventing and/or minimizing complications

All patients with PBC and abnormal liver biochemistries should be considered for specific therapy, which is the focus of this review. Many therapeutic agents have been tested for PBC, but establishing statistically significant long-term benefits for a disease with such a variable and protracted natural history has been challenging. Liver transplantation is the only definitive life-saving procedure for patients who progress to end-stage liver disease.

URSODEOXYCHOLIC ACID

Ursodeoxycholic acid (UDCA) is the only drug approved by the Food and Drug Administration (FDA) for the treatment of PBC. It has been shown to work through different pathways, including stimulation of hepatocellular and ductular secretion, cytoprotection against bile acid–induced injury, and immunomodulatory, anti-inflammatory, and antiapoptotic effects.[8,9]

A study comparing 3 different dosages showed that a dose of 13 to 15 mg/kg per day appeared to be optimal when compared with dosages of either 5 to 7 mg/kg per day or 23 to 25 mg/kg per day.[10] The biochemical response to UDCA in PBC is a strong predictor of long-term outcome and thus facilitates the rapid identification of patients in need of new therapeutic approaches. Biochemical response has been defined in variable ways using different sets of criteria. Regardless of how biochemical response is defined, approximately 30% to 40% of patients with PBC respond incompletely to treatment with UDCA[11,12] (**Table 1**).[13–19]

Various unknown factors could be associated with nonresponse to therapy, but these are not completely elucidated to date. Poor response to UDCA has a major effect on outcome, substantially increasing the risk of death or need for liver transplantation.[14]

A recent meta-analysis evaluated the role of levels of alkaline phosphatase (ALP) and bilirubin as noninvasive surrogate markers for long-term outcomes (death and liver transplantation). Fifteen cohort studies including 4845 patients, most of them treated with UDCA (85%), showed that increased serum ALP and bilirubin levels are strongly associated with reduced transplant-free survival in patients with PBC. The reported 10-year survival rate without a liver transplant was significantly different between patients with ALP levels less than or equal to 2 times the upper limit of normal (ULN) and those with levels greater than 2 times ULN: 84% versus 62%. Similar findings were seen with bilirubin levels: 86% survival free of liver transplantation for patients with bilirubin less than or equal to 1.0 times ULN compared with 41% for patients with bilirubin levels greater than 1.0 times ULN. These results were independent of age, gender, or treatment with UDCA. The reported data

Table 1
UDCA biochemical response criteria

Criteria	Definition	Evaluation Time
Barcelona[11]	Decrease in ALP level >40% of the baseline level or a normal level	1 y
Paris[14]	ALP level ≤3 times ULN together with AST level ≤2 times ULN and a normal bilirubin level	1 y
Rotterdam[15]	Normal bilirubin and/or albumin concentrations when 1 or both parameters are abnormal before treatment	1 y
Toronto[16]	ALP level ≤1.67 times ULN	2 y
Ehime[17]	Decrease in GGT level >70% of the baseline level or a normal level	6 mo
Mayo[18]	ALP level <2 times ULN	2 y
Lammers[19]	ALP level ≤2 times ULN and/or bilirubin ≤1 time ULN	1 y

Abbreviations: ALP, alkaline phosphatase; AST, aspartate amino transferase; GGT, gamma gluta-myltransferase; UDCA, ursodeoxycholic acid; ULN, upper limit of normal.

unequivocally show that both increased serum ALP and bilirubin levels are strongly associated with reduced transplant-free survival in patients with PBC and that a combination of both variables improves prognostic prediction for patients independent of use of UDCA.[19]

FUTURE DIRECTIONS AND EMERGING TREATMENTS

At present, no second-line therapies for patients with inadequate response to UDCA therapy have been approved. This review provides a current perspective on potential new approaches to treatment in PBC, and highlights some of the challenges we face in evaluating and effectively implementing those treatments (**Fig. 1**).

Farnesoid X Receptor Agonists/Obeticholic Acid

Obeticholic acid (OCA; 6-alpha-ethyl-chenodeoxycholic acid) is a novel derivative of the primary human bile acid chenodeoxycholic acid (CDCA) that has been chemically modified to make it 100 times more active. It works mainly by activating the farnesoid X receptor (FXR), which controls bile acid homeostasis and the entero-hepatic circulation of bile acids. In the gut, OCA inhibits uptake of bile acids by repressing the apical sodium bile acid transporter (ASBT) and inducing the baso-lateral organic solute transporters. In the liver, activation of FXR limits entry of bile acids by repressing the sodium taurocholate cotransporter polypeptide (NTCP) and induces their secretion through the canalicular membrane by upregulating bile salts, bilirubin, and phospholipid export pumps (BSEP, MRP2 and MDR3). Furthermore, FXR activation leads to increased expression of fibroblast growth factor (FGF)-19, which in turn leads to further repression of ASBT in the gut and inhibition of CYP7A1 in the hepatocyte, thus decreasing bile acid synthesis.[20] Therefore, by activating FXR, OCA reduces production of bile in the liver and increases bile flow in cholestatic conditions, thus protecting the hepatocytes from accumulation of cytotoxic bile acids.[21]

An international, double-blind, placebo-controlled, dose-response study was conducted to evaluate the effects of OCA on serum ALP, other liver enzymes, and safety in patients with PBC with persistently high ALP levels (>1.5–10.0 times ULN) while on stable dose of UDCA. A total of 165 patients were randomized to placebo or OCA

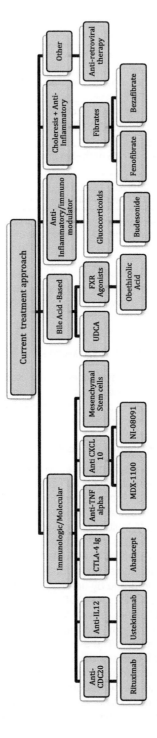

Fig. 1. Potential approaches to treatment in PBC.

10 mg, 25 mg, or 50 mg once daily for 12 weeks, given in addition to their previous UDCA therapy.[22] Daily dosages of OCA, ranging from 10 to 50 mg, significantly reduced levels of ALP, γ-glutamyl transpeptidase (GGT), and alanine aminotransferase (ALT), compared with placebo. Pruritus was the main adverse event, occurring in up to 70% of patients receiving 50 mg per day of OCA. The incidence and severity of pruritus were lowest among patients who received 10 mg per day of OCA. Biochemical responses to OCA were maintained in a 12-month open-label extension trial. In this study, OCA treatment was associated with decreases in total and high-density lipoprotein (HDL) cholesterol.[22]

A second study evaluated OCA as monotherapy, comparing the effects of 10 and 50 mg OCA versus placebo.[23] Significant reductions in ALP with both doses of OCA versus placebo were reported as well as significant improvements in GGT, conjugated bilirubin, C-reactive protein, immunoglobulin (Ig)M, and tumor necrosis factor alpha (TNF-α). Pruritus was the only clinically meaningful adverse event that differed between OCA treatment and placebo. In both studies, the severity of pruritus and the incidence of discontinuations due to pruritus were dose-related, being reported more often among patients treated with higher doses.

Results of the only phase III study of OCA, the PBC OCA International Study of Efficacy (POISE), have recently been presented. OCA, at both 10 mg per day and a 5 mg per day titrated to 10 mg per day as tolerated, met the trial's primary endpoint of achieving a reduction in ALP to less than 1.67 times ULN with a 15% or more reduction from baseline and a normal bilirubin level after 12 months of therapy. The proportion of patients meeting the POISE primary endpoint was 10% in the placebo group, 47% in the 10 mg OCA group, and 46% in the 5 to 10 mg OCA group (both dose groups $P<.0001$ vs placebo) in an intention to treat analysis. The placebo group experienced a mean decrease in ALP from baseline of 5%, compared with a significant mean decrease of 39% in the 10 mg OCA dose group and 33% in the 5 to 10 mg OCA titration group (both dose groups $P<.0001$ vs placebo).[24]

In addition, both OCA dose groups met prespecified secondary endpoints of improvements in other liver function parameters, including GGT, ALT, aspartate aminotransferase (AST), and total bilirubin (both dose groups $P<.0005$ vs placebo). Pruritus, generally mild to moderate, was the most frequently reported adverse event associated with OCA treatment (38% placebo, 68% OCA 10 mg, 56% OCA 5–10 mg titration). Eight patients discontinued due to pruritus: none in the placebo group, 7 (10%) in the 10 mg OCA group, and only 1 (1%) in the OCA 5 to 10 mg titration group. Patients with PBC typically have significantly elevated HDL cholesterol levels and modest decreases in HDL were observed in both OCA dose groups, similar to those seen in the prior PBC clinical trials with OCA. In addition, slight decreases in triglycerides but no change in low-density lipoprotein cholesterol were observed in the OCA dose groups.[24] See **Table 2** for review on OCA studies.

The results of the POISE trial are revolutionary in the management of PBC, and the biochemical response is expected to result in improved clinical outcomes. However, the long-term efficacy of OCA and its benefit in patients with advanced disease will need to be confirmed in longer prospective studies.

Fibrates

Fibrates (fenofibrate/bezafibrate) are used for the treatment of hyperlipidemia. The mechanism of action of fibric acid derivatives in PBC is probably related to anti-inflammatory and choleretic effects via peroxisome proliferator-activated receptor alpha (PPAR alpha), a member of the nuclear hormone receptor superfamily, and

Table 2
Studies using obeticholic acid in patients with primary biliary cirrhosis

Author	Study Design	Inclusion Criteria	Duration	No. Subjects Enrolled/ Completed	OCA Dose, mg	Use of UDCA	Main Result
Hirschfield et al,[22] 2015	DB, PBO, randomized, controlled	ALP ↑ 1.5–10 times ULN while stable on UDCA	12 wk	165	10, 25, 50	Yes	Decrease in ALP, GGT, and ALT in all OCA patients vs PBO
Hirschfield et al,[22] 2015	Open label	Long-term safety extension	Mean 353 d (6–607)	78/48	10 -> 25 -> 50	Yes	Decrease in ALP in 10-mg and 25-mg groups
Kowley et al,[23] 2011	DB, PBO, randomized, controlled	ALP ↑ 1.5–10 times ULN not taking UDCA >6 mo	12 wk	59	10, 50	No	Significant improvement in ALP compared with PBO; 10-mg group had the greatest decrease in ALP
Nevens et al,[24] 2014	DB, PBO, randomized, controlled	ALP ↑ 1.5–10 times ULN while on stable UDCA	12 mo	217/216	10, 5 -> 10	Yes (7% intolerant)	More subjects in OCA groups (47% in 10 mg and 46% in titration 5 -> 10 mg) achieved primary endpoint compared with PBO (10%)

Abbreviations: ALP, alkaline phosphatase; ALT, alanine aminotransferase; DB, double blind; GGT, gamma glutamyltransferase; OCA, obeticholic acid; PBO, placebo; UDCA, ursodeoxycholic acid; ULN, upper limit of normal.

possibly through increase in the expression of multiple drug resistance gene-3, both of which ameliorate hepato-biliary inflammation in PBC.[25,26]

Bezafibrate increases biliary phospholipid secretion into the bile by upregulating the expression of phosphatidyl-choline flippase on the canalicular membrane and restoring the ratio of phospholipid and bile salts to a harmless level.[27] Although bezafibrate is not available in the United States, fenofibrate is currently FDA-approved for the management of hyperlipidemia. Although most studies have been limited by small sample sizes and short duration, a number of clinical trials have assessed the potential efficacy of fibrates in patients with PBC, in particular in combination with UDCA, with encouraging results in terms of biochemical response[25-40] (**Table 3**).

In 2009, Walker and colleagues[41] reported the first European experience with a fibric acid derivative in PBC. The investigators reviewed the effect of fenofibrate 200 mg per day given to 16 patients who previously failed to respond to UDCA 13 to 15 mg/kg per day. These patients received combination therapy for a mean of 22.8 months. Both ALP and IgM levels dropped significantly with 89% of patients normalizing serum ALP levels.

Only one study has been conducted in the United States. In this open-label trial, 20 patients with PBC and incomplete response to UDCA (ALP >2 times ULN despite ongoing UDCA therapy for longer than 1 year) were treated with fenofibrate 160 mg per day in addition to UDCA (13–15 mg/kg per day) for 48 weeks. More than half of the study subjects achieved biochemical response, defined as a more than 40% reduction in serum ALP. Likewise, serum AST and IgM also decreased significantly, whereas bilirubin and albumin remained unchanged.[40] The decrease in serum IgM supports the hypothesis that fenofibrate altered the biology of PBC, as production of IgM in PBC is thought to be disease-specific. A rebound in ALP occurred on drug discontinuation. Interestingly, similar results were obtained in a Spanish study using bezafibrate.[34] More recently, a systematic review including 6 studies of fenofibrate in patients with PBC and incomplete response to UDCA revealed a consistent beneficial effect on serum ALP and total bilirubin.[42] Notably, most of the 102 patients included in this study had early PBC. Thus, the effect of fenofibrate in patients with more advanced PBC is still unclear. Further addressing this issue, Komori and colleagues[43] found that patients with advanced fibrosis and marked ductopenia were more likely to show lack of response to fibrates.

Adding to the controversy, a recent randomized study compared the safety, efficacy, and long-term outcomes of combination therapy with UDCA/bezafibrate (n = 13) versus UDCA monotherapy (n = 14) in 27 patients with PBC and dyslipidemia. In this study, combination therapy given for up to 8 years significantly improved serum ALP levels and the PBC Mayo risk score compared with the monotherapy group. However, the survival rate was not significantly different between groups; in fact, investigators noted a trend toward increased mortality in the UDCA plus bezafibrate group compared with the UDCA monotherapy group. In addition, long-term combination therapy significantly increased serum creatinine levels. Interpretation of these results requires caution, as they are based on a very small sample size and might have been caused by differences between the groups or sampling error.[44] Furthermore, results may not be generalized to all patients with PBC since recruitment was limited to patients with dyslipidemia.

Other than increased creatinine levels, side effects of fibrates have included heartburn,[40] pruritus,[45] and a transient elevation of transaminases.[38] Gallstone formation (possibly due to repression of bile acid synthesis) and paradoxic hypercholesterolemia, which have been reported in patients with PBC on clofibrate,[46,47] were not confirmed during fenofibrate or bezafibrate treatment in PBC.

Table 3
Prospective studies using fibrates in patients with primary biliary cirrhosis

Author	Study Design	Duration, mo	N	Daily Dose		UDCA	Main Results
Honda et al,[26] 2013	Open label bezafibrate + UDCA for patients with incomplete response to UDCA	3	19	Bezafibrate 400 mg		600 mg	Significant improvement of serum liver enzymes, IgM, cholesterol, TG concentrations in patients treated with bezafibrate; reduction of 7α-hydroxy-4-cholesten-3-one (C4), a marker of bile acid synthesis.
Kurihara et al,[28] 2000	Randomized comparative study using bezafibrate monotherapy vs UDCA monotherapy	12	24	Bezafibrate 400 mg		600 mg	ALT, ALP, GGT, and IgM decreased significantly at 1, 3, 6, and 12 mo in the bezafibrate group compared with pretreatment levels; bezafibrate monotherapy was more effective than UDCA monotherapy.
Kanda et al,[29] 2003	Randomized open-label study using bezafibrate + UDCA vs UDCA monotherapy for patients with incomplete response to UDCA	6	22	Bezafibrate 400 mg		600 mg	ALP levels were significantly lower than pretreatment levels in patients receiving UDCA + bezafibrate. Normalization of ALP was observed in 45% patients given bezafibrate and in 18% patients not given bezafibrate.
Akbar et al,[30] 2005	Open label using bezafibrate + UDCA or bezafibrate monotherapy for patients with incomplete response to UDCA	16	10	Bezafibrate 400 mg		600 mg	ALP, GGT, cholesterol, and IgM levels decreased significantly compared with pretreatment levels.
Kita et al,[31] 2006	Open label bezafibrate + UDCA for patients with incomplete response to UDCA	6	22	Bezafibrate 400 mg		600 mg	Decrease in ALP, GGT, IgM levels.
Nakai et al,[32] 2000	Randomized open-label study using bezafibrate + UDCA vs UDCA monotherapy for patients with incomplete response to UDCA	12	23	Bezafibrate 400 mg		600 mg	Combination therapy showed greater improvement of ALP, GGT, IgM levels.

						Results
Hazzan & TurKaspa,[33] 2010	Open label bezafibrate + UDCA for patients with incomplete response to UDCA	4–12	8	Bezafibrate 400 mg	900–1500 mg	ALP levels decreased in all patients and normalized in 6 patients. GGT decrease was also noted.
Lens et al,[34] 2014	Open label bezafibrate + UDCA for patients with incomplete response to UDCA	12	30	Bezafibrate 400 mg	13–15 mg/kg	Significant decrease in, or normalization of, ALP, ALT, GGT, cholesterol, TG, and pruritus. Liver stiffness unchanged.
Iwasaki et al,[35] 2008	Study 1: bezafibrate vs UDCA monotherapy and Study 2: bezafibrate + UDCA for patients with incomplete response to UDCA	12	67	Bezafibrate 400 mg	600 mg	Study 1 showed that bezafibrate monotherapy is as effective as UDCA in the treatment of PBC. Study 2 showed that the combination therapy of bezafibrate and UDCA improved biliary enzymes in noncirrhotic patients.
Itakura et al,[36] 2004	Randomized, cross over, bezafibrate + UDCA compared with UDCA monotherapy	12	16	Bezafibrate 400 mg	600 mg	Decrease in ALP, GGT, IgM, and TG levels.
Ohmoto et al,[37] 2006	Open label bezafibrate + UDCA for patients with incomplete response to UDCA	12	10	Bezafibrate 400 mg	600 mg	ALP, GGT, ALT, and IgM were significantly reduced after 12 mo of treatment. Fatigue and pruritus also improved.
Ohira et al,[38] 2002	Open label fenofibrate + UDCA for patients with incomplete response to UDCA	6	7	Fenofibrate 150–200 mg	600–900 mg	In all 7 patients, there were substantial reductions in levels of ALP, GGT, and IgM.
Liberpoulus et al,[39] 2010	Randomized open-label study using fenofibrate + UDCA vs UDCA monotherapy for patients with incomplete response to UDCA	2	10	Fenofibrate 200 mg	600 mg	Reductions in cholesterol, TG, and non-HDL cholesterol in the combination treatment group. ALP, GGT, ALT also decreased compared with baseline.
Levy et al,[40] 2011	Open-label pilot study using fenofibrate + UDCA for patients with incomplete response to UDCA	12	20	Fenofibrate 160 mg	13–15 mg/kg	Median ALP decreased significantly at 48 wk compared with baseline values, rebound occurred on fenofibrate discontinuation. AST and IgM also decreased significantly. Bilirubin and albumin remained unchanged.
Dohmen et al,[25] 2004	Open-label pilot study using fenofibrate + UDCA for patients with incomplete response to UDCA	3	9	Fenofibrate 100–150 mg	600 mg	ALP and IgM significantly decreased. AMA titers also decreased in 4/9 patients.

Abbreviations: ALP, alkaline phosphatase; ALT, alanine amino transferase; AMA, antimitochondrial antibody; AST, aspartate amino transferase; GGT, Gamma glutamyl transferase; HDL, high-density lipoprotein; Ig, immunoglobulin; TG, triglycerides; UDCA, Ursodeoxycholic acid.

A large phase III, randomized, double-blind placebo-controlled trial of bezafibrate and UDCA treatment in patients with PBC with incomplete biochemical response to UDCA therapy is ongoing (NCT01654731) and will hopefully consolidate, or refute, the role of fibrates in patients with PBC.

Glucocorticoids/Budesonide

Although combination of UDCA with a glucocorticoid might have more favorable results compared with UDCA monotherapy,[48] initial trials with prednisolone resulted in a high incidence of adverse effects, especially loss of bone density, which precluded its use.[49] As a result, clinical trials of budesonide, a nonhalogenated glucocorticoid absorbed in the small bowel, have been conducted in PBC.

Budesonide is a glucocorticoid receptor/pregnane X receptor agonist. Of an oral dose, 90% is metabolized during the first liver pass in healthy individuals. After hepatic uptake, budesonide is metabolized to 2 major metabolites: 16-hydroxy-prednisolone and 6-hydroxy-budesonide. Glucocorticoid activity of these metabolites is only 1% to 10%. Compared with prednisolone, the glucocorticoid receptor binding activity of budesonide is 15 to 20 times higher, so its effect on liver inflammation may be greater.[50–54] Studies have shown positive effects of short-term combination therapy in selected patients with early-stage disease and overlapping features of autoimmune hepatitis.

The beneficial effect of combination therapy with UDCA was first shown in a prospective, controlled, double-blind trial of 20 patients with mainly early-stage disease PBC. One arm was treated with UDCA 10 to 15 mg/kg per day in addition to 3 mg budesonide 3 times daily and the other with UDCA alone. Liver enzymes, and IgM and IgG levels decreased significantly in both groups. Liver histology (inflammation and fibrosis, but not ductular damage) improved by 30% in the combination group.[50]

These results were later replicated by a 3-year multicenter randomized open-label study, which showed that budesonide (6 mg per day) combined with UDCA 15 mg/kg per day showed to be more effective in improving and stabilizing histologic stage compared with UDCA alone, in patients with PBC stages I to III. Fibrosis, assessed by both liver histology and serum PIIINP (serum aminoterminal propeptide of type III procollagen), decreased significantly in the combination group.[44] In contrast, an open-label, pilot study of 22 patients with PBC and a suboptimal response to UDCA showed only a marginal improvement in ALP, but a significant increase in the PBC Mayo risk score and a significant loss of bone mass.[52]

Last, Rabahi and colleagues[53] aimed to assess the benefit of the UDCA/budesonide combination in association with mycophenolate mofetil (MMF) in patients with PBC at a high risk for cirrhosis or liver failure and reported that of 15 patients, 6 (41%) normalized biochemistries and 7 (47%) had a partial but significant biochemical response. Histologic activity and fibrosis were markedly improved. Side effects were minimal or absent, suggesting that triple therapy may provide benefit in patients with PBC without cirrhosis with features of severe disease not responding to UDCA. See **Table 4** for review on budesonide studies.

Thus, combination therapy might be beneficial for some patients with PBC with pre-cirrhotic liver disease, but, for asymptomatic patients with stable early PBC on UDCA therapy, the potential systemic glucocorticoid effect would carry an unnecessary risk for diabetes and osteoporosis during long-term use. Patients with stage IV PBC are no longer considered for combination therapy, as significant increases in budesonide plasma levels were observed in late-stage PBC and were associated with serious side effects. In addition, concern exists with the possibility increasing the risk of portal vein thrombosis in patients with cirrhosis.[54]

Table 4
Studies using budesonide in patients with primary biliary cirrhosis

Author	Study Design	Inclusion Criteria	Duration	n	Budesonide Dose	Main Result
Leuschner et al,[50] 1999	DB, PBO UDCA + budesonide vs UDCA alone	Early-stage disease	2 y	20	3 mg 3 times daily	Significant improvement in liver biochemistries in UDCA + budesonide group; improvement in liver histology
Rautiainen et al,[51] 2005	Randomized UDCA + budesonide vs UDCA alone	Stages I to III	3 y	77	6 mg	Combination therapy improved liver histology
Angulo et al,[52] 2000	Open label UDCA + budesonide	Suboptimal response to UDCA with ALP >2 times ULN	1 y	22	9 mg	Budesonide conferred minimal, if any, additional benefit to UDCA, and it is associated with a significant worsening of osteoporosis
Rabahi et al,[53] 2010	Open label UDCA + budesonide + MFM	Suboptimal biochemical response to 1-year UDCA	3 y	15	6 mg	41% experienced complete normalization of LFTs; improvement in liver histology

Abbreviations: ALP, alkaline phosphatase; DB, double blind; LFTs, liver function test; MFM, mycophenolate mofetil; PBO, placebo; UDCA, ursodeoxycholic acid; ULN, upper limit of normal.

A phase III trial is currently under way for the evaluation of budesonide in UDCA-refractory patients with PBC (NCT00746486).

Immunologic/Molecular Therapies

Anti-CD20/rituximab

Rituximab is a genetically engineered chimeric murine/human monoclonal antibody against protein CD20, which is primarily found on the surface of B cells and selectively depletes B cells via complement-dependent and antibody-dependent, cell-mediated cytotoxicity.[55] Preliminary data suggest a benefit in patients with autoimmune hepatitis,[56] and in a small proof-of-concept pilot study of patients with PBC with an incomplete response to UDCA, reductions in serum AMA, IgM, and ALP were reported.[57]

In a subsequent Canadian study, 14 patients with PBC refractory to UDCA (13–15 mg/kg per day for 6 months) received 2 rituximab infusions (1 g at days 1 and 15) and were followed for up to 12 months. The primary outcome of this study was the proportion of patients with normalization and/or 25% improvement in ALP at 6 months. Twelve and 8 patients completed 6 and 12 months of follow-up, respectively. Although rituximab was well tolerated, 1 patient withdrew due to asthma exacerbation during the first infusion. Effective B-cell depletion was observed in all patients. Rituximab resulted in significant reductions in AMA titers and serum IgM concentration. Nevertheless, the efficacy of rituximab based on biochemical response in their cohort was limited; a median serum ALP reduction of 16% of the baseline value was observed at 24 weeks, and this difference did not persist at week 72. The primary outcome was achieved in 25% of patients at week 24; however, biochemical responses were not maintained at 72 weeks. Pruritus and fatigue improved.[58]

In summary, B-cell depletion with rituximab appears to be safe and associated with a significant decrease in autoantibody production in patients with PBC who have had an incomplete response to UDCA. Modest and transient reductions in serum ALP have been reported, but larger controlled studies are necessary to confirm its long-term benefits.

Anti–interleukin-12/ustekinumab

The identification of 3 interleukin (IL)-12–related genes (IL-12A, IL-12RB2, and STAT4) strongly associated to PBC raised the possibility of targeting IL-12 as a therapeutic approach in PBC.[59,60] The characterization of the nature and functional implication of the HLA and IL12A, IL12RB2 variants that confer a risk of PBC remain under evaluation. The association of PBC with variants at these loci confirms the critical role of immunogenic factors in the genesis of this disease and points to the possibility that modulation of signaling by IL-12 and its receptor may be beneficial in the treatment of patients with PBC.

The binding of IL-12 to its receptor is thought to modulate autoimmune responses by evoking interferon (IFN)-γ production, which may in turn inhibit IL-23–driven induction of IL-17–producing helper T lymphocytes.[61,62] As a proof of concept, a phase II study on the efficacy and safety of ustekinumab administered as 90 mg subcutaneously at week 0, 4, and thereafter every 8 weeks through week 20 was conducted in 20 patients with PBC who had an inadequate response to UDCA. By week 28, serum ALP decreased by 11.25% ± 17.46%. Liver biochemistries, ALT, AST, and bilirubin concentrations decreased by 9.21% ± 32.36%, 7.22% ± 27.18%, and 4.61% ± 14.18%, respectively. These changes were modest at best. One patient (5%) had a serious adverse event (gastrointestinal hemorrhage) and 18 (90%) reported minor events.[63]

The observed lack of efficacy may have been due to the role of IL-12 in the initial break of immune tolerance to PDC-E2 and suggests that IL-12 has little role in disease progression once established.[64]

Cytotoxic T-lymphocyte antigen 4/abatacept

The pathogenesis of PBC is primarily attributed to autoreactive T cells that require costimulatory signaling of CD28 by engagement with CD80 or CD86 on antigen-presenting cells.[58] Due to its greater affinity to CD28, Cytotoxic T-lymphocyte antigen 4 (CTLA-4) Ig attenuates CD28-mediated costimulation and prevents binding of CD28 to CD80 or CD86.[65]

Abatacept (marketed as Orencia) is a fusion protein composed of the Fc region of the immunoglobulin IgG1 fused to the extracellular domain of CTLA-4. Abatacept binds to the CD80 and CD86 molecules, and prevents the costimulatory signal without which the T cell cannot be activated. Abatacept is currently licensed in the United States for the treatment of rheumatoid arthritis in cases of inadequate response to anti–TNF-α therapy.[66]

An open-label, active treatment trial to assess the efficacy and safety of abatacept in subjects with PBC who have had an incomplete biochemical response to UDCA is currently ongoing (NCT02078882). In this trial, 20 subjects with PBC who have had an incomplete biochemical response to UDCA are assigned to treatment with weekly subcutaneous injections of 125 mg abatacept. The treatment phase of the study lasts 24 weeks with an off-treatment follow-up at week 36; the primary outcome is normalization of ALP or decrease of ALP by greater than 40% from baseline at 24 weeks of treatment.

Anti-CXCL10/MDX-1100, NI-08091

C-X-C motif ligand (CXCL10) belongs to the ELR (–) CXC subfamily chemokine. CXCL10 exerts its function through binding to chemokine (C-X-C motif) receptor 3 (CXCR3), a 7-transmembrane receptor coupled to G proteins. CXCL10 and its receptor, CXCR3, appear to contribute to the pathogenesis of many autoimmune diseases, including PBC. The secretion of CXCL10 by cluster of differentiated CD4+, CD8+, natural killer (NK), and NK-T cells is dependent on IFN-γ, which is itself mediated by the IL-12 cytokine family.[67] In patients with PBC, serum levels of CXCL10 are higher, as is the frequency of peripheral blood cells expressing CXCR3 compared with healthy controls.[68]

Neutralizing CXCL10 with a fully monoclonal antibody (MDX-1100) seems to be an attractive therapeutic strategy that is currently under investigation for patients with ulcerative colitis and rheumatoid arthritis.[69] However, 40 patients with PBC and incomplete response to UDCA were included in an open-label study with NI-0801, another fully human anti-CXCL10 monoclonal antibody. The trial was terminated early due to lack of clinically significant improvement in liver biochemistries (NCT01430429).

Mesenchymal stem cells

Mesenchymal stem cells (MSCs) represent a promising tool for cell-based therapies of autoimmune diseases due to their immunosuppressive properties on both innate and adaptive immunity and multiple differentiations into cells of mesoderm lineage as well as endoderm and neuroectoderm lineages, such as hepatocytes and neurons.[70] The cells directly suppress overactivated T-cell proliferation in an antigen-independent and dose-dependent fashion.[71] These characteristics support the possibility of exploiting universal MSCs for clinical therapeutic applications.

A study performed in mice suggested that bone marrow-MSC transplantation could regulate systemic immune response and enhance recovery in liver inflammation of

PBC mice, raising the possibility for clinical application of allogeneic MSC in treatment of patients with early-stage to moderate-stage PBC.[72] It seemed that the infused MSC could not restore the entire liver in the late stage of fibrosis.

A single-arm trial that included 10 patients with UDCA-resistant PBC was conducted in China. Umbilical cord–derived MSCs were infused 3 times at 4-week intervals, and patients were followed for 48 weeks. There was a significant decrease in serum ALP and GGT levels at the end of the follow-up period compared with baseline; the Mayo score prognostic index was also stable during this period. Symptoms such as fatigue and pruritus were alleviated in most patients after treatment. No significant changes were observed in AST, ALT, bilirubin, albumin, prothrombin time activity, international normalized ratio, or IgM levels.[73] Long-term effects of MSCs in PBC remain to be seen.

Antiretroviral therapy

Several bacteria, viruses, and xenobiotics have been implicated in the pathogenesis of PBC. Several years ago, a human beta-retrovirus closely related to the mouse mammary tumor virus was directly cloned from biliary epithelium of patients with PBC.[74]

In previous uncontrolled pilot studies, lamivudine monotherapy was of little utility in treating PBC, whereas significant but not substantial improvements were observed using a twice-daily combination therapy of zidovudine 300 mg and lamivudine 150 mg. This regimen was associated with normalization of hepatic biochemistries in a small proportion of patients with near normal liver tests as well as a reduction in mean necro-inflammatory scores, bile duct damage, and ductopenia.[75] In a subsequent study, Mason and colleagues[76] randomized, 59 patients with a serum ALP level greater than 1.5 times ULN despite being on UDCA therapy to either 300 mg zidovudine and 150 mg lamivudine twice daily or placebo for 6 months. None of the patients normalized ALP and no significant differences were observed in rates of normalization of serum aminotransferase level.

Additional studies using triple regimen of antiretrovirals (tenofovir/emtricitabine and lopinavir/ritonavir) for patients with PBC are currently ongoing (NCT01614405).

SUMMARY

In conclusion, treatment of incomplete responders to UDCA remains an unmet need in the field of PBC. Eventually, we should be able to identify patients at early disease stage and who are at high risk of progression, and target these individuals for immune-modulatory, disease-modifying therapy. At the present time, however, we are unable to clearly identify these patients, nor do we have an early marker of nonresponse. Serum ALP and bilirubin levels are surrogate markers easy to use in clinical practice, which have been shown to correlate with increased risk of progression. New drugs are currently under investigation for the treatment of such nonresponders to UDCA; combination therapy targeting several disease pathways may be necessary.

REFERENCES

1. Pares A. Old and novel therapies for primary biliary cirrhosis. Semin Liver Dis 2014;34:341–51.
2. Lazaridis KN, Talwalkar JA. Clinical epidemiology of primary biliary cirrhosis: incidence, prevalence, and impact of therapy. J Clin Gastroenterol 2007;41(5): 494–500.

3. Selmi C, Mayo MJ, Bach N, et al. Primary biliary cirrhosis in monozygotic and dizygotic twins: genetics, epigenetics, and environment. Gastroenterology 2004;127(2):485–92.
4. Lindor KD, Gershwin ME, Poupon R, et al, American Association for Study of Liver Diseases. Primary biliary cirrhosis. Hepatology 2009;50:291–308.
5. Kim KA, Jeong SH. The diagnosis and treatment of primary biliary cirrhosis. Korean J Hepatol 2011;17:173–9.
6. European Association for the Study of Liver Diseases (EASL). Clinical practice guidelines. Primary biliary cirrhosis. Available at: http://www.easl.eu/research/our-contributions/clinical-practice-guidelines/detail/management-of-cholestatic-liver-diseases/report/3. Accessed June 22, 2015.
7. Czul F, Peyton A, Levy C. Primary biliary cirrhosis: therapeutic advances. Clin Liver Dis 2013;17(2):229–42.
8. Beuers U. Drug insight: mechanisms and sites of action of ursodeoxycholic acid in cholestasis. Nat Clin Pract Gastroenterol Hepatol 2006;3(6):318–28.
9. Poupon R. Ursodeoxycholic acid and bile-acid mimetics as therapeutic agents for cholestatic liver diseases: an overview of their mechanisms of action. Clin Res Hepatol Gastroenterol 2012;36(Suppl 1):S3–12.
10. Angulo P, Dickson ER, Therneau TM, et al. Comparison of three doses of ursodeoxycholic acid in the treatment of primary biliary cirrhosis: a randomized trial. J Hepatol 1999;30(5):830–5.
11. Kaplan MM, Poupon R. Treatment with immunosuppressives in patients with primary biliary cirrhosis who fail to respond to ursodiol. Hepatology 2009;50(2):652.
12. Zhang LN, Shi TY, Shi XH, et al. Early biochemical response to ursodeoxycholic acid and long-term prognosis of primary biliary cirrhosis: results of a 14-year cohort study. Hepatology 2013;58:264–72.
13. Pares A, Caballeria L, Rodes J. Excellent long-term survival in patients with primary biliary cirrhosis and biochemical response to ursodeoxycholic acid. Gastroenterology 2006;130:715–20.
14. Corpechot C, Abenavoli L, Rabahi N, et al. Biochemical response to ursodeoxycholic acid and long-term prognosis in primary biliary cirrhosis. Hepatology 2008; 48:871–7.
15. Kuiper EM, Hansen BE, de Vries RA, et al. Improved prognosis of patients with primary biliary cirrhosis that have a biochemical response to ursodeoxycholic acid. Gastroenterology 2009;136:1281–7.
16. Kumagi T, Guindi M, Fischer SE, et al. Baseline ductopenia and treatment response predict long-term histological progression in primary biliary cirrhosis. Am J Gastroenterol 2010;105:2186–94.
17. Azemoto N, Kumagi T, Abe M, et al. Biochemical response to ursodeoxycholic acid predicts long-term outcome in Japanese patients with primary biliary cirrhosis. Hepatol Res 2011;41:310–7.
18. Angulo P, Lindor KD, Therneau TM, et al. Utilization of the Mayo risk score in patients with primary biliary cirrhosis receiving ursodeoxycholic acid. Liver 1999;19:115–21.
19. Lammers WJ, van Buuren HR, Hirschfield GM, et al. Levels of alkaline phosphatase and bilirubin are surrogate end points of outcomes of patients with primary biliary cirrhosis: an international follow-up study. Gastroenterology 2014;147:1338–49.
20. Pelliciari R, Fiorucci S, Camaioni E, et al. 6 alpha-ethyl-chenodeoxycholic acid (6-ECDCA), a potent and selective FXR agonist endowed with anticholestatic activity. J Med Chem 2002;45:3569–72.

21. Gadaleta RM, van Erpecum KJ, Oldenburg B, et al. Farnesoid X receptor activation inhibits inflammation and preserves the intestinal barrier in inflammatory bowel disease. Gut 2011;60(4):463–72.

22. Hirschfield GM, Mason A, Luketic V, et al. Efficacy of obeticholic acid in patients with primary biliary cirrhosis and inadequate response to ursodeoxycholic acid. Gastroenterology 2015;148(4):751–61.

23. Kowdley KV, Jones D, Luketic V, et al. An international study evaluating the farnesoid X receptor agonist obeticholic acid as monotherapy in PBC. J Hepatol 2011;54:S13.

24. Nevens F, Andreone P, Mazzella G, et al. The first primary biliary cirrhosis phase 3 trial in two decades—an international study of the FXR agonist obeticholic acid in PBC patients. J Hepatol 2014;60:S525–6.

25. Dohmen K, Mizuta T, Nakamuta M, et al. Fenofibrate for patients with asymptomatic primary biliary cirrhosis. World J Gastroenterol 2004;10(6):894–8.

26. Honda A, Ikegami T, Nakamuta M, et al. Anticholestatic effects of bezafibrate in patients with primary biliary cirrhosis treated with ursodeoxycholic acid. Hepatology 2013;57(5):1931–41.

27. Iwasaki S, Akisawa N, Saibara T, et al. Fibrate for treatment of primary biliary cirrhosis. Hepatol Res 2007;37(Suppl 3):S515–7.

28. Kurihara T, Niimi A, Maeda A, et al. Bezafibrate in the treatment of primary biliary cirrhosis: comparison with ursodeoxycholic acid. Am J Gastroenterol 2000; 95(10):2990–2.

29. Kanda T, Yokosuka O, Imazeki F, et al. Bezafibrate treatment: a new medical approach for PBC patients. J Gastroenterol 2003;38(6):573–8.

30. Akbar SM, Furukawa S, Nakanishi S, et al. Therapeutic efficacy of decreased nitrite production by bezafibrate in patients with primary biliary cirrhosis. J Gastroenterol 2005;40(2):157–63.

31. Kita R, Takamatsu S, Kimura T, et al. Bezafibrate may attenuate biliary damage associated with chronic liver diseases accompanied by high serum biliary enzyme levels. J Gastroenterol 2006;41(7):686–92.

32. Nakai S, Masaki T, Kurokohchi K, et al. Combination therapy of bezafibrate and ursodeoxycholic acid in primary biliary cirrhosis: a preliminary study. Am J Gastroenterol 2000;95(1):326–7.

33. Hazzan R, TurKaspa R. Bezafibrate treatment of primary biliary cirrhosis following incomplete response to ursodeoxycholic acid. J Clin Gastroenterol 2010;44(5): 371–3.

34. Lens S, Leoz M, Nazal L, et al. Bezafibrate normalizes alkaline phosphatase in primary biliary cirrhosis patients with incomplete response to ursodeoxycholic acid. Liver Int 2014;34(2):197–203.

35. Iwasaki S, Ohira H, Nishiguchi S, et al. The efficacy of ursodeoxycholic acid and bezafibrate combination therapy for primary biliary cirrhosis: a prospective, multicenter study. Hepatol Res 2008;38:557–64.

36. Itakura J, Izumi N, Nishimura Y, et al. Prospective randomized crossover trial of combination therapy with bezafibrate and UDCA for primary biliary cirrhosis. Hepatol Res 2004;29:216–22.

37. Ohmoto K, Yoshioka N, Yamamoto S. Long-term effect of bezafibrate on parameters of hepatic fibrosis in primary biliary cirrhosis. J Gastroenterol 2006;41: 502–3.

38. Ohira H, Sato Y, Ueno T, et al. Fenofibrate treatment in patients with primary biliary cirrhosis. Am J Gastroenterol 2002;97(8):2147–9.

39. Liberopoulos EN, Florentin M, Elisaf MS, et al. Fenofibrate in primary biliary cirrhosis: a pilot study. Open Cardiovasc Med J 2010;4:120–6.

40. Levy C, Peter JA, Nelson DR, et al. Pilot study: fenofibrate for patients with primary biliary cirrhosis and an incomplete response to ursodeoxycholic acid. Aliment Pharmacol Ther 2011;33(2):235–42.
41. Walker LJ, Newton J, Jones DE, et al. Comment on biochemical response to ursodeoxycholic acid and long-term prognosis in primary biliary cirrhosis. Hepatology 2009;49(1):337–8.
42. Grigorian AY, Mardini HE, Corperchot C, et al. Fenofibrate is effective adjunctive therapy in the treatment of primary biliary cirrhosis: a meta-analysis. Clin Res Hepatol Gastroenterol 2015;39(3):296–306.
43. Komori A, Nakamura M, Aiba Y, et al. Who may have treatment benefits with fibrates in primary biliary cirrhosis: a single center retrospective observational cohort analysis. J Hepatol 2013;58:S387.
44. Hosonuma K, Sato K, Yamazaki Y, et al. A prospective randomized controlled study of long-term combination therapy using ursodeoxycholic acid and bezafibrate in patients with primary biliary cirrhosis and dyslipidemia. Am J Gastroenterol 2015;110(3):423–31.
45. Han XF, Wang QX, Liu Y, et al. Efficacy of fenofibrate in Chinese patients with primary biliary cirrhosis partially responding to ursodeoxycholic acid therapy. J Dig Dis 2012;13:219–24.
46. Summerfield JA, Elias E, Sherlock S. Effects of clofibrate in primary biliary cirrhosis hypercholesterolemia and gallstones. Gastroenterology 1975;69:998–1000.
47. Schaffner F. Paradoxical elevation of serum cholesterol by clofibrate in patients with primary biliary cirrhosis. Gastroenterology 1969;57:253–5.
48. Leuschner M, Güldütuna S, You T, et al. Ursodeoxycolic acid and prednisolone versus ursodeoxycholic acid and placebo in the treatment of early stages of primary biliary cirrhosis. J Hepatol 1996;25(1):49–57.
49. Mitchison HC, Bassendine MF. A pilot, double blinded, controlled 1-year trial of prednisolone treatment in PBC. Hepatology 1989;10(4):420–9.
50. Leuschner M, Maier KP, Schlichting J, et al. Oral budesonide and ursodeoxycholic acid for treatment of primary biliary cirrhosis: results of a prospective double-blind trial. Gastroenterology 1999;117(4):918–25.
51. Rautiainen H, Karkkainen P, Karvonen AL, et al. Budesonide combined with UDCA to improve liver histology in primary biliary cirrhosis: a three-year randomized trial. Hepatology 2005;41(4):747–52.
52. Angulo P, Jorgensen RA, Keack JC, et al. Oral budesonide in the treatment of patients with primary biliary cirrhosis with suboptimal response to ursodeoxycholic acid. Hepatology 2000;31(2):318–23.
53. Rabahi N, Chretien Y, Gaouar F, et al. Triple therapy with ursodeoxycholic acid, budesonide and mycophenolate mofetil in patients with features of severe primary biliary cirrhosis not responding to ursodeoxycholic acid alone. Gastroenterol Clin Biol 2010;34(4–5):283–7.
54. Hempfling W, Grunhage F, Dilger K, et al. Pharmacokinetics and pharmacodynamic action of budesonide in early- and late-stage primary biliary cirrhosis. Hepatology 2003;38(1):196–202.
55. Reff ME, Carner K, Chambers KS, et al. Depletion of B cells in vivo by a chimeric mouse human monoclonal antibody to CD20. Blood 1994;83:435–45.
56. Burak KW, Swain MG, Lee SS, et al. Rituximab for the treatment of patients with autoimmune hepatitis who are refractory to or intolerant of standard therapy. Can J Gastroenterol 2013;27(5):273–80.

57. Tsuda M, Moritoki Y, Lian ZX, et al. Biochemical and immunologic effects of ritux-imab in patients with primary biliary cirrhosis and an incomplete response to ur-sodeoxycholic acid. Hepatology 2012;55:512–21.
58. Myers RP, Swain MG, Lee SS, et al. B-cell depletion with rituximab in patients with primary biliary cirrhosis refractory to ursodeoxycholic acid. Am J Gastroenterol 2013;108:933–41.
59. Liu X. Genome wide meta-analyses identify three loci associated with primary biliary cirrhosis. Nat Genet 2010;42:658–60.
60. Mells GF. Genome-wide association identifies 12 new susceptibility loci for pri-mary biliary cirrhosis. Nat Genet 2011;43:329–32.
61. Hirshfield GM. Primary biliary cirrhosis associated with HLA, IL12A and IL 12RB2 variants. N Engl J Med 2009;360:2544–55.
62. Lleo A. Towards common denominators in primary biliary cirrhosis: the role of IL-12. J Hepatol 2012;56:731–3.
63. Hirschfield GM, Gershwin ME, Strauss R, et al. Phase 2 study evaluating the efficacy and safety of ustekunumab in patients with primary biliary cirrhosis who had an inadequate response to ursodeoxycholic acid. J Hepatol 2014; 60(1):S189–90.
64. Floreani A, Franceshet I, Perini L, et al. New therapies for primary biliary cirrhosis. Clin Rev Allergy Immunol 2015;48(2–3):263–72.
65. Collins AV, Brodie DW, Gilbert RJ, et al. The interaction properties of co-stimulatory molecules revisited. Immunity 2002;17:201–10.
66. Moreland L, Bate G, Kirkpatrick P. Abatacept. Nat Rev Drug Discov 2006;5(3): 185–6.
67. Antonelli A, Ferrari SM, Giuggioli D, et al. Chemokine (C-X-C motif) ligand (CXCL) 10 in autoimmune diseases. Autoimmun Rev 2014;13(3):272–80.
68. Chuang YH, Lian ZX, Cheng CM, et al. Increased levels of chemokine receptor CXCR3 and chemokines IP-10 and MIG in patients with primary biliary cirrhosis and their first degree relatives. J Autoimmun 2005;25(2):126–32.
69. Mayer L, Sandborn WJ, Stepanov Y, et al. Anti-IP-10 antibody (BMS-936557) for ulcerative colitis: a phase II randomized study. Gut 2014;63(3):442–50.
70. Saulnier N, Lattanzi W, Puglisi MA, et al. Mesenchymal stromal cells multipotency and plasticity: induction toward the hepatic lineage. Eur Rev Med Pharmacol Sci 2009;13:71–8.
71. Aggarwal S, Pittenger MF. Human mesenchymal stem cells modulate allogeneic immune cell responses. Blood 2005;105(4):1815–22.
72. Wang D, Zhang H, Liang J, et al. Effect of allogeneic bone marrow–derived mesenchymal stem cells transplantation in a polyl: C-induced primary biliary cirrhosis mouse model. Clin Exp Med 2011;11(1):25–32.
73. Wang L, Li J, Liu H, et al. Pilot study of umbilical cord-derived mesenchymal stem cell transfusion in patients with primary biliary cirrhosis. J Gastroenterol Hepatol 2013;28(Suppl 1):85–92.
74. Mason AL, Zhang G. Linking human beta retrovirus infection with primary biliary cirrhosis. Gastroenterol Clin Biol 2010;34(6–7):359–66.
75. Mason AL, Farr GH, Xu L, et al. Pilot studies of single and combination antiretro-viral therapy in patients with primary biliary cirrhosis. Am J Gastroenterol 2004; 99(12):2348–55.
76. Mason AL, Lindor KD, Bacon BR, et al. Clinical trial: randomized controlled trial of zidovudine and lamivudine for patients with primary biliary cirrhosis stabilized on ursodiol. Aliment Pharmacol Ther 2008;28(7):886–94.

Understanding and Treating Fatigue in Primary Biliary Cirrhosis and Primary Sclerosing Cholangitis

Laura Jopson, MBChB, Jessica K. Dyson, MBBS, David E.J. Jones, MD, PhD*

KEYWORDS

- Fatigue • Primary biliary cirrhosis • Primary sclerosing cholangitis • Cholestasis
- Quality of life

KEY POINTS

- In primary biliary cirrhosis fatigue is unrelated to the severity of the underlying liver disease and unresponsive to ursodeoxycholic acid therapy.
- Further work is warranted to understand the pathogenesis of fatigue in primary sclerosing cholangitis and the development of disease-specific quality of life measures to assess fatigue is needed.
- Despite the lack of specific therapies for fatigue there are several management strategies that can be implemented to improve fatigue severity and quality of life in patients with cholestatic liver disease.

INTRODUCTION

The most common cholestatic liver diseases are primary biliary cirrhosis (PBC) and primary sclerosing cholangitis (PSC). Fatigue in cholestatic liver disease represents a real challenge for patients and clinicians. It is the commonest problem reported by patients with PBC, is not related to the severity of the underlying liver disease, does not improve with conventional disease treatments, and has no recognized specific treatment.[1,2] Fatigue in PSC has been much less studied but seems to be a significant problem in a minority of patients.[3] The normal disease management paradigm for patients with cholestatic liver diseases is the prevention and treatment of

The UK-PBC research Consortium to which the authors are affiliated receives research funding from Intercept, GSK, and Lumena. Dr D.E.J. Jones has acted as an advisor to Intercept.
Institute of Cellular Medicine, Newcastle University, Level 3 William Leech Building, Medical School, Framlington Place, Newcastle upon Tyne NE24HH, UK
* Corresponding author. Medical School, Institute of Cellular Medicine, 4th Floor, William Leech Building, Framlington Place, Newcastle Upon Tyne NE2 4HH, UK.
E-mail address: david.jones@ncl.ac.uk

progressive liver injury and cirrhosis. Clinicians treating these patients often find the management of severely fatigued patients with complex problems challenging. This article summarizes current thinking regarding the epidemiology, pathogenesis, and treatment of this important clinical problem.

THE CLINICAL SCENARIO

The classic clinical scenario is of a young patient with PBC who has mild disease that has responded well to ursodeoxycholic acid (UDCA) therapy in terms of liver biochemistry, but who is still experiencing profound fatigue. This classic fatigue has two elements. The first is a sense of "brain fog," clouded thinking and poor concentration that may have been bad enough to cause problems at work. Patients may feel the need to sleep during the day but fight against it. The second is a sense of profound peripheral weakness, like the "batteries have run down" in their muscles. Patients have good days and bad days but sense that they "pay the price" the following day if they exert themselves. Typically, patients feel less fatigued in the morning and get progressively worse during the day. This makes evenings difficult and shift work challenging. Fatigued patients often decrease their activity, particularly nonessential activities, such as paid employment or caring for children, with a knock-on effect on social life and relationships that can lead to increasing social isolation. A sense that this will never end can lead to frustration and depression. Being told by clinicians how well they are doing because their biochemical tests are good, and by friends and families how well they are looking, can add to the frustration.

THE SCALE OF THE PROBLEM

Current studies suggest that up to 50% of patients with PBC experience clinically significant fatigue[4] and it is more common in younger patients presenting with the disease.[5] The problem seems to be less frequent in PSC (although severe fatigue is still reported) and the phenomenon has been little studied in other cholestatic conditions.[3] Fatigue was not reported as a problem in PBC before 1980 (when the first mention was made of "lethargy" in patients with PBC).[6] Since that time the reported prevalence of fatigue has risen. There are two factors that are likely to underpin this apparent change in disease phenotype. The first is the changing spectrum of disease. In the 1950s, when the first case series of PBC was reported and the phenotype of the condition established, PBC was a rare disease of patients typically in the end stages of disease.[7] The problems a patient experienced, therefore, were likely to be dominated by those of end-stage disease. With the advent of serologic testing and its widespread use in the assessment of cholestatic liver function tests, patients are now typically diagnosed in the early stages of disease. Furthermore, effective treatment approaches are now available for pruritus, which can result in an "unmasking" of fatigue (when present, pruritus tends to predominate in a patient's experience).[8,9] In simple terms, the typical patient with PBC diagnosed in the modern era is well enough in relation to the other aspects of the disease for their fatigue to be their predominant problem.

The second factor is the advent of effective tools to measure fatigue (covered in detail in the next section), and the awareness among clinicians and patients that fatigue is part of the patient experience. These tools are increasingly used in normal clinical practice. The definitive study is the UK-PBC Study, which uses the PBC-40, a patient-derived, disease-specific quality of life (QoL) tool in a very large sample of patients who are representative of the PBC patient population in the United Kingdom as a whole.[10] Using defined PBC-40 fatigue domain cut-offs, severe fatigue was found to affect approximately 20% of patients with PBC and moderate or severe fatigue more than 50% of patients.[5] The problem is therefore substantial. A similar study, UK-PSC, is currently recruiting and will enable the clinical phenotypes in PSC to be described. At present, there is no equivalent disease-specific QoL assessment tool for use in PSC but one is under development.

ASSESSMENT OF FATIGUE

There are three broad approaches to the assessment of fatigue: the use of subjective measures (in essence questionnaires addressing aspects of the problem), objective measures (a biologic measurement of some aspects directly or indirectly related to the symptom), and impact measures (an approach to assessing the impact or sequelae of the symptom). In the context of fatigue in cholestatic liver disease the three categories are fatigue impact scores, physical activity monitoring, and higher QoL or functional status assessment tools. In terms of fatigue assessment tools, the fatigue impact score has been validated and is widely used.[11] However, the PBC-40 fatigue domain, which was derived exclusively in patients with PBC, has greater sensitivity (although it cannot be cross-applied in other diseases).[10] Both are appropriate for patient self-completion and are acceptable to patients. The fatigue impact scores have been used effectively in PSC.[3]

Objective measurement of physical activity is in reality an indirect measure of fatigue. It must be remembered that there are confounding factors in chronic disease that are unrelated to fatigue but that cause reduced activity. Physical activity monitoring has been done in PBC (but not PSC) and correlates well with perceived fatigue.[12] It has no application other than in the clinical trial setting, however, when objective outcome measures have a particular value. In terms of global function and QoL scores, such measures as the PROMIS-HAQ have been used and, perhaps unsurprisingly, show that fatigue is one of the major contributing factors to life quality impairment in PBC.[13] Detailed analysis of the UK-PBC data set reveals that social isolation symptoms (as assessed by the social domain of the PBC-40) are also critical and contextualize fatigue.[4] There is a danger that patients use reduced activity levels as a way of mitigating against the impact of fatigue but with the unintended consequence that they withdraw from normal social activities to the detriment of their overall life quality.

UNDERSTANDING FATIGUE IN PRIMARY BILIARY CIRRHOSIS AND PRIMARY SCLEROSING CHOLANGITIS

Fatigue is a complex symptom across populations and within individual patients, with several pathogenetic processes contributing to a single "headline" phenotype. This adds significant complexity to the understanding of fatigue and attempts to improve treatments for it. One aspect that seems to be clear in PBC fatigue is that, with the exception of a small group of patients with advanced disease in which end-stage liver failure prevails, its severity and impact are unrelated to the severity of underlying liver disease or to the use and response to UDCA treatment.[1,2] Thus, although clearly highly prevalent in PBC (and to a lesser degree in PSC) fatigue is an associated feature of the disease rather than a phenomenon directly resulting from liver injury. The lack of association between conventional parameters of liver disease severity and degree of fatigue has important implications for management. Clinicians may assume a link between disease severity and symptoms leading to a dichotomy between clinician and patient perception as to treatment efficacy in patients showing good biochemical response to UDCA but ongoing severe fatigue.[14] It also has implications for liver transplantation given the evidence that classic non-stage-related PBC fatigue (as opposed to the symptoms associated with end-stage disease) does not improve following transplantation.[1] Fatigue therefore should not be considered an indication for liver transplantation in PBC no matter how severe.

The advent of clinical tools to quantify fatigue has enabled the study of pathogenetic processes for PBC in particular with additional data coming from animal models of cholestasis. There are data to support central and peripheral processes in PBC, and clinicians can now begin to develop a model for fatigue pathogenesis.

Central Fatigue

There are data from animal models of cholestasis and from human studies in PBC to implicate central nervous system (CNS) pathways in fatigue. Most animal studies have used the bile duct ligated (BDL) rodent.[15,16] Although clearly cholestatic, the model is also a severe acute one, a caveat that should be borne in mind when considering the extent to which findings can be extrapolated to human cholestatic patients. Cholestatic rodents exhibit clinical features suggestive of fatigue and cognitive dysfunction.[15] They also exhibit reduced socialization. Specific behavioral features include reduced physical activity, tendency to futility (the animals become frustrated and give up tasks more quickly), impaired memory (animals show latency changes suggesting that they cannot recall painful stimuli and thus avoid them), and reduction in the extent to which they show normal socialized behavior. All these phenomena are redolent of the problems and behavior changes exhibited by fatigued patients. Work undertaken by the Swain group in the BDL model has identified mechanisms underpinning fatigue and linked cognitive impairment, including abnormality in the hypothalamic-pituitary-adrenal axis.[17] Strikingly, CNS inflammation has been implicated, with BDL animals showing increased recruitment of inflammatory leucocytes into the brain. Furthermore, knock-out models lacking either tumor necrosis factor-α or selectins (and thus CNS cell recruitment) show mitigation of key behavioral aspects, such as impaired socialization.[18] As a result, therapies targeting these pathways have been proposed for PBC.

In patients with PBC the evidence to support a central component to fatigue includes the clinical associations seen in the disease, imaging findings, and neurophysiologic abnormalities. In terms of clinical associations, fatigue in PBC is associated with sleep abnormality (in the absence of any association with obstructive sleep apnea) and depression (although the potential for this to be a secondary phenomenon is important to remember).[2,4] Fatigue also has a circadian rhythm in PBC, which is redolent of other centrally mediated phenomena, with fatigue typically being worse later in the day.[19] The sleep abnormality association is with sleep initiation, with increased sleep latency typically being accompanied by significant daytime somnolence.[20] Stimulant agents, such as modafinil, are effective for reducing daytime somnolence and where this benefit is seen fatigue severity is also typically reduced.[21,22] These agents have significant side effects and their use should only be considered in highly selected patients following assessment in specialist centers.

Autonomic dysfunction is also seen in PBC and can be a significant clinical problem through increasing susceptibility to falls (increased risk of vasomotor-mediated falls is as important a contributor to risk of fractures in PBC as osteoporosis) and through a strong association with fatigue and cognitive impairment.[23–25] Indeed, the presence of autonomic dysfunction at baseline is associated with increased risk of progressive deterioration in cognitive function over follow-up.[26] Autonomic dysfunction is associated with impaired cerebral autoregulation, and the areas of the brain demonstrated to show significant change are those where the autonomic centers are located, suggesting that the clinical phenomenon of autonomic dysfunction is also centrally mediated.[26]

In terms of imaging, patients with PBC exhibit dense white matter lesions on MRI, with lesion load associating with degree of cognitive impairment and, anatomically, with autonomic regulatory centers.[26] Functional MRI approaches have also shown abnormality, with decreased magnetization transfer ratio being seen across brain centers from early in the disease course (and certainly before the onset of encephalopathy, which is a rare clinical event in PBC).[27] The association of this change with specific symptoms remains, however, unclear. Study of the functional and neurophysiologic basis of fatigue in PSC has been more limited. Overt cognitive impairment with, in particular, impaired executive function is seen even in patients with no cirrhosis with a severity that correlates with perception of cognitive symptoms and perceived fatigue.[26] Patients with PBC also exhibit reduced neural drive to exercise before and after fatiguing exercise, and an increase in intracortical inhibition modeled using transcranial magnetic stimulation.[28] Both phenomena were associated with degree of daytime somnolence and seen in pretransplant and posttransplant patients. This further supports the concept of irreversible brain change in the disease potentially being linked to symptom pathogenesis.

Fewer data are currently available regarding the presence of any CNS processes in fatigue in PSC. The only study to look at clinical associations found an association between fatigue severity in PSC and autonomic dysfunction but not sleep disturbance.[3] Both fatigue and autonomic symptom severity were, however, most marked in patients with PSC with inflammatory bowel disease (IBD), and in particular those who had a colectomy suggesting that fluid-balance issues may have a particular impact in such patients. There have been no studies using either CNS imaging or neurophysiology approaches in PSC.

Peripheral Fatigue

Despite clear evidence to support CNS mechanisms there are also data to suggest the presence of a peripheral component to fatigue pathogenesis in PBC. Patient descriptions highlight a perceived lack of energy with such terminology as "batteries running down" frequently being used. Perceived fatigue severity also associates with levels of physical activity, although this could represent effect rather than cause. Fatigued patients with PBC demonstrate, in particular, an impaired ability to sustain repeat physical activity compared with either nonfatigued patients or age-matched community control subjects.[12] MR spectroscopy approaches used to explore the physiologic basis of sustained exercise impairment in PBC demonstrated significant peripheral muscle acidosis with low-level exercise, with postexercise calculated pH levels falling to 6.5 (compared with a minimum of 7.0 in control subjects).[29] Low pH, which is presumed but not confirmed to be a result of increased lactic acid production, seems to be related to impaired mitochondrial function. The impairment in mitochondrial function seems most marked in the patients with the highest level of anti–pyruvate dehydrogenase (PDH) autoantibody (the classic antimitochondrial antibody of PBC).[30] Bioenergetic abnormality was not limited to peripheral muscle, with abnormalities in cardiac muscle bioenergetic function also being seen and shown to be linked with diastolic muscle dysfunction.[31,32] In peripheral muscle, recovery to baseline pH following exercise was also significantly prolonged. Severity of fatigue was strongly associated with the prolongation of pH recovery time and, strikingly, with the area under the curve for pH suggesting that the duration and degree of exposure to excess intracellular proton levels significantly contributes to the expression of fatigue. Although muscle acidosis was seen in some patients with minimal or no fatigue, this group shared the characteristic of a very rapid recovery to baseline pH, which was supranormal on repeat exercise.[30] It is normal to show some shortening of the time taken for pH to recover to normal with repeat exercise. This phenomenon is thought to relate to increased muscle blood flow (and thus lactic acid outflow) and, potentially, sympathetic nervous system activation of muscle lactate and proton outflow transporters. Fatigued patients, in contrast, showed no shortening of recovery time with repeat exercise. The opposite effect was in fact seen with significant prolongation of recovery time and several patients unable to complete the repeat exercise protocol.[30]

One interpretation of these findings is that there are two processes occurring in peripheral muscle in PBC. A presumably acquired propensity to impaired mitochondrial dysfunction may lead to increased use of the lactate dehydrogenase pathway. A failure of a normal adaptation pathway to anaerobic metabolism ("deconditioning") may mean that many patients are unable to cope with the lactic acid load. If correct, this model opens the way to approaches to therapy. It may be possible to alter the balance of aerobic and anaerobic metabolism through approaches that increase PDH function. This could plausibly be achieved through reduction of PDH kinase activity, which reduces PDH activity by phosphorylating it or by decreasing PDH dysfunction. Alternatively, it may be possible to increase the adaptive response to anaerobic acidosis through exercise intervention, which is known to increase muscle acid outflow in part through increased expression of transporters, such as the lactate cell membrane transporter MCT4.[33,34] A pilot study of exercise intervention has shown clinical benefit and good uptake by participants, although patients remain concerned about their potential ability to undertake such programs.[30]

A Model for Pathogenesis

Is it possible to reconcile the seemingly conflicting observations regarding peripheral and central components to fatigue in PBC? There are two potential scenarios. The first is that the symptom of fatigue represents a perception that can result from different processes in different patients, and the experimental data suggesting different processes reflect this. In this model fatigue would behave rather like pain; another symptom in which a single perception can have multiple different causes in different patients. There would thus not be one single cause of fatigue in PBC in the same way that there is no single cause of pain.

The second scenario would be that peripheral and central processes are seen because they synergize to give rise to the specific form of fatigue seen in PBC. There are potential mechanisms for a central/peripheral interaction (**Fig. 1**). Autonomic dysfunction, and in particular impairment of vasomotor function, may be responsible for the interaction. Impaired vasomotor function is strongly associated with fatigue in

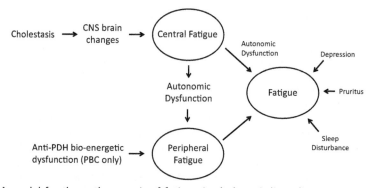

Fig. 1. A model for the pathogenesis of fatigue in cholestatic liver disease.

PBC (and several other chronic conditions characterized by fatigue).[24,35,36] Although the origin of vasomotor autonomic dysfunction in PBC remains unclear there is evidence to suggest a central component, including a link between autonomic dysfunction and overtly CNS symptoms, such as cognitive dysfunction.[26] There are structural abnormalities in areas of the brain linked to autonomic regulation in PBC and an association between lesion load and degree of cognitive impairment and a loss of cerebral autoregulation, which is associated with autonomic dysfunction.[26] The autonomic nervous system plays a key role in regulation of peripheral blood flow in muscles and the function of proton and/or lactate transporters, which allow muscle to cope with the acidosis resulting from overuse of anaerobic pathways. Thus autonomic dysfunction of central origin could play a key role in reducing the peripheral adaptation to the upregulated anaerobic metabolism seen in PBC. An alternative potential peripheral/central link could be through the release by stressed muscle of inflammatory cytokines and myokines, including interleukin-6.[37,38] The data in this regard are, however, very limited.

With regard to PSC it is more difficult to develop a model because of lack of experimental data. The most likely scenario is that PSC fatigue is specifically driven by autonomic dysfunction (potentially of central cholestatic origin but also, probably, exacerbated by fluid issues in extensive colitis) but not exacerbated by any direct bioenergetics effect (a PBC-specific phenomenon). This lack of a direct peripheral component could explain why fatigue is less of an issue in PSC than in PBC.

TREATMENT OF FATIGUE IN PRIMARY BILIARY CIRRHOSIS AND PRIMARY SCLEROSING CHOLANGITIS

Despite the complexity of fatigue in cholestatic liver disease, the questions that still remain about its pathogenesis, and the lack of any specific therapy, there are strategies that can be adopted to manage this symptom and improve fatigue severity and the impact it has on QoL. This section reviews therapies that have been trialed in the past, outline current management strategies, and explore future opportunities.

In PBC, fatigue is unresponsive to the only licensed therapy for disease progression (UDCA)[5] and remains largely unchanged after transplantation.[1] Emerging second-line therapies are effective at improving liver biochemistry in those patients that have a suboptimal response to UDCA but do not seem to have any effect on symptoms (although data are currently limited in this area).

One of the first challenges in managing fatigue is understanding what it means to the patient, and appreciating the impact that it has on their life and the lives of their family and friends. The *TRACE* algorithm was developed to provide a structured approach to managing fatigue in PBC. It was developed for use in PBC but could be easily adapted for use in other chronic diseases, including PSC. This approach focuses on managing treatable or associated factors that can contribute to fatigue and helping patients to develop techniques to manage their fatigue (**Box 1**).

The first step is to screen for and treat any symptoms or associated conditions that can directly cause or exacerbate fatigue, and which may be contributing to the overall clinical picture. Pruritus, another commonly experienced symptom in cholestatic liver disease, can cause sleep disturbance and can thereby worsen fatigue. Unlike fatigue, there are several recognized therapies available for cholestatic pruritus and it should therefore be screened for, and treatment initiated if present.[8,9] Other autoimmune disorders, such as thyroid dysfunction and celiac disease, can cause fatigue, as can anemia and vitamin D deficiency. These conditions, all of which are associated in some way with PBC, can be easily tested for and if present, treated. Treating these

---

Box 1
The TRACE approach to managing fatigue in primary biliary cirrhosis

- *TR*eatment
  - Pruritus
  - Autoimmune conditions
    - Thyroid dysfunction
    - Celiac disease
    - Anemia
  - Other comorbidities
    - Diabetes
    - Heart failure
    - Renal failure
- *A*melioration
  - Sleep disturbance
  - Depression
  - Autonomic dysfunction
- *C*oping strategies
  - Explanation
  - Maintain social interactions
  - Physical activity
- *E*mpathy

---

conditions may not completely alleviate fatigue but even small improvements in fatigue severity can have a significant impact on QoL and can help create a positive cycle where small reductions in fatigue lead to increased confidence to undertake activity. This can reduce deconditioning and lead to positive reinforcement.

Autonomic dysfunction, sleep disturbance, and depression are all associated with fatigue in PBC[4] (and to a lesser extent PSC) and attempts should be made to ameliorate these processes if possible. Screening tools are available that can be used in the clinical setting and can identify at-risk patients who warrant further investigation and potentially treatment. The Orthostatic Grading Scale can identify patients with autonomic dysfunction and this can be confirmed with 24-hour blood pressure monitoring and tilt-testing as appropriate.[39] Simple lifestyle measures, such as increasing fluid intake, drinking up to five cups of caffeinated drinks per day (although timing needs to be considered to avoid an unwanted sleep impact), and taking care when standing from sitting or lying can be initiated in the clinical setting. It is important to undertake a medication review because patients may be taking unnecessary antihypertensives or taking preparations associated with fatigue. More complex or resistant cases of autonomic dysfunction may need referral to a specialist falls service. Sleep disturbance can be assessed by the Epworth Sleepiness Scale.[40] This can identify patients that warrant referral to a sleep service. However, simple causes, such as nocturnal pain, pruritus, or nocturia, can be identified and addressed in the clinic. Obstructive sleep apnea is not specifically associated with PBC, unlike in nonalcoholic fatty liver disease, but should be considered because fatigue can improve after treatment.[20,41] Prominent daytime somnolence can be identified in a minority of patients with PBC and it is important to recognize this because the stimulant modafinil is useful in this setting.[21,22] Modafinil should not be used as a treatment of fatigue per se, but can be trialed in patients with marked daytime somnolence. It should only be considered in patients with pronounced daytime somnolence and following formal sleep assessment, and only under specialist supervision. Its use is often limited by side effects, the most common being headaches. Depression should be treated if present, regardless of whether it is thought to be the cause or consequence of fatigue.

The efforts made by clinicians can only go part of the way to managing fatigue. Patients should be encouraged to take ownership of the symptom and clinicians need to assist patients in finding strategies to cope and live with their fatigue. Patients often reduce social activities to try and preserve energy. However, this reduction in social interactions has a significant negative impact on QoL. The importance of maintaining social functioning should be stressed to patients. Educating patients and their relatives can help increase understanding and development of coping strategies. Discussions need to take place about available treatment options and to set realistic expectations about what can be achieved. Patients are often concerned about increasing activity levels and exercising because of concerns about "paying" for it with even lower energy levels afterward. Pilot data, however, suggest that a moderate and tailored exercise program is beneficial in improving fatigue and QoL.[30] This also has the appeal of a management strategy that patients can initiate themselves, which can empower them and give them ownership of their fatigue. Fatigue in PBC is typically worse later in the day and this information is useful to patients allowing them to time their activities during the day to maximize function.

The final step in the *TRACE* algorithm is empathy. Patients do not need sympathy, they need understanding, empathetic clinicians who work with them to try to improve fatigue severity and QoL.

The treatment approach previously described, although largely designed for use in PBC, can also be adopted for use in PSC given that many of the contributing factors and associations are seen in both conditions. PSC and the strong association with IBD adds another layer of complexity to fatigue. Uncontrolled, active IBD can contribute to fatigue and should be the primary target for therapy in patients with PSC.

Novel Therapies

There are currently no licensed therapies for fatigue in cholestatic liver disease. However, Bio-Quinone Q10, an antioxidant, demonstrated an improvement in fatigue and itch in patients with PBC in an open-label pilot study and this can be bought from health food stores and supermarkets in the United Kingdom.[42]

The first randomized controlled trial of a treatment of fatigue in PBC has been running in Newcastle Upon Tyne in the United Kingdom and is due to close to recruitment in October 2015 (Clinicaltrials.gov NCT02376335). The phase II trial, RITPBC is a trial of rituximab versus placebo to treat moderate to severe fatigue in PBC. This landmark trial has demonstrated that it is possible to undertake trials with fatigue as a primary outcome measure and it is hoped will encourage further trials in cholestatic liver disease and other chronic diseases.

Prescribed exercise therapy as a treatment of fatigue warrants further evaluation, particularly to evaluate whether the bioenergetic abnormalities seen in peripheral muscle can be modified following exercise. Pilot data suggested an improvement in fatigue, social, and emotional symptoms in patients with PBC following an exercise program and a trial to further investigate this is in the design stage.[30]

There is a strong association between social dysfunction and impaired QoL in fatigued patients with PBC, which identifies a potential management approach.[4] Targeting social dysfunction through improving social support networks and providing group therapy sessions to provide psychological support may prove beneficial.

Future Perspectives

Newer therapies are being developed to treat high-risk patients with PBC and modify disease progression in PSC. In parallel with this it is important to assess and have treatment options for the symptoms associated with these diseases because they have a significant impact on patients' QoL. Development and validation of the PBC-40 has changed the way that fatigue is assessed and enabled trials to be performed with symptoms as a primary outcome. A similar tool is being developed for use in PSC. The pathogenesis of fatigue in PBC has been the subject of extensive study and the mechanisms underpinning this debilitating symptom are the ongoing focus of therapeutic trials. Recent work has highlighted that fatigue is also a dominant problem for some patients with PSC but further attention is needed to understand the complex issues involved for these patients to guide future studies and therapeutic development.

REFERENCES

1. Goldblatt J, Taylor PJS, Lipman T, et al. The true impact of fatigue in primary biliary cirrhosis: a population study. Gastroenterology 2002;122:1235–41.
2. Cauch-Dudek K, Abbey S, Stewart DE, et al. Fatigue in primary biliary cirrhosis. Gut 1998;43:705–10.
3. Dyson JK, Elsharkawy AM, Lamb CA, et al. Fatigue in primary sclerosing cholangitis is associated with sympathetic over-activity and increased cardiac output. Liver Int 2015;35(5):1633–41.
4. Mells G, Pells G, Newton JL, et al. The impact of primary biliary cirrhosis on perceived quality of life: the UK-PBC National Study. Hepatology 2013;58:273–83.
5. Carbone M, Mells G, Pells G, et al. Sex and age are determinants of the clinical phenotype of primary biliary cirrhosis and response to ursodeoxycholic acid. Gastroenterology 2013;144:560–9.
6. James OFW, Macklon AF, Watson AF. Primary biliary cirrhosis: a revised clinical spectrum. Lancet 1981;1:1278–81.
7. Sherlock S. Primary biliary cirrhosis (chronic intrahepatic obstructive jaundice). Gastroenterology 1959;37:574–86.
8. Beuers U, Boberg KM, Chazouilleres O, et al. EASL practice guidelines on management of cholestatic liver diseases. J Hepatol 2009;51:237–67.
9. Lindor KD, Gershwin ME, Poupon R, et al. Primary biliary cirrhosis. Hepatology 2009;50(1):291–308.
10. Jacoby A, Rannard A, Buck D, et al. Development, validation and evaluation of the PBC-40, a disease specific health related quality of life measure for primary biliary cirrhosis. Gut 2005;54:1622–9.
11. Prince MI, James OFW, Holland NP, et al. Validation of a fatigue impact score in primary biliary cirrhosis: towards a standard for clinical and trial use. J Hepatol 2000;32:368–73.
12. Newton JL, Bhala N, Burt J, et al. Characterisation of the associations and impact of symptoms in primary biliary cirrhosis using a disease specific quality of life measure. J Hepatol 2006;44:776–82.
13. Newton JL, Elliott C, Frith J, et al. Functional capacity is significantly impaired in primary biliary cirrhosis and related to orthostatic symptoms. Eur J Gastroenterol Hepatol 2011;23:566–72.
14. Hale M, Newton JL, Jones DE. Fatigue in primary biliary cirrhosis. BMJ 2013;345:e7004.

15. Swain MG, Le T. Chronic cholestasis in rats induces anhedonia and loss of social interest. Hepatology 1998;28:6–10.
16. Burak KW, Le T, Swain MG. Increased midbrain 5-HT1A receptor number and responsiveness in cholestatic rats. Brain Res 2001;892:376–9.
17. Burak KW, Le T, Swain MG. Increased sensitivity to the locomotor-activating effects of corticotrophin-releasing hormone in cholestatic rats. Gastroenterology 2002;122:681–8.
18. Kerfoot SM, D'Mello C, Nguyen H, et al. TNF-alpha secreting monocytes are recruited into the brain of cholestatic mice. Hepatology 2006;43:154–62.
19. Montagnese S, Nsemi LM, Cazzagon N, et al. Sleep wake profiles in patients with primary biliary cirrhosis. Liver Int 2013;33(2):203–9.
20. Newton JL, Gibson JG, Tomlinson M, et al. Fatigue in primary biliary cirrhosis is associated with excessive daytime somnolence. Hepatology 2006;44:91–8.
21. Hardy T, McDonald C, Jones DEJ, et al. A follow-up study of modafinil for the daytime somnolence and fatigue in PBC. Liver Int 2010;30:1551–2.
22. Ian Gan S, de Jongh M, Kaplan MM. Modafinil in the treatment of debilitating fatigue in primary biliary cirrhosis: a clinical experience. Dig Dis Sci 2009;54(10):2242–6.
23. Newton JL, Hudson M, Tachtatzis P, et al. The population prevalence and symptom associations of autonomic dysfunction in primary biliary cirrhosis. Hepatology 2007;45:1496–505.
24. Newton JL, Davidson A, Kerr S, et al. Autonomic dysfunction in primary biliary cirrhosis correlates with fatigue severity. Eur J Gastroenterol Hepatol 2007;19:125–32.
25. Frith J, Kerr S, Robinson L, et al. Primary biliary cirrhosis is associated with falls and significant fall related injury. QJM 2010;103:153–61.
26. Newton JL, Hollingsworth KG, Taylor R, et al. Cognitive impairment in primary biliary cirrhosis: symptom impact and potential aetiology. Hepatology 2008;48:541–9.
27. Forton D, Patel N, Prince M, et al. Fatigue and primary biliary cirrhosis: association of globus pallidus magnetization transfer ratio measurements with fatigue severity and blood manganese levels. Gut 2004;53:587–92.
28. McDonald C, Newton JL, Ming Lai H, et al. Central nervous system dysfunction in primary biliary cirrhosis patients and its relationship to symptoms. J Hepatol 2010;53:1095–100.
29. Hollingsworth KG, Newton JL, Taylor R, et al. A pilot study of peripheral muscle function in primary biliary cirrhosis: potential implications for fatigue pathogenesis. Clin Gastroenterol Hepatol 2008;6:1041–8.
30. Hollingsworth KG, Newton JL, Robinson L, et al. Loss of capacity to recover from acidosis in repeat exercise is strongly associated with fatigue in primary biliary cirrhosis. J Hepatol 2010;53:155–61.
31. Hollingsworth KG, MacGowan GA, Morris L, et al. Cardiac torsion-strain relationships in fatigued primary biliary cirrhosis patients show accelerated ageing: a pilot cross-sectional study. J Appl Physiol 2012;112(12):2043–8.
32. Jones DEJ, Hollingsworth K, Fattakhova G, et al. Impaired cardiovascular function in primary biliary cirrhosis. Am J Physiol Gastrointest Liver Physiol 2010;298:G764–73.
33. Coles L, Litt J, Hatta H, et al. Exercise rapidly increases expression of the monocarboxylate transporters MCT1 and MCT4 in rat muscle. J Physiol 2004;561(Pt 1):253–61.
34. Pilegaard H, Domino K, Noland T, et al. Effect of high-intensity exercise training on lactate/H+ transport capacity in human skeletal muscle. Am J Physiol 1999;276:E255–61.

35. Flackenecker P, Rufer A, Bihler I, et al. Fatigue in MS is related to sympathetic vasomotor dysfunction. Neurology 2003;61(6):851–3.
36. Mathias CJ, Mallipeddi R, Bleasdale-Barr K. Symptoms associated with orthostatic hypotension in pure autonomic failure and multiple system atrophy. J Neurol 1999;246(10):893–8.
37. Kiecolt-Glaser JK, Preacher KJ, MacCallum RC, et al. Chronic stress and age related increase in the pro inflammatory cytokine IL-6. Proc Natl Acad Sci U S A 2003;100(15):9090–5.
38. Keller P, Keller C, Carey AL, et al. Interleukin-6 production by contracting human skeletal muscle: autocrine regulation by IL-6. Biochem Biophys Res Commun 2003;310:550–4.
39. Schrezenmaier C, Gehrking JA, Hines SM, et al. Evaluation of orthostatic hypotension: relationship of a new self-report instrument to laboratory-based measures. Mayo Clin Proc 2005;80:330–4.
40. Johns MW. A new method for measuring daytime sleepiness: the Epworth Sleepiness Scale. Sleep 1991;14(6):540–5.
41. Sookoian S, Pirola CJ. Obstructive sleep apnea is associated with fatty liver and abnormal liver enzymes: a meta-analysis. Obes Surg 2013;23(11):1815–25.
42. Watson JP, Jones DE, James OF, et al. Case report: oral antioxidant therapy for the treatment of primary biliary cirrhosis: a pilot study. J Gastroenterol Hepatol 1999;14(10):1034–40.

Utility of Noninvasive Markers of Fibrosis in Cholestatic Liver Diseases

Christophe Corpechot, MD[a,b],*

KEYWORDS

- Primary biliary cirrhosis • Primary sclerosing cholangitis • Surrogate markers
- Elastography • Liver biopsy • Prognosis

KEY POINTS

- In classical histologic systems, fibrosis is only partly addressed through stages 3 and 4 (ie, bridging fibrosis and cirrhosis), making them poorly appropriate for an accurate staging of fibrosis.
- In cholestatic liver diseases, noninvasive markers of hepatic fibrosis have been studied much more in primary biliary cirrhosis (PBC) than in primary sclerosing cholangitis (PSC).
- In PBC the best compromise between reported performance, data robustness, validation status, and prognostic relevance is vibration-controlled transient elastography.
- Liver stiffness as measured by vibration-controlled transient elastography is the only credible noninvasive marker of liver fibrosis in PSC.
- Liver stiffness measurement and enhanced liver fibrosis score are both able to provide independent long-term prognostic information in PBC and PSC.

Since their first description in the 1980s, major advances were made in the development of noninvasive markers of liver fibrosis. Whether generated from biochemical analyses or imaging techniques, surrogate indices of liver fibrosis have progressively replaced liver biopsy in the management of the most prevalent chronic liver diseases, including viral hepatitis infections and alcoholic and nonalcoholic fatty liver diseases. As yet, however, chronic cholestatic liver diseases, namely primary biliary cirrhosis and primary sclerosing cholangitis, do remain a branch of hepatology in which the

[a] Hepatology Department, Reference Center for Chronic Inflammatory Biliary Diseases (MIVB), French Network for Childhood and Adult Rare Liver Diseases (FILFOIE), Saint-Antoine Hospital, Assistance Publique - Hôpitaux de Paris (APHP), 184 rue du Faubourg Saint-Antoine, 75571, Paris Cedex 12, France; [b] Inserm UMR_S938, Faculty of Medicine Pierre et Marie Curie, Saint-Antoine Site, Paris 6 University, 27 rue de Chaligny, Paris 75012, France
* Hepatology Department, Reference Center for Chronic Inflammatory Biliary Diseases (MIVB), French Network for Childhood and Adult Rare Liver Diseases (FILFOIE), Saint-Antoine Hospital, Assistance Publique - Hôpitaux de Paris (APHP), 184 rue du Faubourg Saint-Antoine, 75571, Paris Cedex 12, France
E-mail address: christophe.corpechot@sat.aphp.fr

Clin Liver Dis 20 (2016) 143–158
http://dx.doi.org/10.1016/j.cld.2015.08.013
1089-3261/16/$ – see front matter © 2016 Elsevier Inc. All rights reserved.
liver.theclinics.com

use of such markers does not command consensus. Yet, a large body of evidence now supports the reliability and efficiency of noninvasive fibrosis markers in both primary biliary cirrhosis and primary sclerosing cholangitis, even though histologic examination of the liver has probably not said its last word.

WHY EVALUATE FIBROSIS IN CHRONIC CHOLESTATIC LIVER DISEASES?

Chronic cholestatic diseases can be defined as liver conditions for which progression and prognosis are impacted to a large extent by the effects of bile acid accumulation in the liver, regardless of the mechanisms involved.[1] In adults, primary biliary cirrhosis (PBC) and primary sclerosing cholangitis (PSC) account for more than 90% of all patients. Despite different phenotypes and courses, progression of both diseases is characterized histologically by progressive loss of bile ducts, periportal ductular reaction, extensive fibrosis, and eventually cirrhosis. Therefore, as observed in most chronic liver diseases, the extent of fibrotic scares within the hepatic parenchyma marks the progression and severity of chronic cholestatic liver diseases. The progression of fibrosis is closely linked to the parallel processes of bile duct loss and periportal biliary or lymphocytic interface hepatitis, thus likely resulting from a dual cholestatic and necro-inflammatory mechanism.[2] Progressive hyperbilirubinemia, which characterizes severe cholestatic liver diseases, has been recognized as a major predictor of clinical outcomes in both PBC and PSC.[3,4] However, most patients with PBC and PSC are now diagnosed at an early asymptomatic stage, underlying the need for more sensitive prognostic indices. Studies in the 1980s clearly pointed out the importance of fibrosis stage as an independent prognostic factor of these disease conditions.[5,6] However, with the development of popular prognostic models built on noninvasive measurements,[7,8] the use of liver biopsy fell into disgrace. Yet, several recent studies have revived the interest in liver histology to assess prognosis, highlighting the independent and additive prognostic value of histologic stage and, more specifically, of advanced fibrosis and cirrhosis.[9–11] **Fig. 1** shows the significant impact of fibrosis stage (expressed here as stages III or IV of the Ludwig's histologic system) on the survival of patients with either PBC or PSC. Fibrosis stage is,

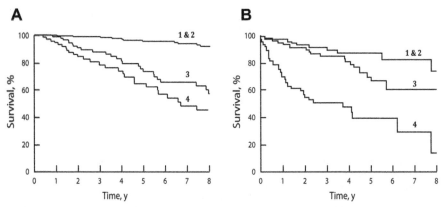

Fig. 1. Impact on survival of histologic stage in PBC and PSC. Kaplan-Meier estimated survival by Ludwig's histologic stage on initial liver biopsy. (*A*) Personal data derived from 292 patients with PBC receiving ursodeoxycholic acid therapy. (*B*) Data from 174 patients with PSC. (*Data from* Corpechot C, Abenavoli L, Rabahi N, et al. Biochemical response to ursodeoxycholic acid and long-term prognosis in primary biliary cirrhosis. Hepatology 2008;48:871–7; and Wiesner RH, Grambsch PM, Dickson ER, et al. Primary sclerosing cholangitis: natural history, prognostic factors and survival analysis. Hepatology 1989;10:430–6.)

therefore, a determinant of severity and prognosis of chronic cholestatic liver diseases. Its determination in PBC and PSC is of major relevance, in particular in asymptomatic patients for whom prognostic markers are sorely lacking. Consequently, the question is not whether fibrosis should be assessed in PBC and PSC, but how it should be. Clearly, that is a key point in the current context of new emerging therapeutic agents for which fibrosis assessment will likely play a major role in future clinical trials.[12]

HISTOLOGY AS A GOLD STANDARD FOR ASSESSING FIBROSIS: RELEVANCE AND LIMITATIONS

Since the recognition in the 1960s of histologic lesions associated with PBC,[13] several staging systems were proposed to grade the histologic severity of the disease (**Table 1**).

Table 1
Histologic scoring systems of liver fibrosis in PBC and PSC

System	Disease Stage/Fibrosis Score	Comments
Scheuer,[14] 1967	Stage 1: No septal fibrosis. Florid bile duct lesions. Stage 2: No septal fibrosis. Periportal ductular reaction Stage 3: Septal fibrosis Stage 4: Cirrhosis	• Primarily designed for PBC • Similar to the Popper & Schaffner's system[59] • Mixes inflammation, bile duct changes and fibrosis • Unknown reproducibility
Ludwig et al,[15] 1978	Stage 1: No septal fibrosis. Portal hepatitis Stage 2: No septal fibrosis. Periportal hepatitis Stage 3: Septal fibrosis or bridging necrosis or both Stage 4: Cirrhosis	• Primarily designed for PBC • Probably the most popular among pathologists • Mixes together inflammation and fibrosis • Unknown reproducibility • Linked to clinical outcome in both PBC and PSC[9,10]
Nakanuma et al,[16] 2010	Score 0: No fibrosis or fibrosis limited to portal tract Score 1: Periportal fibrosis or incomplete septal fibrosis Score 2: Bridging fibrosis Score 3: Cirrhosis	• Primarily designed for PBC • Fibrosis, cholestasis, and bile duct loss are combined for final staging • Fair reproducibility[16] • Linked to clinical outcome in both PBC and PSC[10,18]
Wendum et al,[17] 2015	Score 0: No fibrosis Score 1: Portal/periportal fibrosis without septa Score 2: Periportal fibrosis with a few septa Score 3: Numerous septa Score 4: Cirrhosis	• Primarily designed for PBC • Separate scores for fibrosis, bile duct ratio, and interface hepatitis (FBI system) • Derived from the widely used METAVIR fibrosis score[19] • Better reproducibility than for classical systems[17]
Ishak et al,[60] 1995	Score 0: No fibrosis Score 1: Fibrous expansion of some portal areas Score 2: Fibrous expansion of most portal areas Score 3: Occasional portal-portal or portal-central bridging Score 4: Marked bridging Score 5: Occasional nodules Score 6: Definite cirrhosis	• Not primarily designed for but applicable to PBC and PSC[10,22] • Individual fibrosis score • Unknown reproducibility in chronic cholestatic diseases • Linked to clinical outcome in both PBC and PSC[10,22]

It is noteworthy that, by contrast, no such histologic classifications have specifically been designed in PSC, although the Ludwig's staging system has been applied by extension in numerous studies. The 2 most widely used staging systems are the Scheuer's and the Ludwig's histologic systems.[14,15] Both have the characteristic to combine either simultaneously or sequentially different kinds of histologic lesions (ie, inflammation, fibrosis, with or without bile duct changes) deemed to differentiate between recognizable progression stages. These 2 staging systems were found to be linked to clinical outcome.[9,10] Of note, the Ludwig's system was originally designed to reduce the risk of misleading conclusion because of the segmental distribution of bile duct lesions in the liver. However, in both systems, fibrosis is only partly addressed through stages 3 and 4 (ie, bridging fibrosis and cirrhosis), making them poorly appropriate for an accurate staging of fibrosis. Moreover, although routinely used by pathologists, these histologic classifications have never been validated in terms of intra- and interobserver reproducibility. In this context, 2 new PBC staging systems have recently been developed.[16,17] The Japanese staging system includes a separate fibrosis score, which together with bile duct loss and cholestasis assessment contributes to the definition of disease stage. This new system has shown quite fair interobserver agreement[16] and significant links with clinical outcomes.[10,18] The French staging system, called FBI (fibrosis, bile duct ratio, interface hepatitis) system, has the characteristic and, possibly, the advantage to evaluate separately 3 histologic features known to be associated with clinical outcomes, namely fibrosis (based on the METAVIR fibrosis score[19]), interface hepatitis,[11,20] and bile duct ratio.[21] The intra- and interobserver reproducibility of this system was found to be superior to those of the Scheuer's and Ludwig's classical systems. Its prognostic relevance, however, remains to be confirmed. Finally, although not primarily designed for the assessment of cholestatic liver diseases, the Ishak fibrosis score has been applied with success not only in the evaluation of fibrosis but also of clinical outcomes in PBC and PSC.[10,22] Besides the invasiveness and potentially dangerous nature of liver biopsy, which hold limited applicability and repeatability in practice, the sampling variability of small-size specimens seems particularly high in chronic cholestatic liver diseases, as considerable variation in the degree of fibrosis is described within explant livers.[23,24] If histology remains a gold-standard for assessing fibrosis in cholestatic liver diseases with established links with clinical outcomes, there is currently no consensus regarding the best staging system, although it can be speculated that individual generic fibrosis scores (METAVIR, Ishak) are more reliable and reproducible than historical staging systems. On the other hand, in a context of noninvasive medicine, the issue is rather whether we do have credible alternative methods to evaluate fibrosis in these diseases.

THE (LONG) STORY OF FIBROSIS MARKERS IN CHRONIC CHOLESTATIC LIVER DISEASES

Since the late 1980s, several steps have punctuated the long march of noninvasive fibrosis markers in chronic liver diseases. Early studies focused on individual candidate biomarkers, including serum markers of connective tissue, like hyaluronic acid and procollagen III peptide,[25] and quantitative liver function tests, like indocyanine green and sulfobromophtalein.[26] Around the 2000s, composite scores generated from large serum biomarker databases using multiple logistic regression analyses were developed and validated.[27-29] Finally, over the last 10 years, new functional imaging techniques, including ultrasound elastography–based methods and MRI assessment of the liver have further emerged.[30,31] It is noticeable that, in cholestatic liver diseases, noninvasive markers of hepatic fibrosis have been much more studied in PBC than in PSC. Serum components of extracellular matrix have been assessed widely in PBC with consistent results. Hyaluronic acid and procollagen III were found to be significantly increased in late stages of the disease compared with early stages or controls.[32,33] Unfortunately, only a few studies have estimated with accuracy the diagnostic performance and reliability of the latter 2 markers.[34,35] Consequently, they have not been used widely in clinical practice. Of note, both hyaluronic acid and procollagen III peptide are part, with tissue inhibitor of metalloproteinase 1, of the enhanced liver fibrosis (ELF) score,[36] a paying algorithm that has shown good performance for the detection of significant fibrosis or cirrhosis in PBC.[22] Recently, a novel biomarker named *hyperglycosylated Wisteria floribunda agglutinin-positive Mac-2 binding protein* (WFA(+)-M2BP), which has relevance in cell-cell and cell-extracellular matrix adhesion, has shown promising ability for the determination of fibrosis stages in PBC.[37] However, at the moment, these results remain anecdotal and have to be validated. Whether based on classical biochemistries or on more specific markers, as connective tissue compounds or bile acids, only few specific composite scores have been designed in cholestatic liver diseases.[38–40] None of them have been extensively studied in spite of fairly good estimated accuracy to discriminate advanced from less severe fibrosis stages. Regarding generic composite scores, aspartate aminotransferase/platelet ratio index (APRI)[29] and fibrosis-4 (FIB-4) score[41] have been the most investigated in chronic cholestatic liver diseases. Both in PBC and PSC, APRI and FIB-4 have exhibited acceptable performance for the diagnosis of advanced fibrosis.[35,42,43] Whereas applicability of serum fibrosis markers is virtually optimal, reproducibility in cholestatic liver diseases remains uncertain, and causes of misleading results still understudied. Vibration-controlled transient elastography (VCTE, Fibroscan) has been, to date, the most widely used physical method of fibrosis assessment in cholestatic liver diseases. VCTE is a simple and rapid bedside method allowing the physician to capture an instant estimate of liver stiffness, a parameter that has been validated as a robust surrogate marker of liver fibrosis in different large populations of patients with various chronic liver diseases.[44] Unlike serum markers, however, VCTE has an incomplete applicability with a significant 15% rate of failure results or failure.[45] In PBC and PSC, VCTE has been confirmed to have very high accuracy for the detection of severe fibrosis and cirrhosis.[35,42,43,46] Yet, diagnostic thresholds of liver stiffness measurement remain to be refined, and large-scale replication studies are needed. There are currently only anecdotal reports on other imaging-based techniques, including acoustic radiation force impulse (ARFI) elastography[47] and contrast-enhanced or diffusion-weighted MRI[48–50] for the assessment of fibrosis in cholestatic liver diseases.

NONINVASIVE EVALUATION OF FIBROSIS IN PRIMARY BILIARY CIRRHOSIS: TOWARD A RATIONAL CHOICE

In the absence of comparative studies and meta-analyses, it is difficult to get a clear picture of the relative performance of noninvasive fibrosis markers in PBC. A rational approach could be to consider together the cumulative number of biopsy tests assessed, the range of diagnostic accuracy based on area under receiver operating characteristic curve (AUROC), and the existence (or lack) of external validation studies. Concurrent ability in predicting clinical outcomes is also a candidate parameter. **Tables 2** and **3** compile these data. Severe fibrosis, as defined by either bridging fibrosis according to the Ludwig's histologic system, periportal fibrosis with numerous septa (METAVIR fibrosis score 3 or more), or fibrous expansion of most portal areas with occasional portal-to-portal or portal-to-central bridging (Ishak

Table 2
Noninvasive markers of liver fibrosis in PBC

	Cumulated No. of Biopsy Tests	External Validation	References
Serum markers			
APRI score	931	Yes	35,37,39,42,57,61,62
AST/ALT Ratio	670	Yes	35,37,39,42,61,63
FIB-4 score	360	Yes	35,37,42
Hyaluronic acid	394	Yes	32–35,39,64–66
Forns score	334	Yes	37,39,42
Procollagen III peptide	314	Yes	33,34,39,64,65,67,68
Mayo risk score	240	Yes	35,37
ELF test	189	—	22,69
Fibrotest	169	—	62,69,70
Bilirubin-hyaluronan index	153	—	38,39
WFA(+)-M2BP	137	—	37
Cytokeratin-18	130	—	58
Laminin P1	129	—	64,66,68,71
Collagen IV	126	—	66,68,72
FibroIndex	120	—	42
PBC score	77[a]	—	39
H-index	63	—	40
BSP-ICG test	50	—	26
Imaging techniques			
VCTE	351	Yes	35,42,46,62,69
Contrast-enhanced MRI	74	—	48,62
ARFI	61	—	73
Diffusion-weighted MRI	44	—	51

Fibrosis markers are split into serum markers and imaging techniques. They are sorted within both categories by decreasing number of cumulated biopsy-test pairs evaluated reported in the literature.

Abbreviations: ALT, alanine transaminase; AST, aspartate transaminase; BSP-ICG, sulfobromophthalein and indocyanine green.

[a] No cirrhosis.

fibrosis score 3 or more), has been used as a benchmark. These data must be interpreted with caution. Diagnostic performance closely depends on the populations studied and, more specifically, on the distribution of fibrosis stages within each population, which can greatly vary from study to study. Furthermore, not all studies have used an intent-to-diagnose analysis, which consists of adjusting performance estimates for testing applicability in clinical practice,[35] and only a minority of them have provided data on reproducibility. Moreover, large numbers of biopsy tests and available validation studies are not synonymous with reliability and performance. The best compromise to date among reported performance, data robustness, validation status, and prognostic relevance goes to VCTE, then to APRI score, ELF score, and hyaluronic acid level, without marked differences among the latter 3 markers. **Fig. 2** is an illustration of the ability of VCTE in discriminating histologic fibrosis stages. Recent promising, but still anecdotal data, obtained with ARFI elastography

Table 3
Diagnostic and prognostic performance of fibrosis markers in PBC

	Performance to Detect Advanced Fibrosis[a]	Correlation with Clinical Outcomes
VCTE	0.86–0.95	Yes[35]
ARFI	0.93	—
WFA(+)-M2BP	0.93	Yes[37]
Diffusion-weighted MRI	0.91	—
APRI score	0.67–0.86	Yes[57]
H-index	0.86	—
FIB-4 score	0.63–0.83	—
Contrast-enhanced MRI	0.83	—
Fibrotest	0.72–0.80	—
ELF test	0.75–0.79	Yes[22]
Hyaluronic acid	0.63–0.79	Yes[55,65]
Bilirubin-hyaluronan index	0.79	—
Mayo risk score	0.73–0.75	Yes[7]
Cytokeratin-18	0.61–0.73	Yes[58]
FibroIndex	0.69	—
Procollagen III peptide	0.68	Yes[55,67]
Forns score	0.61–0.67	—
AST/ALT ratio	0.57–0.66	—
PBC score	ND[b]	—
Laminin P1	ND	Yes[55]
Collagen IV	ND	—
BSP-ICG test	ND	—

Abbreviations: ALT, alanine transaminase; AST, aspartate transaminase; BSP-ICG, sulfobromophthalein and indocyanine green; ND, nondetermined.

[a] As based on AUROC(s) reported in the literature. Advanced fibrosis is defined by either cirrhosis or bridging fibrosis according to the Ludwig's histologic staging system, periportal fibrosis with numerous septa (METAVIR fibrosis score 3 or more), or fibrous expansion of most portal areas with occasional portal to portal and/or portal to central bridging (Ishak fibrosis score 3 or more). Fibrosis markers are sorted by decreasing order of the most elevated AUROC.

[b] 0.75 for discriminating F0F1 from F2F3 METAVIR stages.[39]

or diffusion-weighted MRI suggest that these techniques offer high comparable performance.[47,51] Results recently reported on the new biomarker WFA(+)-M2BP are also encouraging, but independent confirmation studies are certainly required.[52] VCTE currently is the best choice among all noninvasive methods available for the detection of advanced fibrosis and cirrhosis in PBC. Its practice, easily achievable at outpatient clinics with instant results, is a real asset compared with other options. As with many other fibrosis indices, liver stiffness measured by VCTE exhibits a nonlinear relationship with fibrosis stage, explaining better performance for extreme ends of the fibrosis spectrum and poorer discriminative capacity for intermediate fibrosis stages. In addition, its reproducibility and variability deserve further evaluation. APRI score, ELF score, and hyaluronic acid level seem to be good alternative options but with lower diagnostic accuracy. All of these noninvasive tests have established ability in predicting clinical outcomes.

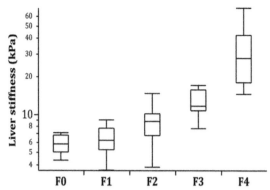

Fig. 2. Distribution of liver stiffness measurement in PBC according to the METAVIR fibrosis score. Box plot of liver stiffness measured by VCTE depending on biopsy score (logarithm scale). The bottom and top of the boxes are the first and third quartiles (interquartiles), and the band inside the boxes is the median. The ends of the whiskers are the minimum and maximum of the data. (*Adapted from* Corpechot C, Carrat F, Poujol-Robert A, et al. Noninvasive elastography-based assessment of liver fibrosis progression and prognosis in primary biliary cirrhosis. Hepatology 2012;56:202; with permission.)

NONINVASIVE EVALUATION OF FIBROSIS IN PRIMARY SCLEROSING CHOLANGITIS: NOTHING BUT LIVER STIFFNESS MEASUREMENT?

The context in PSC is much easier than in PBC because studies of noninvasive markers of fibrosis in this disease are scarce. As for PBC in the previous section, **Tables 4** and **5** summarize the (few) data currently available in PSC. It is clear from these tables that liver stiffness, as measured by VCTE, is currently the only credible noninvasive marker of liver fibrosis in PSC. As in other chronic liver diseases, VCTE in PSC has been found to show excellent performance (AUROC >0.90) for the diagnosis of cirrhosis or advanced fibrosis.[43,53] **Fig. 3** illustrates the discriminative ability

Table 4			
Noninvasive markers of liver fibrosis in PSC			
	Cumulated No. of Biopsy Tests	**External Validation**	**References**
Serum markers			
AST/ALT Ratio	154	—	[74]
Hyaluronic acid	73	—	[43]
APRI score	73	—	[43]
FIB-4 score	73	—	[43]
Mayo risk score	73	—	[43]
Imaging techniques			
VCTE	129	Yes	[43,53]
Diffusion-weighted MRI	38	—	[50]

Fibrosis markers are split into serum markers and imaging techniques. They are sorted within both categories by decreasing number of cumulated biopsy-test pairs evaluated reported in the literature.

Abbreviations: ALT, alanine transaminase; AST, aspartate transaminase.

Table 5		
Diagnostic and prognostic performance of fibrosis markers in PSC		
	Performance to Detect Advanced Fibrosis[a]	**Correlation with Clinical Outcomes**
VCTE	0.93	Yes[43]
Hyaluronic	0.93	—
Diffusion-weighted MRI	0.89	—
Mayo risk score	0.83	—
APRI score	0.81	—
FIB-4	0.76	—
AST/ALT ratio	ND	—
ELF test	ND[b]	Yes[56]

Abbreviations: ALT, alanine transaminase; AST, aspartate transaminase.

  [a] As based on AUROC reported in the literature. Advanced fibrosis is defined by either cirrhosis or bridging fibrosis according to the Ludwig's histologic staging system, periportal fibrosis with numerous septa (METAVIR fibrosis score 3 or more), or fibrous expansion of most portal areas with occasional portal to portal and/or portal to central bridging (Ishak fibrosis score 3 or more). Fibrosis markers are sorted by decreasing order of the most elevated AUROC reported.

  [b] Closely correlated with liver stiffness as measured by VCTE or shear wave elastography (ARFI, Supersonic Shear wave Imaging [SSI]).[56]

of VCTE for the detection of advanced (F3–F4) fibrosis stages in PSC. However, as yet, these results are supported by only 2 midsize studies, bringing together less than 130 biopsy tests, thus necessitating large-scale validation. Of note, taking into consideration the known patchy distribution of liver fibrosis within the liver in PSC, intercostal

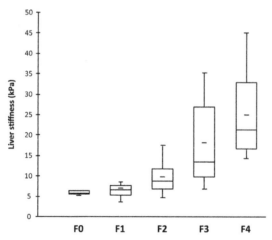

Fig. 3. Distribution of liver stiffness measurement in PSC according to the METAVIR fibrosis score. Box plot of liver stiffness measured by VCTE depending on biopsy score. The bottom and top of the boxes are the first and third quartiles (interquartiles), and the band inside the boxes is the median. The ends of the whiskers are the minimum and maximum of the data. (*From* Corpechot C, Gaouar F, El Naggar A, et al. Baseline values and changes in liver stiffness measured by transient elastography are associated with severity of fibrosis and outcomes of patients with primary sclerosing cholangitis. Gastroenterology 2014;146:973; with permission.)

variability of liver stiffness has been specifically evaluated, showing only few changes in measurements and acceptable reproducibility.[43] Progression rates of liver stiffness in PSC have been estimated as a specific function of time and fibrosis stage, and global pattern of liver stiffness increase could be established as a continuous time process, as shown in **Fig. 4**. The course of liver stiffness measurement indicates that, after an approximate 10-year period of slow increase, the hardening of the liver sharply accelerates, and stiffness exponentially increases once significant fibrosis develops. These data strongly suggest that liver stiffness, whether measured by VCTE or any other technique, could be used as a continuous quantitative surrogate marker of fibrosis in chronic cholestatic liver diseases. It is important to remember, however, that VCTE results should always be interpreted within a given clinical, biochemical, and radiologic context, taking into account all factors (food intake, weight change, acute hepatitis, acute cholangitis, right heart failure) likely to alter liver stiffness temporarily. In PSC, special attention must be paid in patients with jaundice to exclude biliary obstruction by dominant strictures of major bile ducts before performing VCTE.[53] By increasing bile pressure within bile ducts, obstructive cholestasis is known to impact liver stiffness significantly, irrespective of fibrosis.[54] In addition to VCTE, hyaluronic acid level, APRI score, FIB-4 score, and diffusion-weighted MRI have been used as potential markers of fibrosis in PSC, but the level of confidence for these markers is low. Of note, the accuracy of ELF score as a marker of fibrosis in PSC remains undetermined. VCTE is currently the only noninvasive tool that can decently compete with liver biopsy to assess fibrosis in PSC. Large-scale validation of its diagnostic accuracy is awaited.

PROGNOSTIC SIGNIFICANCE OF FIBROSIS MARKERS IN CHOLESTATIC LIVER DISEASES

Being able to determine fibrosis stage noninvasively is a good thing, but predicting outcome at the same time is even better. Some efficient noninvasive markers of liver fibrosis in cholestatic liver diseases have further been found to separate patients into

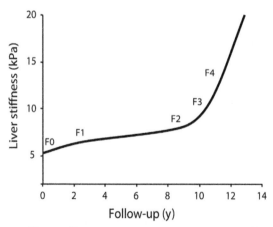

Fig. 4. Natural course of liver stiffness measurement in PSC as assessed by VCTE. Modeling of liver stiffness progression as a continuous-time function derived from data of 142 patients with PSC repeatedly assessed with VCTE. (*Adapted from* Corpechot C, Gaouar F, El Naggar A, et al. Baseline values and changes in liver stiffness measured by transient elastography are associated with severity of fibrosis and outcomes of patients with primary sclerosing cholangitis. Gastroenterology 2014;146:975; with permission.)

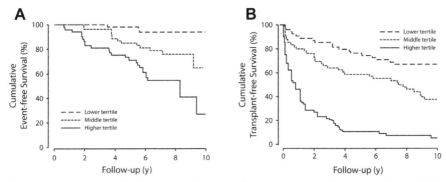

Fig. 5. Impact on survival of ELF score in PBC and PSC. Kaplan-Meier estimated survival by ELF score in (A) 161 patients with PBC receiving ursodeoxycholic acid therapy and (B) 167 patients with PSC. (*Data from* Mayo MJ, Parkes J, Adams-Huet B, et al. Prediction of clinical outcomes in primary biliary cirrhosis by serum enhanced liver fibrosis assay. Hepatology 2008;48:1549–57; and Vesterhus M, Hov JR, Holm A, et al. Enhanced liver fibrosis score predicts transplant-free survival in primary sclerosing cholangitis. Hepatology 2015;62:188–97.)

significant risk groups. Serum level of hyaluronic acid was the first noninvasive marker of fibrosis to show significant association with clinical outcome in PBC.[32,55] Since then, several other fibrosis indices have exhibited similar predictive aptitudes. It is particularly true for ELF score and liver stiffness assessed by VCTE, whose baseline values are able to provide independent long-term prognostic information in both PBC and PSC.[22,35,43,56] ELF score has been found to stratify patients efficiently into low-, intermediate-, and high-risk groups for liver-related death, liver complications, or liver transplantation (**Fig. 5**). Likewise, baseline values of liver stiffness highly suggestive of advanced fibrosis or of definite cirrhosis have been found to discriminate patients according to their survival rates without adverse outcomes (**Fig. 6**). Dynamic

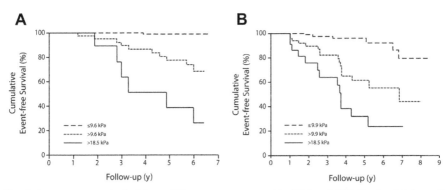

Fig. 6. Impact on survival of liver stiffness measurement in PBC and PSC. Kaplan-Meier estimated survival by liver stiffness measurement as assessed with VCTE in (A) 150 patients with PBC and (B) 168 patients with PSC, all receiving ursodeoxycholic acid therapy. (*Data from* Corpechot C, Carrat F, Poujol-Robert A, et al. Noninvasive elastography-based assessment of liver fibrosis progression and prognosis in primary biliary cirrhosis. Hepatology 2012;56:198–208; and Corpechot C, Gaouar F, El Naggar A, et al. Baseline values and changes in liver stiffness measured by transient elastography are associated with severity of fibrosis and outcomes of patients with primary sclerosing cholangitis. Gastroenterology 2014;146:970–9; [quiz: e15–6].)

changes in these markers may even show stronger disposition to predict clinical outcomes, as shown by longitudinal study of liver stiffness measurement in PBC and PSC patients.[35,43] These results must be confirmed in prospective studies (FICUS study). Among other fibrosis markers, APRI score has been validated as an independent prognostic factor of PBC,[57] and both serum levels of WFA(+)-M2BP and cytokeratin 18 have also shown prognostic ability in this disease.[37,58] For now, no surrogate markers of fibrosis have been found to predict the development of esophageal varices in cholestatic liver diseases. In a nutshell, there is now growing evidence showing that noninvasive markers of liver fibrosis are valid prognostic indicators in chronic cholestatic liver diseases that could reasonably be used as surrogate endpoints in clinical trials.

SUMMARY

Assessing fibrosis is a key step in the prognosis evaluation of PBC and PSC. If liver biopsy is still regarded as a gold standard for these diseases, physicians now have several noninvasive alternative methods to achieve this aim. In PBC, VCTE has the best diagnostic accuracy to detect advanced fibrosis and cirrhosis, followed by APRI score, ELF score, and hyaluronic acid level. In PSC, VCTE is currently the only well-documented noninvasive method of fibrosis assessment. Both VCTE and ELF score have proven prognostic value in PBC and PSC, whereas APRI score and hyaluronic acid level have only in PBC.

REFERENCES

1. Poupon R, Chazouilleres O, Poupon RE. Chronic cholestatic diseases. J Hepatol 2000;32:129–40.
2. Poupon R, Chazouilleres O, Balkau B, et al. Clinical and biochemical expression of the histopathological lesions of primary biliary cirrhosis. J Hepatol 1999;30: 408–12.
3. Shapiro JM, Smith H, Schaffner F. Serum bilirubin: a prognostic factor in primary biliary cirrhosis. Gut 1979;20:137–40.
4. Helzberg JH, Petersen JM, Boyer JL. Improved survival with primary sclerosing cholangitis. A review of clinicopathologic features and comparison of symptomatic and asymptomatic patients. Gastroenterology 1987;92:1869–75.
5. Roll J, Boyer JL, Barry D, et al. The prognostic importance of clinical and histologic features in asymptomatic and symptomatic primary biliary cirrhosis. N Engl J Med 1983;308:1–7.
6. Wiesner RH, Grambsch PM, Dickson ER, et al. Primary sclerosing cholangitis: natural history, prognostic factors and survival analysis. Hepatology 1989;10: 430–6.
7. Dickson ER, Grambsch PM, Fleming TR, et al. Prognosis in primary biliary cirrhosis: model for decision making. Hepatology 1989;10:1–7.
8. Kim WR, Therneau TM, Wiesner RH, et al. A revised natural history model for primary sclerosing cholangitis. Mayo Clin Proc 2000;75:688–94.
9. Corpechot C, Abenavoli L, Rabahi N, et al. Biochemical response to ursodeoxycholic acid and long-term prognosis in primary biliary cirrhosis. Hepatology 2008; 48:871–7.
10. de Vries EM, Verheij J, Hubscher SG, et al. Applicability and prognostic value of histologic scoring systems in primary sclerosing cholangitis. J Hepatol 2015. [Epub ahead of print].

11. Carbone M, Sharpe SJ, Heneghan MA, et al. Histological stage is relevant for risk-stratification in primary biliary cirrhosis. J Hepatol 2015;62:S805.
12. Beuers U, Trauner M, Jansen P, et al. New paradigms in the treatment of hepatic cholestasis: from UDCA to FXR, PXR and beyond. J Hepatol 2015;62:S25–37.
13. Rubin E, Schaffner F, Popper H. Primary biliary cirrhosis. Chronic non-suppurative destructive cholangitis. Am J Pathol 1965;46:387–407.
14. Scheuer P. Primary biliary cirrhosis. Proc R Soc Med 1967;60:1257–60.
15. Ludwig J, Dickson ER, McDonald GS. Staging of chronic nonsuppurative destructive cholangitis (syndrome of primary biliary cirrhosis). Virchows Arch A Pathol Anat Histol 1978;379:103–12.
16. Nakanuma Y, Zen Y, Harada K, et al. Application of a new histological staging and grading system for primary biliary cirrhosis to liver biopsy specimens: Interobserver agreement. Pathol Int 2010;60:167–74.
17. Wendum D, Boelle PY, Bedossa P, et al. Primary biliary cirrhosis: proposal for a new simple histological scoring system. Liver Int 2015;35:652–9.
18. Kakuda Y, Harada K, Sawada-Kitamura S, et al. Evaluation of a new histologic staging and grading system for primary biliary cirrhosis in comparison with classical systems. Hum Pathol 2013;44:1107–17.
19. Bedossa P, Poynard T. An algorithm for the grading of activity in chronic hepatitis C. The METAVIR cooperative study group. Hepatology 1996;24:289–93.
20. Corpechot C, Carrat F, Poupon R, et al. Primary biliary cirrhosis: incidence and predictive factors of cirrhosis development in ursodiol-treated patients. Gastroenterology 2002;122:652–8.
21. Kumagi T, Guindi M, Fischer SE, et al. Baseline ductopenia and treatment response predict long-term histological progression in primary biliary cirrhosis. Am J Gastroenterol 2010;105:2186–94.
22. Mayo MJ, Parkes J, Adams-Huet B, et al. Prediction of clinical outcomes in primary biliary cirrhosis by serum enhanced liver fibrosis assay. Hepatology 2008;48:1549–57.
23. Garrido MC, Hubscher SG. Accuracy of staging in primary biliary cirrhosis. J Clin Pathol 1996;49:556–9.
24. Olsson R, Hagerstrand I, Broome U, et al. Sampling variability of percutaneous liver biopsy in primary sclerosing cholangitis. J Clin Pathol 1995;48:933–5.
25. Engstrom-Laurent A, Loof L, Nyberg A, et al. Increased serum levels of hyaluronate in liver disease. Hepatology 1985;5:638–42.
26. Vaubourdolle M, Gufflet V, Chazouilleres O, et al. Indocyanine green-sulfobromophthalein pharmacokinetics for diagnosing primary biliary cirrhosis and assessing histological severity. Clin Chem 1991;37:1688–90.
27. Imbert-Bismut F, Ratziu V, Pieroni L, et al. Biochemical markers of liver fibrosis in patients with hepatitis C virus infection: a prospective study. Lancet 2001;357:1069–75.
28. Cales P, Oberti F, Michalak S, et al. A novel panel of blood markers to assess the degree of liver fibrosis. Hepatology 2005;42:1373–81.
29. Wai CT, Greenson JK, Fontana RJ, et al. A simple noninvasive index can predict both significant fibrosis and cirrhosis in patients with chronic hepatitis C. Hepatology 2003;38:518–26.
30. Ziol M, Handra-Luca A, Kettaneh A, et al. Noninvasive assessment of liver fibrosis by measurement of stiffness in patients with chronic hepatitis C. Hepatology 2005;41:48–54.
31. Lewin M, Poujol-Robert A, Boelle PY, et al. Diffusion-weighted magnetic resonance imaging for the assessment of fibrosis in chronic hepatitis C. Hepatology 2007;46:658–65.

32. Nyberg A, Engstrom-Laurent A, Loof L. Serum hyaluronate in primary biliary cirrhosis–a biochemical marker for progressive liver damage. Hepatology 1988; 8:142–6.
33. Remmel T, Remmel H, Salupere V. Aminoterminal propeptide of type III procollagen and hyaluronan in patients with primary biliary cirrhosis: markers of fibrosis in primary biliary cirrhosis. J Gastroenterol Hepatol 1996;11:1016–20.
34. Guéchot J, Poupon R, Giral P, et al. Relationship between procollagen III aminoterminal propeptide and hyaluronan serum levels and histological fibrosis in primary biliary cirrhosis and chronic viral hepatitis C. J Hepatol 1994;20:388–93.
35. Corpechot C, Carrat F, Poujol-Robert A, et al. Noninvasive elastography-based assessment of liver fibrosis progression and prognosis in primary biliary cirrhosis. Hepatology 2012;56:198–208.
36. Rosenberg WM, Voelker M, Thiel R, et al. Serum markers detect the presence of liver fibrosis: a cohort study. Gastroenterology 2004;127:1704–13.
37. Umemura T, Joshita S, Sekiguchi T, et al. Serum wisteria floribunda agglutinin-positive Mac-2-binding protein level predicts liver fibrosis and prognosis in primary biliary cirrhosis. Am J Gastroenterol 2015;110:857–64.
38. Corpechot C, Poujol-Robert A, Wendum D, et al. Biochemical markers of liver fibrosis and lymphocytic piecemeal necrosis in UDCA-treated patients with primary biliary cirrhosis. Liver Int 2004;24:187–93.
39. Farkkila M, Rautiainen H, Karkkainen P, et al. Serological markers for monitoring disease progression in noncirrhotic primary biliary cirrhosis on ursodeoxycholic acid therapy. Liver Int 2008;28:787–97.
40. Ma JL, Wang R, Zhang FK, et al. A noninvasive diagnostic model of liver fibrosis using serum markers in primary biliary cirrhosis. Zhonghua Nei Ke Za Zhi 2012; 51:618–22 [in Chinese].
41. Sterling RK, Lissen E, Clumeck N, et al. Development of a simple noninvasive index to predict significant fibrosis in patients with HIV/HCV coinfection. Hepatology 2006;43:1317–25.
42. Floreani A, Cazzagon N, Martines D, et al. Performance and utility of transient elastography and noninvasive markers of liver fibrosis in primary biliary cirrhosis. Dig Liver Dis 2011;43:887–92.
43. Corpechot C, Gaouar F, El Naggar A, et al. Baseline values and changes in liver stiffness measured by transient elastography are associated with severity of fibrosis and outcomes of patients with primary sclerosing cholangitis. Gastroenterology 2014;146:970–9 [quiz: e15–6].
44. Friedrich-Rust M, Ong MF, Martens S, et al. Performance of transient elastography for the staging of liver fibrosis: a meta-analysis. Gastroenterology 2008; 134:960–74.
45. Castera L, Foucher J, Bernard PH, et al. Pitfalls of liver stiffness measurement: a 5-year prospective study of 13,369 examinations. Hepatology 2010;51:828–35.
46. Gomez-Dominguez E, Mendoza J, Garcia-Buey L, et al. Transient elastography to assess hepatic fibrosis in primary biliary cirrhosis. Aliment Pharmacol Ther 2008; 27:441–7.
47. Pfeifer L, Strobel D, Neurath MF, et al. Liver stiffness assessed by acoustic radiation force impulse (ARFI) technology is considerably increased in patients with cholestasis. Ultraschall Med 2014;35:364–7.
48. Meng Y, Liang Y, Liu M. The value of MRI in the diagnosis of primary biliary cirrhosis and assessment of liver fibrosis. PLoS One 2015;10:e0120110.
49. Takeyama Y, Tsuchiya N, Kunimoto H, et al. Gadolinium-ethoxybenzyl-diethylene-triamine pentaacetic acid-enhanced magnetic resonance imaging as a useful

detection method for advanced primary biliary cirrhosis. Hepatol Res 2015. [Epub ahead of print].

50. Kovac JD, Jesic R, Stanisavljevic D, et al. MR imaging of primary sclerosing cholangitis: additional value of diffusion-weighted imaging and ADC measurement. Acta Radiol 2013;54:242–8.

51. Kovac JD, Jesic R, Stanisavljevic D, et al. Integrative role of MRI in the evaluation of primary biliary cirrhosis. Eur Radiol 2012;22:688–94.

52. Toshima T, Shirabe K, Ikegami T, et al. A novel serum marker, glycosylated Wisteria floribunda agglutinin-positive Mac-2 binding protein (WFA(+)-M2BP), for assessing liver fibrosis. J Gastroenterol 2015;50:76–84.

53. Ehlken H, Lohse AW, Schramm C. Transient elastography in primary sclerosing cholangitis-the value as a prognostic factor and limitations. Gastroenterology 2014;147:542–3.

54. Millonig G, Reimann FM, Friedrich S, et al. Extrahepatic cholestasis increases liver stiffness (FibroScan) irrespective of fibrosis. Hepatology 2008;48:1718–23.

55. Poupon RE, Balkau B, Guechot J, et al. Predictive factors in ursodeoxycholic acid-treated patients with primary biliary cirrhosis: role of serum markers of connective tissue. Hepatology 1994;19:635–40.

56. Vesterhus M, Hov JR, Holm A, et al. Enhanced liver fibrosis score predicts transplant-free survival in primary sclerosing cholangitis. Hepatology 2015;62: 188–97.

57. Trivedi PJ, Bruns T, Cheung A, et al. Optimising risk stratification in primary biliary cirrhosis: AST/platelet ratio index predicts outcome independent of ursodeoxycholic acid response. J Hepatol 2014;60:1249–58.

58. Sekiguchi T, Umemura T, Fujimori N, et al. Serum cell death biomarkers for prediction of liver fibrosis and poor prognosis in primary biliary cirrhosis. PLoS One 2015;10:e0131658.

59. Popper H, Schaffner F. Nonsuppurative destructive chronic cholangitis and chronic hepatitis. Prog Liver Dis 1970;3:336–54.

60. Ishak K, Baptista A, Bianchi L, et al. Histological grading and staging of chronic hepatitis. J Hepatol 1995;22:696–9.

61. Alempijevic T, Krstic M, Jesic R, et al. Biochemical markers for non-invasive assessment of disease stage in patients with primary biliary cirrhosis. World J Gastroenterol 2009;15:591–4.

62. Friedrich-Rust M, Muller C, Winckler A, et al. Assessment of liver fibrosis and steatosis in PBC with FibroScan, MRI, MR-spectroscopy, and serum markers. J Clin Gastroenterol 2010;44:58–65.

63. Nyblom H, Bjornsson E, Simren M, et al. The AST/ALT ratio as an indicator of cirrhosis in patients with PBC. Liver Int 2006;26:840–5.

64. Plebani M, Giacomini A, Floreani A, et al. Biochemical markers of hepatic fibrosis in primary biliary cirrhosis. Ric Clin Lab 1990;20:269–74.

65. Nyberg A, Lindqvist U, Engstrom-Laurent A. Serum hyaluronan and aminoterminal propeptide of type III procollagen in primary biliary cirrhosis: relation to clinical symptoms, liver histopathology and outcome. J Intern Med 1992;231:485–91.

66. Voumvouraki A, Koulentaki M, Notas G, et al. Serum surrogate markers of liver fibrosis in primary biliary cirrhosis. Eur J Intern Med 2011;22:77–83.

67. Babbs C, Smith A, Hunt LP, et al. Type III procollagen peptide: a marker of disease activity and prognosis in primary biliary cirrhosis. Lancet 1988;1:1021–4.

68. Niemela O, Risteli L, Sotaniemi EA, et al. Serum basement membrane and type III procollagen-related antigens in primary biliary cirrhosis. J Hepatol 1988;6: 307–14.

69. Friedrich-Rust M, Rosenberg W, Parkes J, et al. Comparison of ELF, FibroTest and FibroScan for the non-invasive assessment of liver fibrosis. BMC Gastroenterol 2010;10:103.
70. Munteanu M, Gaouar F, Corpechot C, et al. Non-invasive assessment of liver fibrosis in primar y biliar y cirrhosis (PBC) patients using transient elastography by fibroscan, fibrotest (FT) and liver biopsy as reference method. Hepatology 2013;58:797A.
71. van Zanten RA, van Leeuwen RE, Wilson JH. Serum procollagen III N-terminal peptide and laminin P1 fragment concentrations in alcoholic liver disease and primary biliary cirrhosis. Clin Chim Acta 1988;177:141–6.
72. Fukutomi T, Sakamoto S, Isobe H, et al. Clinical significance of the serum levels of the 7S domain of type IV collagen in patients with primary biliary cirrhosis. J Gastroenterol Hepatol 1992;7:596–601.
73. Zhang DK, Chen M, Liu Y, et al. Acoustic radiation force impulse elastography for non-invasive assessment of disease stage in patients with primary biliary cirrhosis: a preliminary study. Clin Radiol 2014;69:836–40.
74. Nyblom H, Nordlinder H, Olsson R. High aspartate to alanine aminotransferase ratio is an indicator of cirrhosis and poor outcome in patients with primary sclerosing cholangitis. Liver Int 2007;27:694–9.

Total Parenteral Nutrition–Induced Cholestasis

Prevention and Management

Sue V. Beath, BSc, MB.BS*, Deirdre A. Kelly, MD

KEYWORDS

- PNALD • PNAC • IFALD • Liver disease • Intravenous nutrition • Lipids • Cytokines
- Microbiota

KEY POINTS

- Intestinal failure–associated liver disease (IFALD) encompasses a wide spectrum of disease from steatosis to jaundice, although currently available biochemical monitoring tests are unreliable in detecting pathology such as inflammation and fibrosis in the hepatic parenchyma.
- Improvements in management of IFALD in the past 15 years have led to fewer patients developing end-stage liver failure.
- The management IFALD has been improved by multiprofessional working and better collaborations between expert groups, including surgeons, intestinal rehabilitation teams, and transplant centers.
- The use of line locks and additional hygiene measures for central venous catheters and amelioration in toxicity of PN solutions by addition of fish oil and reductions in omega 6 fats (linoleic acid) has been important in minimizing cholestasis.

INTRODUCTION

Terminology

Total parenteral nutrition (TPN)-induced cholestasis is a description of the onset of liver disease in the context of administration of intravenous nutrition in patients with temporary and/or permanent intestinal failure. Other terms in common usage are:

- Parenteral nutrition–associated cholestasis (PNAC)
- Intestinal failure–associated liver disease (IFALD)
- Parenteral nutrition–associated liver disease (PNALD).

The authors have nothing to disclose.
The Liver Unit, Birmingham Children's Hospital, Steelhouse Lane, Birmingham, West Midlands, B4 6NH, UK
* Corresponding author.
E-mail address: Sue.beath@nhs.net

Clin Liver Dis 20 (2016) 159–176
http://dx.doi.org/10.1016/j.cld.2015.08.009   liver.theclinics.com

All 3 terms are often used interchangeably. IFALD is used in this article because it is a more broadly based term encompassing not only the TPN solutions, but also the patient-related factors that increase the risk of liver disease developing.

Definition

The term TPN-induced cholestasis or IFALD encompasses a wide range of disruption to liver function. It is often defined biochemically as an elevation of liver enzymes 1.5 times the upper limit of normal that persist for at least 6 months (6 weeks in children), in the absence of another cause such as viral hepatitis or drug-induced changes. Detecting TPN-induced cholestasis at this early stage of modest biochemical disturbance depends on regular monitoring, as clinical signs are usually absent. It is important to recognize these biochemical signs of liver stress, so that steps can be taken to prevent progression to more severe forms of liver disease[1] (see Management section later in this article). IFALD has been arbitrarily subdivided according to severity into 3 stages as follows (**Box 1**):

- Mild/early/type 1
- Moderate/established/type 2
- Advanced/late/type 3

Frequency and Spectrum of Disease

Most adults do not progress beyond type 1 IFALD,[2] but those who do may develop significant fibrosis as a consequence of chronic steato-hepatitis.[3] Although it is rare for adult patients to become jaundiced, up to 50% of children become overtly jaundiced (bilirubin in excess of 2 or 3 mg/L) at some point during the administration of TPN[4–6] (**Fig. 1**). Paradoxically some children with ongoing need for TPN may develop fibrosis after an episode of cholestatic jaundice has resolved.[7–9] The absence of a major disturbance to liver function tests does not mean that the hepatic acinus is free of inflammation and fibrosis; a study of the liver histology in 66 children with short bowel syndrome found that 8 had cirrhosis and in 3 of these, there was no biochemical cholestasis.[10] Because it is not always possible to obtain liver histology, other forms of screening and monitoring for liver disease are needed (see later in this article).

Box 1
Criteria for categories of intestinal failure–associated liver disease (IFALD)

Type 1 IFALD is defined as an elevation of liver enzymes alkaline phophatase and γ-glutamyl transferase 1.5 times above upper limit reference range, combined with an echogenic appearance of the liver on ultrasound; and liver histology will show steatosis (up 25% of the acinus) and some periportal fibrosis.

Type 2 IFALD is defined as alkaline phophatase and γ-glutamyl transferase 1.5 times above the normal range, bilirubin 3 to 6 g/L, abdominal ultrasound shows enlarged spleen, liver biopsy will show fatty change (more than 25% of the acinus), fibrosis affecting more than 50% of portal tracts.

Type 3 IFALD is defined when liver function tests are 3 times above normal range, platelet count less than 100×10^9, bilirubin more than 6 g/L, international normalized ratio worse than 1.5, and occurrence of spider naevi, ascites, varices, gastrointestinal bleeding from erosions or varices.

Adapted from Beath S, Pironi L, Gabe S, et al. Collaborative strategies to reduce mortality and morbidity in patients with chronic intestinal failure including those who are referred for small bowel transplantation. Transplantation 2008;85:1379; with permission.

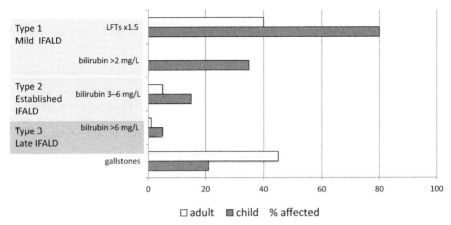

Fig. 1. Categories of IFALD and frequency of disease in children and adults. LFT, liver function test. (*Data from* Refs.[2,5,6,11-13])

However, once the bilirubin has climbed above 6 g/L, as in type 3 IFALD, it is associated with major disruption to the structure and function of the liver. The resistance to blood flow across the sinusoids caused by fibrosis leads to a rise in sinusoidal pressures above 12 mm Hg at which point the spleen enlarges and varices start to form, and ascites becomes more likely.[14] The capacity of hepatocytes to synthesize adequate amounts of albumin and coagulation factors, and respond to glucose, fatty acids, glucagon, and insulin carried to the liver in the portal vein, all become compromised leading to the well-recognized symptoms of end-stage liver disease: ascites, prolonged prothrombin time, hypoglycemia, and hypercholesterolemia.

Gallstones are not associated with a specific stage of IFALD and can develop at any time. They are common in adults,[11] and some centers will perform cholecystectomy electively if it is clear that the patient is going to remain on PN for many years. With home PN becoming more common in children[15] (a fourfold increase has occurred in the United Kingdom between 1995 and 2015) the incidence of cholelithiasis has been reported as 22% (15/67 patients in one program[12]) and a quarter of these children had cholecystectomy because of acute cholangitis after a median of 11.9 years on TPN.[12]

Differences Between Children and Adults in Pathophysiology and Risk Factors for Intestinal Failure–Associated Liver Disease

It hardly needs to be stated that there are a vast number differences between children and adults, but there are some highly relevant distinctions in anatomy and physiology that offer insights into how IFALD develops and explain why children are so much more susceptible to IFALD. These aspects are summarized in **Table 1**.

At birth, the hepatic acinus has not yet acquired the well-ordered adult-pattern sinusoids in which the adult plates of hepatocytes are just 2 cells thick, which allow for optimal transfer of nutrients from incoming portal blood.[16] Absorption of amino acids, glucose, free fatty acids, and subsequent secretion of complex synthesized molecules into blood around the central hepatic vein is relatively inefficient in the first few weeks and months of life. Also, the passage of bilirubin from the sinusoidal surface to the canalicular surface may be incomplete and the immature conjugation reactions also mean that cholestasis is much more likely if any added stress occurs in the first few weeks of life.

Table 1
Comparisons between children and adults and the evolution of intestinal failure–associated liver disease

Parameter	Child	Adult
Anatomy	At birth, hepatocytes are in transition from the fetal organization of plates 3–5 cells thick to the adult pattern of where hepatocytes have a sinusoidal surface over which blood from the portal vein and hepatic artery flows, and a basolateral canalicular surface from which bile is secreted.[16]	Well-developed portal tracts are connected to the central veins by plates of hepatocytes in layers that are 2 cells thick.
Physiology	Impaired transsulfuration in the first few months of life because of lack of cystathionase, especially in preterm infants[17] High energy requirements for growth (80–100 kcal/kg per day)	Normal transsulfuration pathway for methionine is bypassed when amino acids are delivered systemically rather than enterally via the portal vein[16] Energy requirements 20–30 kcal/kg per day
Clinical scenarios associated with IFALD	Prematurity[18] Necrotizing enterocolitis[19] Bowel <25 cm[20]	Malignancy[2,13] Age >40[21] Hepatitis C[3] Bowel <100 cm[13] Crohn disease[22]
Risk factors for IFALD	Lack of taurine[23] Excess calories[21] Excess lipid >3.5 g/kg/d[24] Phytosterols[25] Exposure to soya oil fat emulsions[26] Excess w6 fatty acids[27,28] Catheter infections >3 episodes[5,29] Inflammation in the bowel[30] Lack of ICV[28]	Lack of choline[31] Excess calories[32] Excess lipid >1 g/kg/d[3] Phytosterols[2] Inflammation in the bowel[22] Small bowel bacterial overgrowth[22] Lack of ICV[11]
Histology of IFALD	Cholestasis: frequent Portal fibrosis and bridging Pericellular fibrosis Bile ductular proliferation Pigmented Kupffer cells Nonprogressive cirrhosis[7–10,33]	Steatosis Steatohepatitis Cholestasis rarely[2,34] Fibrosis and cirrhosis rarely
Natural history of IFALD	Septic episodes leading to cholestasis and high risk of hepatic decompensation in first year of life unless risk factors are addressed. Nonprogressive cirrhosis, even when cholestasis resolves[7,9]	Elevated liver enzymes in association with steatosis for years, followed by steatohepatitis in some. Nonprogressive cirrhosis in a small minority. When cholestasis occurs, there is a favorable response to ω-3 supplemented fat emulsions[35]

Abbreviations: ICV, ileo-caecal valve; IFALD, intestinal failure–associated liver disease.

The transsulfuration pathway is an important one in adults and children. In adults, the normal pathway is compromised by the administration of amino acids through a large systemic vein (eg, the subclavian vein) rather than the portal vein, which means that methionine is metabolized in other tissues before eventually reaching the liver via the hepatic artery.[36] Methionine is a precursor for cysteine, serine, and taurine and aids the synthesis of choline and carnitine, all of which are important for ameliorating oxidation events associated with injury and sepsis. In children on TPN, the transsulfuration pathway is further compromised by a relative lack the enzyme cystathionase at birth, which may take many months to reach adult activities.[17]

The requirement for energy for growth in children places them at extra risk from imperfectly balanced intravenous nutrition. The dangers of excess calories are now well recognized and several recently published consensus publications are available containing recommendations on daily amounts of carbohydrates and lipids, with an upper limit of 3.5 g/kg per day of lipid in infants and 1 g/kg per day lipid in adults.[3,21,24]

These key differences in anatomy, hepatocellular physiology, and energy requirements account for many of the observed differences in risk factors, histology, and natural history listed in **Table 1**.

Biological Mechanisms for Intestinal Failure–Associated Liver Disease

There is a complex biology associated with IFALD, and many interesting mechanisms have been proposed in recent years (**Box 2**). These include the concept of a "fibrogenic microbiotome" in which in animal models it has been possible to induce hepatic fibrosis by transplanting the microbiotome from one group of mice with bacterial bowel overgrowth and hepatic fibrosis, to a second group that then develops fibrosis.[37] An overabundance of Lactobacilli, Proteobacteria, and Actinobacteria was observed in the microbiota of a group of 21 patients with intestinal failure and this correlated with steatosis and fibrosis.[38] The role of bacterial overgrowth of Proteobacteria was linked to liver injury via the proinflammatory lipopolysaccharides produced by these bacteria.

Exacerbations of Crohn disease and necrotizing enterocolitis are also associated with inflammation caused by bacterial overgrowth and an increased risk of IFALD,[19,22,45] possibly via the phenomenon of homing of activated gut lymphocytes to the liver. The homing of activated lymphocytes is mediated via vascular adhesion protein 1, which is strongly expressed by hepatic endothelium cells and encourages adhesion of the migrating leukocytes released by an inflamed bowel.[46,47]

The inhibitory effects of endotoxin on bile salt transporters are well described and the secondary effect of cholestasis is ductular proliferation.[30,18] Proliferating cholangiocytes secrete proinflammatory and chemotactic cytokines (interleukin-6 [IL-6], IL-8 and monocyte chemoattractant protein-1), which in turn drive the fibrogenic process.[43] This explains the association of sepsis, especially gram-negative bacteria, which have a large amount of lipopolysaccharide (synonymous with endotoxin), with jaundice and changes to liver histology seen in children. Other cytokines (neopterin, tumor necrosis factor-alpha, soluble IL-2 receptors) are also elevated during inflammatory events, and concentrations of these cytokines correlate with erythrocyte sedimentation rate, and hepatic enzymes gamma glutamyl transferase and alkaline phosphatases.[32]

Intracellular metabolism also plays a role in the evolution of IFALD; for example, inefficient transsulfuration of methionine reduces the supply of choline and carnitine, cysteine, serine, taurine, and glutathione, which act to neutralize free radicals produced during sepsis and may magnify the effects of endotoxin.[17,36] The resilience

Box 2
Biological mechanisms in IFALD

Processes leading to steatosis and fibrosis

- Fibrogenic microbiotome

- Gut inflammation

- Endotoxin/lipopolysaccharide

- Cholestasis

- Short bowel syndrome (SBS)

- Proinflammatory parenteral nutrition (excess w6 lipids)

Inhibition of bile acid transporters by endotoxin (as in sepsis) leads to cholestasis and through TLR4 increased activity of transforming growth factor b1, the most potent fibrogenic cytokine to activate hepatic stellate cells[39]

Disrupted enterohepatic circulation in SBS and lack of fibroblast growth factor-19 results in reduced Farnesoid X, which in turn causes lipogenesis and bile salt synthesis to continue unchecked[40–42]

Impaired transsulfuration, reduced anti-oxidant reserve, endoplasmic reticulum stress triggers cell death and promotion of fibrosis.[31,36,43,44]

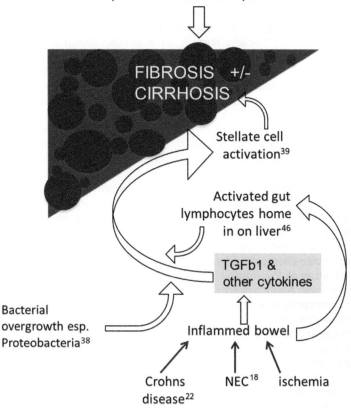

Cholestasis causes cholangiocyte proliferation which induces Il-6, IL-8 and monocyte chemo attractant protein-1 and TGFb1 cytokines[33,43]

FIBROSIS +/- CIRRHOSIS

Stellate cell activation[39]

Activated gut lymphocytes home in on liver[46]

TGFb1 & other cytokines

Bacterial overgrowth esp. Proteobacteria[38]

Inflammed bowel

Crohns disease[22]   NEC[18]   ischemia

of the endoplasmic reticulum (ER) may also be important; this was evaluated by measuring the glucose-regulated chaperone protein 94 (GRP94 is a member of the heat shock protein 90 family contributing to protein folding in the ER) in a rabbit model of IFALD,[49] and then in archived liver tissue from 20 adult patients with early and late IFALD and normal liver (n = 3). Much higher mean relative RNA levels of ER stress markers (GRP 78 and ERDj4) were found in those with advanced IFALD.[44]

The disrupted enterohepatic circulation and the reduced levels of the ileal fibroblast growth factor-19 (FGF-19) found in short bowel syndrome are other mechanisms for inducing fibrosis and IFALD.[40] FGF-19 appears to be important in the activation of the nuclear transcription factor receptor Farnesoid X (FXR), and because FXR inhibits lipogenesis and bile salt synthesis,[41,42] its relative lack in short bowel syndrome may be key to the development of steatosis and fibrosis seen in IFALD.[50]

Cytokine activation of stellate cells combined with immature or depleted antioxidant capacity appears to be the common pathway to hepatic fibrosis (see **Box 2**).[39]

PREVENTION

Recent studies demonstrate that severe IFALD type 3 can be prevented.[51–54] The prevalence of mild type 1 IFALD remains unchanged,[6] but the number of children and adults requiring liver and bowel transplantation has decreased.[55] This has occurred for a myriad of reasons, which include better appreciation of high-risk clinical scenarios, a willingness to change PN prescriptions when early signs of IFALD are detected, and improved care of the feeding catheters.

In addition to the high-risk clinical scenarios and risk factors that are listed in **Table 1**, the following features should put clinicians on alert for IFALD: dysmotility, especially if it makes enteral feeding impossible[12,56]; lack of ileocecal valve; ultrashort bowel; comorbid conditions; physiologic immaturity; and need for emergency abdominal surgery.[2,28,29,32]

Monitoring

The key to preventing IFALD is in early detection of liver dysfunction through focused monitoring, but because the standard liver function tests are neither discriminatory nor totally reliable,[7–10] better methods are required (**Table 2**). Furthermore, these tests do not quantify fibrosis or measure dynamic liver function until in advanced liver failure when rising prothrombin time and lactate are associated with imminent mortality.

Tests that measure the functional reserve of the liver are in development and are promising because they correlate well with liver functional capacity and provide a tool to evaluate new interventions, as well as a means of staging IFALD more precisely. For example, [13 C] methionine breath test (13 C-MBT) has been used to evaluate the methionine oxidative capacity of the liver by detecting the carbon 13 isotope enrichment of expired air after injecting 2 mg/kg intravenous dose of 13 C-MBT.[57] In a group of 14 children with IFALD and liver histology available, the 13 C-MBT differentiated those with cirrhosis (n = 5) from those with fibrosis/cholestasis only (n = 9) at a significance level of $P = .04$.[57] Follow-up tests with 13 C-MBTs in 5 patients found a relationship between changing pediatric end-stage liver disease scores and 13 C-MBTs.

The important role of inflammation in the genesis of IFALD means that monitoring inflammatory markers such as erythrocyte sedimentation rate (ESR) may be useful. In a study of 17 adult patients, the ESR and tumor necrosis factor-alpha (but not C-reactive protein) were found to correlate with alkaline phosphatase, and soluble IL-2 receptor and tumor necrosis factor-alpha correlated with gamma glutamyl transferase.[32]

Abdominal ultrasound can be useful in detecting increased echogenicity in livers with steatosis, gall stones, and biliary sludge and in tracking an enlarging spleen in portal hypertension, particularly in children, and it is good practice to carry out an annual abdominal ultrasound when following patients on home TPN.[12]

Table 2
Intestinal failure–associated liver disease monitoring methodologies compared

Methodology	Advantages	Disadvantages
Liver function tests in serum	Cheap and convenient Well standardized	Do not always correlate with fibrosis; may underestimate liver disease; bilirubin fluctuates widely according to sepsis and inflammatory states
Prothrombin time	Cheap and convenient Well standardized	Detects end-stage liver disease, not helpful for monitoring early or mild IFALD
Inflammatory markers ESR, Tumor necrosis factor-α[32]	ESR is cheap Tumor necrosis factor-α is a useful marker for research studies	ESR is sensitive but not specific to IFALD Tumor necrosis factor-α is still being evaluated as a clinical tool
Serum markers of collagen synthesis[a]	Relatively cheap Correlates with fibrosis better than LFTs/bilirubin	Not yet standardized for use in IFALD Still being evaluated as a clinical tool
[13 C] methionine breath test[57]	Provides a more precise measure of metabolic capacity of the liver Can differentiate between fibrosis and cirrhosis	The carbon-labeled methionine has to be injected, although this can be done via CVL in patients on TPN Not yet standardized for use in IFALD Still being evaluated as a clinical tool
Abdominal ultrasound	Noninvasive Well standardized, can detect biliary sludge and gall stones Indirect measures of portal hypertension (spleen size) and echogenicity of liver	Requires sonographic expertise Moderately expensive to perform
FibroScan	Noninvasive, sound attenuation correlates well with fibrosis Less sonographic expertise required	Not yet standardized for use in IFALD; still being evaluated as a clinical tool; high capital costs
CT	CT provides good quantification of established steatosis	Radiation exposure in CT not as accurate in detecting grade 1 steatosis Signal may be affected by excess iron and glycogen amiodarone and methotrexate
MRI	MRI can evaluate the entire liver within a short breath hold	Not as accurate as MRS Not yet standardized for use in IFALD; still being evaluated as a clinical tool; high capital costs

(continued on next page)

Table 2 (continued)		
Methodology	Advantages	Disadvantages
MRS[58–60]	MRS has a higher diagnostic accuracy than US or CT and shows best correlation with the results of liver biopsy	Expensive, acquisition and analysis of MRS information requires expertise and is time-consuming and complex Single-voxel MRS acquires data from a small portion of the liver and may be subject to sampling error
Liver biopsy	Provides detailed information on severity and structural changes in IFALD	Invasive Risk of bleeding May be subject to sampling error

Abbreviations: CT, computed tomography; CVL, central venous line; ESR, erythrocyte sedimentation rate; IFALD, intestinal failure–associated liver disease; LFT, liver function test; MRS, multiple resonance spectroscopy; TPN, total parenteral nutrition; US, ultrasound.
[a] Cytokeratin 18 fragment levels, hyaluronic acid, matrix metalloproteinase 9.
From Mansoor S, Collyer E, Alkhouri N. A comprehensive review of noninvasive liver fibrosis tests in pediatric nonalcoholic Fatty liver disease. Curr Gastroenterol Rep 2015;17:447; with permission.

Another approach to quantifying fibrosis without resorting to liver biopsy is the use of a specialized sound wave emitted by a FibroScan, which becomes attenuated in the presence of fatty tissue and fibrosis. Liver biopsy may still be required if there is diagnostic uncertainty, but the noninvasive nature of FibroScan (Echosens, France) makes it useful for repeat evaluations in patients with nonalcoholic liver disease as well as IFALD.[59]

Computed tomography, MRI, and magnetic resonance spectroscopy (MRS) have been used to evaluate hepatic changes in IFALD. MRI and MRS avoid irradiation, but the technique is still in the evaluation stage and may not come into routine use because it is relatively expensive and difficult to do in young children.[60] A study in mice showed a good correlation between the MRS signal (using the liver-to-muscle ratio) and hydroxyproline, $r = 0.89$ (ie, collagen), as well as standard Ishak fibrosis scoring of liver biopsy material.[61]

Dedicated Expert Teams

Expert teams dedicated to the welfare of patients on TPN have made a big difference by ensuring that the PN prescription is reviewed and deficiencies of conditionally essential amino acids, taurine and choline, are avoided. The nutrition support team can also provide training in the care of feeding catheter, which reduces the rate of blood stream infections and lead on establishing enteral nutrition that protects the patient from hepatobiliary disease.[28,51,62]

The involvement of dedicated vascular access teams[63] is associated with improved clinical outcomes and their role has been endorsed in a report from Centers for Disease Control and Prevention.[64] Injury to veins minimized through the use of ultrasound for insertion and adherence to recommended hygiene practices has reduced the number of injuries to the cannulated vein (2.4%), and catheter-related bloodstream infections (CRBSIs) fell to 3.16 per 1000 line days in hospitalized children compared with twice this rate of infection.[65]

MANAGEMENT

The management of IFALD should be considered in 3 phases that parallel the stage and severity of IFALD types 1 to 3 (**Table 3**). The general principles are as follows:

- Exclusion of other relevant etiology; for example, biliary obstruction, genetic cholestatic syndromes, viral hepatitis, autoimmune hepatitis, endocrine disorders, drug reactions, and malignancy.
- Screen for sepsis, especially CRBSIs, and treat bacterial overgrowth of the bowel.
- Review the PN prescription: reduce exposure to soybean-derived lipids.
- Attempt rehabilitation: assess potential for advancing enteral nutrition. If enteral nutrition is not possible, evaluate causes such as strictures or dilated dysmotile bowel.

Sepsis

Managing sepsis and the associated systemic inflammatory response is an important and effective way of minimizing IFALD. Infections are particularly damaging in preterm infants and young children.[19,29,73] In a mouse model of bacterial overgrowth in the small bowel, rifaximin treatment led to reversal of fibrosis and angiogenesis, and reduction in portal pressure.[45] In humans, biochemical cholestasis was reversed when the bowel was decontaminated with metronidazole.[22,30]

Components of Parenteral Nutrition

Calories and amino acids

The PN prescription should be scrutinized regularly, even if liver biochemical tests are normal. A link with excess calories and IFALD has been reported many times,[3,32] and expert opinion from Europe[24] and North America[21] advises that exposure to lipid and overall calories be restricted to prevent IFALD. The ideal infusion to start in neonates is not settled, but PN containing added taurine and not too much carbohydrate is recommended.[21,23] In adults, added choline appears to protect from IFALD, especially those with no enteral source of nutrition.[31]

Lipids and fish oil

Adults on long-term PN may benefit from lipid limited to 1 g/kg per day.[3] For patients who become cholestatic, there are numerous case series, mainly in children, demonstrating that fish oils (either Omegaven (Fresenius Kabi, Germany) or multisource lipids) are associated with resolution of jaundice, and this strategy also seems to be useful in reducing hepatobiliary disease.[54,69,74–76] The prevalence of biliary sludge was significantly more likely in children who received pure soya lipid ($P = .01$).[12] In adults, researchers reported on a relatively small cohort of 15 patents who demonstrated improvements in biochemistry and histology within 4 weeks when their lipid source was switched from soybean to one containing omega 3 poly-unsaturated fatty acids.[35] A larger study of 94 liver transplant recipients who received PN postoperatively also suggested that omega 3 lipids were useful in conditions of stress for the liver, such as engraftment and reperfusion.[77] The patients (n = 33) who had part of their intralipid substituted with Omegaven, 10%, 2 mL/kg per day had significantly better alanine aminotransferase levels on day 9 after transplantation, reduced injury of the transplanted liver (less inflammatory cells in sinusoids and less hepatocyte ballooning on day 9), decreases in the incidence of infections, and shortened posttransplant hospital stay, when compared with patients who received standard PN (Intralipid [Baxter Healthcare Inc, USA]) (n = 33) and enterally fed patients (n = 32).

Table 3
Management of intestinal failure–associated liver disease

IFALD – Type 1 ALP & GGT Raised; Bilirubin <3 mg/dL	IFALD – Type 2 Bilirubin 3–6 mg/dL	IFALD – Type 3 Portal Hypertension; Bilirubin >6 mg/dL
Exclude primary liver disease (examine stool pigmentation, Abdo USS, markers for genetic cholestatic syndromes, endocrine disorders, viral hepatitis, autoimmune hepatitis, drug reactions)	*Screen for infection and treat* as indicated, consider replacement of feeding catheter	*May fulfill criteria for isolated liver transplant[56] for children with a realistic chance of achieving intestinal autonomy:*
Give antibiotics if infection likely	*Review hygiene measures* for feeding catheter; consider line lock[64]	Infants <2 y
Review PN prescription – use amino acid solutions containing taurine[23] or choline.[31]	*Discuss with NST to reduce overexposure to PN* calories[21,24]	IFALD (SBR >8.8 mg/dL)
Reduce exposure to lipid and/or switch to emulsion containing less linoleic acid (w6 18:2)	*Limit lipids* – consider emulsion with enhanced tocopherol or enriched with w3 fish oils[19,54,69]	>30 cm functional small bowel remaining intact
Commence enteral nutrition unless concerns about NEC[19,66]	*Consider stopping lipid* infusions for 1–2 wk[52]	>50% daily calorie requirement has been tolerated enterally at some time point before listing
Start *ursodeoxycholic acid* p.o.[67]	*Consider surgical strategies* to enhance intestinal rehabilitation[20,51,70,71]	*Or liver and small bowel transplant[72]:* Children/adults with severely diseased bowel and unacceptable morbidity despite interventions from intestinal rehabilitation MDT team;
Start *cycling PN* as soon as feasible[53]	*Treat possible intestinal bacterial overgrowth* with metronidazole p.o. or neomycin p.o. for 2–4 wk[22,30]	Thrombosis of 3 of 4 upper body central veins;
If enteral nutrition not progressing despite absence of intestinal obstruction *consider trial of erythromycin* for dysmotility[68]	*Consult specialist center* for advice about intestinal rehabilitation, and suitability of liver +/– small bowel Tx[5,20,51]	Persistent hyperbilirubinemia >4.4 mg/dL μmol/L despite lipid strategies:
		Necessity for 2 or more ITU admissions to resuscitate as a result of complications of intestinal failure (infective, fluid balance problems, liver disease)

Abbreviations: Abdo USS, abdominal ultrasound; IFALD, intestinal failure–associated liver disease; ITU, intensive therapy unit; MDT, multi-disciplinary team; NEC, necrotizing enterocolitis; NST, nutrition support team; PN, parenteral nutrition; Tx, transplant.

The role of fish oils in neonates is still being debated[78] and so far no clear benefits have been shown in the short term, although the fish oil emulsions containing a blend of soybean-medium chain triglyceride-olive-fish oil did improve the docosahexaenoic acid in plasma and red cell membranes. However, there are concerns that these infusions provide an overdose of eicosapentaenoic acid (EPA), which may improve pulmonary vasodilation, but at the same time a high EPA status is associated with lower arachidonic acid, which may lead to poorer growth.[79]

In summary, although progression in liver histology cannot be ruled out, the use of fish oils[18,21,24,35,80] and/or reducing overall exposure to omega 6 fats (linoleic acid) found in soy-based infusions[27] is now established practice outside the neonatal period.

Multiprofessional Working

Active management of intestinal failure is essential and should include supervision by a dietician familiar with intestinal failure and a weaning plan for those with short bowel syndrome and strategies to limit hours per day spent receiving PN for all patients with intestinal failure.[54,81] Patients who are not progressing with their enteral nutrition should have intestinal obstruction excluded (or treated surgically if feasible) and symptoms of dysmotility, in the absence of obstruction should be treated with a trial of high-dose erythromycin 12.5 mg/kg per dose.[68]

It is important to avoid intestinal stasis and in combination with encouraging enteral nutrition (by naso-enteral tube if necessary), multidisciplinary review involving the surgical team is advisable so that stomas can be closed as early as possible, and where dysmotile dilated loops of bowel are present, these can be treated with an serial transverse enteroplasty procedure or autologous bowel-lengthening procedures.[20,70,71]

Reducing Intestinal Failure–Associated Liver Disease Through Improvements in Central Venous Catheter Care

The use of a 2% chlorhexidine wash for daily skin cleansing to reduce CRBSI[82] has been endorsed by the Healthcare Infection Control Practices Advisory Committee[64] and the valuable role of the nutrition support team in education of staff and patients about the care of central venous lines[51,82] has been shown to reduce the incidence of CRBSI. There have been several useful developments in the CRBSI prophylaxis, especially in patients who have recurrent infections. These consist of sterilizing solutions, such as ethanol, Taurolidine,[83] and antimicrobials, such vancomycin, which are injected into the dead space of the feeding catheter and left in situ until the line is next used to administer the intravenous nutrition. In a study of more than 200 adult patients, the use of Taurolidine was associated with a fivefold reduction in the incidence of CRBSI.[84]

Intestinal Transplantation

The improvements in management of IFALD, which have led to a change in natural history of IFALD in the past 15 years, has affected the numbers of children and adults being listed for intestinal transplantation.[55] The criteria for intestinal transplantation are also under review. In Canada, the Group for Improvement of Intestinal Function and Treatment (GIFT)[72] has been able to use their comparatively large database and evaluated clinical risk factors for poor outcome (ie, death on the wait list) in children looked after in the old era (n = 99; until 2001) and children who have benefited from improvements in the management of intestinal failure since 2001 (n = 91). They found that ultra-short bowel is no longer a predictor of poor outcome, and the positive predictive power of advanced cholestasis (bilirubin >100 mmol/L or 5.8 mg/dL) has dropped from 64% (odds ratio 12.7) in the old era to 42% (odds ratio 4.7) in the current era.

Table 4
Proposed new transplant criteria for a new era of intestinal failure–associated liver disease

Transplant Criterion	Sensitivity	Specificity	OR	P Value[a]
2 admissions to ICU	26	98	23.6	.0001
Loss of 3 CVC sites	17	100	33.3	.0003
Persistently elevated conjugated bilirubin (>75 mmol/L) following 6 wk of lipid strategies	67	92	24.0	.0003

Abbreviations: CVC, central venous catheter; ICU, intensive care unit.
[a] Chi squared and odds ratio.
Data from Burghaardt KM, Wales PW, de Silva N, et al. Pediatric intestinal transplant listing criteria – a call for a change in the new era of intestinal failure outcomes. Am J Transplant 2015;15:1674–81.

By combining risk factors in the current era, the GIFT team was able to predict death or transplantation in 98% of patients when 2 of the 3 criteria were fulfilled (**Table 4**). Of the 3 criteria, admission to intensive care and loss of 3 central venous access sites had a relatively low specificity (26% and 17%, respectively) and it should be borne in mind that the median age of the patients studied was 12 months and they were all younger than 2 years. These criteria will need wider evaluation with larger numbers, but are an important contribution to the evolving criteria for intestinal transplantation.

Isolated Liver Transplantation in Intestinal Failure–Associated Liver Disease

The role of isolated liver transplantation in IFALD is somewhat controversial. It is a rare operation reserved for the infant with short bowel syndrome who has developed rapidly progressive liver failure who was previously making good progress weaning from PN and judged likely to become independent of PN.[85,86] Criteria for isolated liver transplantation in intestinal failure based on the post liver transplant outcomes of the coexisting intestinal failure are described by Dell-Olio and colleagues.[56]

SUMMARY

The advances in neonatal care and surgery in the past half century have contributed to a steep rise in children receiving PN and also to their long-term survival, when once such an outcome would have been impossible.[15,87] The rise in numbers of adults on long-term home PN has not been as great, but currently adults outnumber the children on long-term PN by approximately 4 to 1 in the United Kingdom.

Adults are less likely to develop TPN-induced cholestasis, and most reports of IFALD are in the context of pediatrics. The susceptibility of children to IFALD is related to a long list of factors of which the most important are prematurity, need for abdominal surgery, necrotizing enterocolitis, and infections, especially CRBSIs,[17,18,26,29,88] and all have in common an inflammatory pathway leading to fibrosis with or without cholestasis. Institutional factors, such as access to a nutrition support team and dedicated venous access team, also influence the risk of complications such as IFALD.[28,51,57,63–65,82]

IFALD is still the main indication for intestinal transplantation and has been the subject of numerous reviews.[1,21,24,26,72,87] IFALD is not a single entity but a continuum from mild reversible disease designated type 1 IFALD, to severe irreversible and life-threatening end-stage liver failure type 3 IFALD. The natural history of IFALD has changed in the past decade with fewer children and adults developing type 3 IFALD as a result of better monitoring and more active management of PN solutions[89] and promoting enteral feeding. Although IFALD may have changed, there is still the possibility that children and adults will develop a slowly developing hepatic cirrhosis in the coming decades,[7–9] and if patients on long-term TPN are to avoid liver transplantation (with or with bowel), then care provided for patients on intravenous nutrition should continue to be critically evaluated and improved.

REFERENCES

1. Beath S, Pironi L, Gabe S, et al. Collaborative strategies to reduce mortality and morbidity in patients with chronic intestinal failure including those who are referred for small bowel transplantation. Transplantation 2008;85:1378–84.
2. Gabe SM. Lipids and liver dysfunction in patients receiving parenteral nutrition. Curr Opin Clin Nutr Metab Care 2013;16:150–5.
3. Cavicchi M, Beau P, Crenn P, et al. Prevalence of liver disease and contributing factors in patients receiving home parenteral nutrition for permanent intestinal failure. Ann Intern Med 2000;132:525–32.
4. Kelly DA. Liver complications of pediatric parenteral nutrition-epidemiology. Nutrition 1998;14:153–7.
5. Gupte GL, Beath SV, Kelly DA, et al. Current issues in the management of intestinal failure. Arch Dis Child 2006;91:259–64.
6. Lauriti G, Zani A, Aufieri R, et al. Incidence, prevention, and treatment of parenteral nutrition-associated cholestasis and intestinal failure-associated liver disease in infants and children: a systematic review. JPEN J Parenter Enteral Nutr 2014;38:70–85.
7. Mercer DF, Hobson BD, Fischer RT, et al. Hepatic fibrosis persists and progresses despite biochemical improvement in children treated with intravenous fish oil emulsion. J Pediatr Gastroenterol Nutr 2013;56:364–9.
8. Matsumoto CS, Kaufman SS, Island ER, et al. Hepatic explant pathology of pediatric intestinal transplant recipients previously treated with omega-3 fatty acid lipid emulsion. J Pediatr 2014;165:59–64.
9. Nandivada P, Chang MI, Potemkin AK, et al. The natural history of cirrhosis from parenteral nutrition-associated liver disease after resolution of cholestasis with parenteral fish oil therapy. Ann Surg 2015;261:172–9.
10. Fitzgibbons SC, Jones BA, Hull MA, et al. Relationship between biopsy-proven parenteral nutrition-associated liver fibrosis and biochemical cholestasis in children with short bowel syndrome. J Pediatr Surg 2010;45:95–9.
11. Nightingale J, Woodward JM. Guidelines for the management of patients with short bowel. Gut 2006;55(Suppl iv):1–12.
12. Pichler J, Watson T, McHugh K, et al. Prevalence of gallstones compared in children with different intravenous lipids. J Pediatr Gastroenterol Nutr 2015;61(2):253–9.
13. Lumen W, Shaffer JL. Prevalence, outcome and associated factors of deranged liver function tests in patients on home parenteral nutrition. Clin Nutr 2002;21:337–43.
14. McKiernan P, Abdel-Hady M. Advances in the management of childhood with portal hypertension. Expert Rev Gastroenterol Hepatol 2015;9(5):575–83.
15. Barclay AR, Henderson P, Gowen H, et al, BIFS Collaborators. The continued rise of paediatric home parenteral nutrition use: implications for service and the improvement of longitudinal data collection. Clin Nutr 2014. [Epub ahead of print].
16. Malhi H, Irani AN, Gagandeep S, et al. Isolation of human progenitor liver epithelial cells with extensive replication capacity and differentiation into mature hepatocytes. J Cell Sci 2002;115:2679–88.

17. Vina J, Vento M, Garcia-Sale F, et al. L-cysteine and glutathione metabolism are impaired in premature infants due to cystathionase deficiency. Am J Clin Nutr 1995;61:1067–9.
18. Hsieh MH, Pai W, Tseng HI, et al. Parenteral nutrition-associated cholestasis in premature babies: risk factors and predictors. Pediatr Neonatol 2009;50: 202–7.
19. Teng J, Arnell H, Bohlin K, et al. Impact of parenteral fat composition on cholestasis in pre-term neonates. J Pediatr Gastroenterol Nutr 2015;60:703–7.
20. Sudan D, DiBaise J, Torres C, et al. A multidisciplinary approach to the treatment of intestinal failure. J Gastrointest Surg 2005;9:165–76.
21. Wales PW, Allen N, Worthington P, et al, the American Society for Parenteral and Enteral Nutrition. A.S.P.E.N. clinical guidelines: support of pediatric patients with intestinal failure at risk of parenteral nutrition-associated liver disease. JPEN J Parenter Enteral Nutr 2014;38:538–57.
22. Capron JP, Herve MA, Gineston JL, et al. Metronidazole in prevention of cholestasis associated with total parenteral nutrition. Lancet 1983;26:446–7.
23. Spencer AU, Yu S, Tracy TF, et al. Parenteral nutrition-associated cholestasis in neonates: multivariate analysis of the potential protective effect of taurine. JPEN J Parenter Enteral Nutr 2005;29:337–43.
24. Lacaille F, Gupte G, Colomb V, et al. Intestinal failure-associated liver disease. A position paper by the ESPGHAN working group of intestinal failure and intestinal transplantation. J Pediatr Gastroenterol Nutr 2015;60:272–83.
25. Mutanen A, Nissinen MJ, Lohi J, et al. Serum plant sterols, cholestanol, and cholesterol precursors associated with histological liver injury in pediatric onset intestinal failure. Am J Clin Nutr 2014;100:1085–94.
26. Hess RA, Welch KB, Brown PI, et al. Survival outcomes of pediatric intestinal failure patients: analysis of factors contributing to improved survival over the past two decades. J Surg Res 2011;170:27–31.
27. Khan FA, Fisher JG, Sparks EA, et al. Preservation of biochemical liver function with low-dose soy-based lipids in children with intestinal failure-associated liver disease. J Pediatr Gastroenterol Nutr 2015;60(3):375–7.
28. Goulet O, Ruemmele F. Causes and management of intestinal failure in children. Gastroenterology 2006;130(2 Suppl 1):16–28.
29. Hermans D, Talbotec C, Lacaille F, et al. Early central catheter infection may contribute to hepatic fibrosis in children receiving long-term parenteral nutrition. J Pediatr Gastroenterol Nutr 2007;44:459–63.
30. Kubota A, Okada A, Imura K, et al. The effect of metronidazole on TPN-associated liver dysfunction in neonates. J Pediatr Surg 1990;25:618–21.
31. Buchman AL, Ament ME, Sohel M, et al. Choline deficiency causes reversible hepatic abnormalities in patients receiving parenteral nutrition: proof of a human choline requirement: a placebo-controlled trial. JPEN J Parenter Enteral Nutr 2001;25(5):260–8.
32. Reimund JM, Duclos B, Arondel Y, et al. Persistent inflammation and immune activation contribute to cholestasis in patients receiving home parenteral nutrition. Nutrition 2001;17:300–4.
33. Beath SV, Needham SJ, Kelly DA, et al. Clinical features and prognosis of children assessed for isolated small bowel (ISBTx) or combined small bowel and liver transplantation (CSBLTx). J Pediatr Surg 1997;32:459–61.
34. Tulikoura I, Huikuri K. Morphological fatty changes and function of the liver, serum free fatty acids and triglycerides during parenteral nutrition. Scand J Gastroenterol 1982;17:177–85.

35. Xu Z, Li Y, Wang J, et al. Effect of omega-3 polyunsaturated fatty acids to reverse biopsy-proven parenteral nutrition-associated liver disease in adults. Clin Nutr 2012;31:217–23.

36. Buchman AL, Iyer K, Fryer J. Parenteral nutrition-associated liver disease and the role of isolated intestine and intestine/liver transplantation. Hepatology 2006;43: 9–19.

37. De Minicis S, Rychlicki C, Agostinelli L, et al. Dysbiosis contributes to fibrogenesis in the course of chronic liver injury in mice. Hepatology 2014;59: 1738–49.

38. Korpela K, Mutanen A, Salonen A, et al. Intestinal microbiota signatures associated with histological liver steatosis in pediatric-onset intestinal failure. JPEN J Parenter Enteral Nutr 2015. [Epub ahead of print].

39. Lee YA, Wallace MC, Friedman SL. Pathobiology of liver fibrosis: a translational success story. Gut 2015;64:830–41.

40. Mutanen A, Lohi J, Heikkilä P, et al. Loss of ileum decreases serum fibroblast growth factor 19 in relation to liver inflammation and fibrosis in pediatric onset intestinal failure. J Hepatol 2015;62(6):1391–7.

41. Ali AH, Carey EJ, Lindor KD, et al. Recent advances in the development of farnesoid X receptor agonists. Ann Transl Med 2015;3:5.

42. Legry V, Schaap FG, Delire B, et al. Yin Yang 1 and farnesoid X receptor: a balancing act in non-alcoholic fatty liver disease. Gut 2014;63:1–2.

43. Svegliati-Baroni G, De Minicis S, Marzioni M. Hepatic fibrogenesis in response to chronic liver injury: novel insights on the role of cell-to-cell interaction and transition. Liver Int 2008;28(8):1052–64.

44. Sharkey LM, Davies SE, Kaser A, et al. Endoplasmic reticulum stress is implicated in intestinal failure-associated liver disease. JPEN J Parenter Enteral Nutr 2015. [Epub ahead of print].

45. Zhu Q, Zou L, Jagavelu K, et al. Intestinal decontamination inhibits TLR4 dependent fibronectin-mediated cross-talk between stellate cells and endothelial cells in liver fibrosis in mice. J Hepatol 2012;56:893–9.

46. Lalor PF, Sun PJ, Weston CJ, et al. Activation of vascular adhesion protein-1 on liver endothelium results in an NF-kappaB-dependent increase in lymphocyte adhesion. Hepatology 2007;45:465–74.

47. Welham ML. VAP-1: a new anti-inflammatory target? Blood 2004;103:3250–1.

48. Kosters A, Karpen SJ. The role of inflammation in cholestasis: clinical and basic aspects. Semin Liver Dis 2010;30:186–94.

49. Zhu X, Xiao Z, Chen X, et al. Parenteral nutrition-associated liver injury and increased GRP94 expression prevented by w-3 fish oil based lipid emulsion supplementation. J Pediatr Gastroenterol Nutr 2014;59:708–13.

50. Pereira-Fantini PM, Lapthorne S, Joyce SA, et al. Altered FXR signalling is associated with bile acid dysmetabolism in short bowel syndrome-associated liver disease. J Hepatol 2014;61:1115–25.

51. Torres C, Sudan D, Vanderhoof J, et al. Role of an intestinal rehabilitation program in the treatment of advanced intestinal failure. J Pediatr Gastroenterol Nutr 2007; 45:204–12.

52. Jakobsen MS, Jørgensen MH, Husby S, et al. Low-fat, high-carbohydrate parenteral nutrition (PN) may potentially reverse liver disease in long-term PN-dependent infants. Dig Dis Sci 2015;60:252–9.

53. Jensen AR, Goldin AB, Koopmeiners JS, et al. The association of cyclic parenteral nutrition and decreased incidence of cholestatic liver disease in patients with gastroschisis. J Pediatr Surg 2009;44:183–9.

54. Muhammed R, Bremner R, Protheroe S, et al. Resolution of parenteral nutrition-associated jaundice on changing from a soybean oil emulsion to a complex mixed-lipid emulsion. J Pediatr Gastroenterol Nutr 2012;54:797–802.
55. Grant D, Abu-Elmagd K, Mazariegos G, et al, Intestinal Transplant Association. Intestinal transplant registry report: global activity and trends. Am J Transplant 2015;15:210–9.
56. Dell Olio D, Beath SV, de VilledeGoyet J, et al. Isolated liver transplant in infants with short bowel syndrome: insights into outcomes and prognostic factors. J Pediatr Gastroenterol Nutr 2009;48:334–40.
57. Duro D, Fitizgibbons S, Valim C, et al. [13C]Methionine breath test to assess intestinal failure-associated liver disease. Pediatr Res 2010;68(4):349–54.
58. Cowles RA, Ventura KA, Martinez M, et al. Reversal of intestinal failure-associated liver disease in infants and children on parenteral nutrition: experience with 93 patients at a referral center for intestinal rehabilitation. J Pediatr Surg 2010;45:84–7.
59. Mansoor S, Collyer E, Alkhouri N. A comprehensive review of noninvasive liver fibrosis tests in pediatric nonalcoholic fatty liver disease. Curr Gastroenterol Rep 2015;17:447.
60. Koplay M, Sivri M, Erdogan H, et al. Importance of imaging and recent developments in diagnosis of nonalcoholic fatty liver disease. World J Hepatol 2015;7:769–76.
61. Fuchs BC, Wang H, Yang Y, et al. Molecular MRI of collagen to diagnose and stage liver fibrosis. J Hepatol 2013;59:992–8.
62. Puntis JW, Holden CE, Smallman S, et al. Staff training: a key factor in reducing intravascular catheter sepsis. Arch Dis Child 1991;66:335–7.
63. Brunelle D. Impact of a dedicated infusion therapy team on the reduction of catheter-related nosocomial infections. J Infus Nurs 2003;26:362–6.
64. O'Grady NP, Alexander M, Burns LA, et al. Guidelines for the prevention of intravascular catheter-related infections. Centers for Disease Control and Prevention. MMWR Recomm Rep 2011;51:1–82.
65. Arul GS, Lewis N, Bromley P, et al. Ultrasound-guided percutaneous insertion of Hickman lines in children. Prospective study of 500 consecutive procedures. J Pediatr Surg 2009;44:1371–6.
66. Brown MR, Thunberg BJ, Golub L, et al. Decreased cholestasis with enteral instead of intravenous protein in the very low-birth-weight infant. J Pediatr Gastroenterol Nutr 1989;9:21–7.
67. Arslanoglu S, Moro GF, Tauschel HD, et al. Ursodeoxycholic acid treatment in preterm infants: a pilot study for the prevention of cholestasis associated with total parenteral nutrition. J Pediatr Gastroenterol Nutr 2008;46:228–31.
68. Ng PC, Lee CH, Wong SP, et al. High-dose oral erythromycin decreased the incidence of parenteral nutrition-associated cholestasis in preterm infants. Gastroenterology 2007;132:1726–39.
69. Puder M, Valim C, Meisel JA, et al. Parenteral fish oil improves outcomes in patients with parenteral nutrition–associated liver injury. Ann Surg 2009;250:395–402.
70. Cusick E, Spicer RD, Beck JM. Small-bowel continuity: a crucial factor in determining survival in gastroschisis. Pediatr Surg Int 1997;12:34–7.
71. Jones BA, Hull MA, Potanos KM, et al, International STEP Data Registry. Report of 111 consecutive patients enrolled in the International Serial Transverse Enteroplasty (STEP) Data Registry: a retrospective observational study. J Am Coll Surg 2013;216(3):438–46.

72. Burghaardt KM, Wales PW, de Silva N, et al. Pediatric intestinal transplant listing criteria–a call for a change in the new era of intestinal failure outcomes. Am J Transplant 2015;15:1674–81.
73. Beath SV, Davies P, Papadopoulou A, et al. Parenteral nutrition related cholestasis in post surgical neonates: multivariate analysis of risk factors. J Pediatr Surg 1996;31:604–6.
74. Antebi H, Mansoor O, Ferrier C, et al. Liver function and plasma antioxidant status in intensive care unit patients requiring total parenteral nutrition: comparison of 2 fat emulsions. JPEN J Parenter Enteral Nutr 2004;28:142–8.
75. Gura KM, Lee S, Valim C, et al. Safety and efficacy of a fish oil-based fat emulsion in the treatment of parenteral nutrition–associated liver disease. Pediatrics 2008; 121:e678–86.
76. Sigalet D, Boctor D, Robertson M, et al. Improved outcomes in paediatric intestinal failure with aggressive prevention of liver disease. Eur J Pediatr Surg 2009; 19:348–53.
77. Zhu X, Wu Y, Qiu Y, et al. Effects of ω-3 fish oil lipid emulsion combined with parenteral nutrition on patients undergoing liver transplantation. JPEN J Parenter Enteral Nutr 2013;37:68–74.
78. Lam HS, Tam YH, Poon TC, et al. A double-blind randomised controlled trial of fish oil-based versus soy-based lipid preparations in the treatment of infants with parenteral nutrition-associated cholestasis. Neonatology 2014;105:290–6.
79. Zhao Y, Wu Y, Pei J, et al. Safety and efficacy of parenteral fish oil containing lipid emulsions in premature neonates. J Pediatr Gastroenterol Nutr 2015;60:708–16.
80. Abu-Wasel B, Molinari M. Liver disease secondary to intestinal failure. Biomed Res Int 2014;2014:968357.
81. Nghiem-Rao TH, Cassidy LD, Polzin EM, et al. Risks and benefits of prophylactic cyclic parenteral nutrition in surgical neonates. Nutr Clin Pract 2013 Dec;28(6): 745–52.
82. Popovich KJ, Hota B, Hayes R, et al. Effectiveness of routine patient cleansing with chlorhexidine gluconate for infection prevention in the medical intensive care unit. Infect Control Hosp Epidemiol 2009;30:959–63.
83. Vassallo M, Dunais B, Roger PM. Antimicrobial lock therapy in central-line associated bloodstream infections: a systematic review. Infection 2015;43(4):389–98.
84. Olthof ED, Versleijen MW, Huisman-de Waal G, et al. Taurolidine lock is superior to heparin lock in the prevention of catheter related bloodstream infections and occlusions. PLoS One 2014;9(11):e111216.
85. Horslen SP, Sudan DL, Iyer KR, et al. Isolated liver transplantation in infants with end-stage liver disease associated with short bowel syndrome. Ann Surg 2002; 235:435–9.
86. Botha JF, Grant WJ, Torres C, et al. Isolated liver transplantation in infants with end-stage liver disease due to short bowel syndrome. Liver Transpl 2006;12: 1062–6.
87. Kelly DA. Intestinal failure-associated liver disease: what do we know today? Gastroenterology 2006;130(2 Suppl 1):S70–7.
88. Bishay M, Pichler J, Horn V, et al. Intestinal failure-associated liver disease in surgical infants requiring long-term parenteral nutrition. J Pediatr Surg 2012;47: 359–62.
89. Nandivada P, Carlson SJ, Chang MI, et al. Treatment of parenteral nutrition-associated liver disease: the role of lipid emulsions. Adv Nutr 2013;4(6):711–7.

New Insights on Intrahepatic Cholestasis of Pregnancy

 CrossMark

Annarosa Floreani, MD[a],*, Maria Teresa Gervasi, MD[b]

KEYWORDS

- Intrahepatic cholestasis of pregnancy • Itching • Bile salts • Ursodeoxycholic acid
- Cholelithiasis

KEY POINTS

- Intrahepatic cholestasis of pregnancy (ICP) is a disorder of pregnancy occurring in the third trimester, characterized by pruritus, elevated serum transaminases and serum bile acids.
- Fetal delivery results in the resolution of symptoms, but recurrence is common.
- The etiology is likely multifactorial, and includes genetic factors and the influence of several environmental factors.
- Elevated serum bile acids have been shown to be correlated with fetal complications, such as anoxia, prematurity, fetal distress, perinatal death, and stillbirth.
- Ursodeoxycholic acid is the current therapy for this condition, owing to its possible benefits on pruritus, liver function tests, safety, and decreased rates of prematurity and fetal adverse.

INTRODUCTION

Intrahepatic cholestasis of pregnancy (ICP) is a specific liver disease with onset during pregnancy. It classically presents in the third trimester with pruritus, increased levels of serum transaminases, and high total serum bile acids (BA).[1] The symptoms and biochemical abnormalities resolve rapidly after delivery, but may recur in subsequent pregnancies.

EPIDEMIOLOGY

The incidence of ICP varies worldwide between 0.2% and 25% with the greatest prevalence up to 25% in the Araucanic race in South America.[2] In Europe, the prevalence

The authors have nothing to disclose.
[a] Department of Surgery, Oncology and Gastroenterology, University of Padova, Via Giustiniani, 2, Padova 35128, Italy; [b] Department of Obstetrics and Gynecology, Azienda Ospedaliera, Via Giustiniani, 2, Padova 35128, Italy
* Corresponding author.
E-mail address: annarosa.floreani@unipd.it

Clin Liver Dis 20 (2016) 177–189
http://dx.doi.org/10.1016/j.cld.2015.08.010   liver.theclinics.com
1089-3261/16/$ – see front matter © 2016 Elsevier Inc. All rights reserved.

is 0.5% to 1.5% of all pregnancies, and the highest incidence has been reported in Sweden.[3] In China, ICP is considered to be common, with an incidence of 2.3% to 6.0%.[4]

RISK FACTORS

The most important risk factors are reported in **Table 1**. A risk for the development of ICP in hepatitis C virus (HCV)-positive mothers has been described. The first retrospective study reported a highly significant incidence of ICP in HCV-positive pregnant women compared with HCV-negative women.[5] Subsequently, another prospective Italian study confirmed these results and suggested the need to investigate the HCV status in women with ICP.[6] In a study population of 21,008 women with ICP identified from the Finnish Hospital Discharge Register from 1972 to 2000, the incidence of hepatitis C was significantly higher than in controls.[7] More recently, a study analyzing data of women with births between 1973 and 2009, registered in the Swedish Medical Birth Registry, confirmed a strong positive association between ICP and hepatitis C both before and after ICP diagnosis.[8] Moreover, women with HCV infection who developed ICP have been found to exhibit a higher HCV viral load compared with those without ICP.[9] The link between ICP and HCV has not been completely explained so far, although several hypotheses can be suggested, including a defect in the transport of sulphated pregnancy hormones in the liver. In fact, it has been suggested that HCV would downregulate the expression of the ABC transporter multidrug-resistance–protein 2 in the liver, thus inducing a failure in the transport of various toxic substances.[10] Furthermore, another link may be with a defect in ABCB11 gene encoding the bile salt export pump (BSEP).[11]

It was reported from Sweden, Finland, and Chile that the incidence of ICP is higher in the winter than in the summer.[12–14] It has also been suggested that other exogenous cofactors, such as low selenium levels, may act in alteration of oxidative metabolism in the liver.[15] A low vitamin D concentration has also been reported in women with ICP, although its role has yet to be defined.[16] It frequently recurs in multiparous women who previously experienced ICP and is more common in multiple gestations.[17–19] In particular, in the Finnish study[19] the incidence of ICP was 14% in twin pregnancies, and 43% in triplets. Moreover, a relatively advanced age (>35 years) has been shown to be a risk for ICP.[20]

GENETICS

Genetic defects in at least 6 canalicular transporters have been found to be associated with ICP (**Table 2**). Genetic variations may implicate heterozygous or homozygous

Table 1 Risk factors related to intrahepatic cholestasis of pregnancy	
Risk Factor	**References**
HCV	5–8
Seasonal onset (winter)	12–14
Low selenium levels	15
Low vitamin D	16
Multiple gestations	17–19
Advanced age	20

Table 2
Genetic defects associated to ICP

Canalicular Transporter	Chromosomal Locus	Biochemical/Histologic Characteristics	Functional Defect	Clinical Spectrum
ATP8B1 (FIC1)	18q 21–22	High serum bile salts; low GGT/ bland cholestasis with coarse and granular bile	Abnormal excretion of aminophospholipids; downregulation of FXR	ICP, PFIC1, BRIC1, Byler disease
ABCB11 (BSEP)	2q24	High serum bile salts; low GGT/ portal tract fibrosis; bile duct proliferation	Abnormal bile acid secretion	ICP, Byler syndrome, PFIC2, BRIC2, drug-induced cholestasis, transient neonatal cholestasis
ABCB4 (MDR3)	7q21	High serum bile salts; elevated GGT/fibrosis, vanishing bile duct syndrome; low phospholipids in bile	Defect in phosphatidylcholine floppase	ICP, PFIC3, LPAC, neonatal cholestasis, drug-induced cholestasis
ABCC2 (MRP2)	10q24	High serum conjugated bilirubin/ black liver pigmentation	Alteration in canalicular transport of conjugated metabolites	ICP, Dubin–Johnson syndrome
NR1H4 (FXR)	12q23.1	High serum bile salts	Altered homeostasis of BSEP and MDR3	ICP, familial gallstone disease, idiopathic infantile cholestasis
FGF19	11q13.3	High serum bile salts	Abnormality in bile acid transport	ICP, Bile acid malabsorption

Abbreviations: BRIC, benign recurrent cholestasis; BSEP, bile salt export pump; FIC, familial intrahepatic cholestasis; FXR, farnesoid X receptor; GGT, gamma-glutamyl transferase; LPAC, low phospholipid cholestasis; MDR, multidrug resistance; MRP, multidrug resistance protein; PFIC, progressive familial intrahepatic cholestasis.

polymorphisms located in different points of the genes. ATP8B1 (or FIC1) gene, located in the chromosomal locus 18q21 to 22, encodes a P-type ATPase. Its functional defects have been identified in ICP, PFIC1, BRIC1, and Byler disease, depending on the localization and functional effect of the variation.[21,22] Mullenbach and colleagues[23] identified 2 ATP8B1 mutations that resulted in an amino acid exchange (D7ON and R867C) after DNA sequencing of 16 ICP cases in the UK. However, in an expanded study including 563 patients with ICP from Western Europe and 642 controls, no significant evidence for association with ATP8B1 was found.[24]

ABCB11 (BSEP, a member of the ABC transporter superfamily) is the high-affinity, liver-specific transporter responsible for the export of conjugated BA into the canaliculus.[25] The gene is located in the 2q24 chromosomal locus; its functional defect causes abnormal BA secretion and a clinical spectrum of diseases including ICP, Byler syndrome, PFIC2, BRIC2, drug-induced cholestasis, and transient neonatal cholestasis. The role of genetic variation at this locus in ICP has been explored in detail, with several recurrent mutations identified. In particular, the European study identified 6 SNIPs (single nucleotide polymorphisms) in ABCB11 significantly associated with risk for ICP.[24]

The ABCB4 (MDR3) is a transporter responsible for bile salt-dependent bile flow. Initial studies identified heterozygous mutations of this gene causing a defect in phosphatidylcholine (PC) floppase in familial and sporadic cases of ICP.[26,27] This susceptibility has been confirmed in large cohort studies.[24,28,29] The gene is located in the 7q21 chromosome and a defect in PC lipase causes low phospholipids in bile with a consequence of different clinical spectrum: ICP, progressive familial intrahepatic cholestasis type 3, juvenile cholelithiasis, neonatal cholestasis, and drug-induced cholestasis.

The ABCC2 (multidrug-resistance–protein 2) is a transporter of bilirubin and BA across the canalicular membrane located in the 10q24 chromosome. Involvement of genetic variants of multidrug-resistance–protein 2 have been reported in association with ICP in South American populations,[30] but not confirmed in the large European cohort study.[24]

The NR1H4 (farnesoid receptor X) is a major BA sensor that protects the liver from the BA toxicity by regulation the transcription genes involved in the BA homeostasis.[31] Genetic variations of farnesoid receptor X have been rarely identified in ICP.[32,33]

All the association studies with these candidate genes stress the complex variability of genotypes, the different penetrance, and the influence of several environmental factors. A recent study using microarray technology in 12 women with ICP and in 12 healthy controls, found that 20 genes were potentially correlated with ICP.[34] Among these, an upregulation of gamma-aminobutyric acid (GABA)2 receptor gene may indicate that GABA may play a role in the pathogenesis of pruritus in this condition.

The placentas of women with ICP displayed significant proteome differences compared with women with a normal pregnancy.[35] In particular, the proteins differentially expressed together with various enzymes comprised proteins in cytoskeleton activity, blood coagulation, platelet and chaperones activation, heat shock proteins, RNA-binding and calcium-binding proteins, and various enzymes. These results indicate that the pathogenic mechanism underlying ICP is rather complex and further verification and research are required to elucidate the exact role of proteins in ICP pathogenesis. Indeed placenta, connecting the developing fetus to the uterine wall allowing fetal and maternal exchanges of blood and nutrients, plays a crucial role in ICP pathogenesis. By a DNA microarray study, it has been found that placenta differentially express genes in mild ICP and severe ICP compared with healthy pregnancies.[36]

DIAGNOSIS

The condition typically occurs during the third trimester of pregnancy with pruritus and increases in both bile salts and transaminases, with rapid resolution immediately after delivery. Some patients may have an early onset during the first trimester as early as in the seventh gestational week.[37,38] A marked increase in maternal serum estrogen levels, as in the case of ovarian hyperstimulation, might trigger ICP in the first trimester of pregnancy.[39] A recent study including 305 patients with ICP (subdivided in early onset [<28 weeks] and late onset [≥28 weeks]) showed that women presenting with early onset had a worse clinical course with a higher rate of preterm labor and fetal distress than women with late onset.[40]

Pruritus typically affects the palm of hands and soles, but can occur anywhere. As the disease progresses and generalizes, secondary skin changes develop from scratching and can range from minor excoriation to severe prurigo nodules. Skin lesions tend to concentrate on the extremities, although they may involve other sites such as buttocks and abdomen.[41] The relationship between the onset of pruritus and deranged liver function tests is unclear, but generally pruritus may precede or follow biochemical alteration.[42] Jaundice with dark urine and pale stools is exceptional.

SERUM BIOCHEMISTRY

Serum BA level is the most sensitive and specific marker for the diagnosis of ICP, after exclusion of other causes of cholestasis.[43] Higher BA levels (>40 mmol/L) have been found to be associated with higher rates of fetal complications in a large cohort series of 690 Swedish women diagnosed with ICP between 1999 and 2002.[44] This study reported an increased incidence of spontaneous preterm delivery, asphyxia events, meconium staining of the amniotic fluid, placenta, or amniotic fluid and placenta, and membranes. However, the increased risk became statistically significant only in 17% of women (having BA >40 μmol/L). Several studies have found that BA increase the sensitivity and expression of oxytocin receptors in the human myometrium, and this can explain the mechanism of preterm labor as a complication of ICP.[45,46] A Dutch group conducted a retrospective study that included women with ICP stratified according to the BA level into mild (10–39 μmol/L), moderate (40–99 μmol/L), and severe (≥100 μmol/L). Spontaneous preterm birth (19%), meconium-stained fluid (47.6%), and perinatal death (9.5%) occurred significantly more often in cases with severe ICP.[47] Moreover, BA levels correlated between mother and fetus, suggesting a causal relationship between levels of BA and fetal complications and adverse outcome.[47]

Despite the high levels of transaminases, gamma-glutamyl transferase (GGT) is commonly normal. GGT might be abnormal only in approximately 10% of cases and it is accompanied by a greater impairment of liver function tests.[48] Increased GGT serum levels suggested the involvement of ABCB4 mutations, whereas genetic BSEP dysfunction was postulated in the low GGT levels.[26] MDR3 is a flippase translocating PC from the cytosolic leaflet of the canalicular membrane to the leaflet facing the bile duct lumen. If MDR3 is not expressed, bile salts are pumped in the canaliculus unaccompanied by PC. Bile without PC is toxic to the bile ducts (bile salts are membranolytic); thus, damaged bile ducts proliferate and with the help of bile salts they shed large amounts of GGT into the circulation.[49] Otherwise, bile salts are pumped into the canaliculus by the BSEP and remove PC from the canalicular membrane to form mixed micelles containing bile salts, PC, and cholesterol. Bile, devoid of bile salts, cannot release GGT from the bile ducts.[49]

Serum autotaxin activity represents a highly sensitive, specific, and robust diagnostic marker distinguishing ICP from other pruritic disorders of pregnancy and pregnancy-related liver disease.[50] Bilirubin is increased only in exceptional cases.

Finally, a small case-control study demonstrated that ICP is characterized by glucose intolerance and dyslipidemia, consistent with the changes seen in the metabolic syndrome, in conjunction with enhanced fetal growth.[51] Further work, however, is required to understand whether these changes may have an influence on the pregnancy outcome and on the long-term morbidity of the offspring of the affected mothers.

Differential diagnosis of ICP include other cause of pruritus, specific or nonspecific to pregnancy, including pruritus gravidarum, atopic eruption of pregnancy, pemphigoid gestationis, atopic dermatitis, allergic or drug reactions, pregnancy-specific causes of hepatic impairment, liver disease preexisting, or coincidental to pregnancy.[1]

FETAL OUTCOME

Initial reports of adverse perinatal outcome associated with ICP focused on increased risk for prematurity, intrapartum fetal distress, and still births. The most alarming sequelae was a 3- to 5-fold increased risk of fetal death in utero.[52] However, a systematic review of a 53-year period found only 14 published cases of unexplained term stillbirths that were associated with ICP-affected pregnancies.[53] Given the relatively low frequency of stillbirths, 3 to 10 per 1000 birth in the general population, the risk of stillbirth in ICP is insignificant clinically without statistical proof. These data have been confirmed also by a cohort study in Australia between 2001 and 2011 including 975,240 births.[54] The adoption of routine active management of ICP has been also investigated.[53] No evidence has been found to support the use of active management of ICP-affected pregnancies; nevertheless, individual patient-centered management with informed decision making under the guidance of health care professionals, rather than routine implementation of an active management protocol, is recommended.[53] In selected cases Doppler investigation of the umbilical artery might be of some value in recognizing the specific risk of fetal compromise in pregnancies complicated by intrahepatic cholestasis.[55]

Numerous studies focused on predictors of fetal complications in ICP, but the majority are not large enough to assess the real risk. A summary of studies including at least 100 cases is presented in **Table 3**.[44,47,56–60] The percentage of fetal

Table 3					
Risk factors associated with fetal complications (observational studies including ≥100 cases)					
Author	No. of Cases	Period	Country	Fetal Complications (%)	Risk Factor
Brouwers et al,[47] 2015	215	2005–2012	Netherlands	64.1	High BA (>100 mmol/L)
Lee et al,[56] 2008	122	2000–2007	USA	34.4	Meconium passage
Glantz et al,[44] 2004	640	1999–2002	Sweden	25	High BA (>40 mmol/L)
Oztekin et al,[57] 2009	187	2004–2008	Turkey	19.2	High BA
Rook et al,[58] 2012	101	2005–2009	USA	33	None
Jin et al,[59] 2015	371	1993–2014	China	23.5	Early-onset ICP
Hu et al,[60] 2014	100	NA	China	43	HBV infection

Abbreviations: BA, bile acids; HBV, hepatitis B virus; ICP, intrahepatic cholestasis of pregnancy; NA, not available.

complications ranged between 19.2% and 64.1%. In a retrospective study including a Hispanic population with ICP, an association was found between meconium passage and moderate/severe ICP.[56] Three studies found that the main risk factor for fetal complications was the high BA concentration.[44,47,57] In a Chinese study early-onset ICP was associated with a greater frequency of adverse fetal outcomes than was in late-onset ICP, especially in severe disease.[59] In another Chinese study, it has been found that the rates of hepatitis B virus infection in the newborn, fetal distress, neonatal asphyxia, and birth defects in the newborns were higher in ICP pregnancies in whom the mother was infected with hepatitis B virus than in either healthy pregnancy or in mother with ICP not infected with hepatitis B virus.[60] Finally, a United States–based retrospective study of women with ICP, of whom 90% were of Hispanic origin, found a 33% rate of perinatal complications, but no risk factor was specifically correlated with fetal complications.[58]

A retrospective study carried out in Finland in 365 sons of mothers with ICP from 1969 to 1988 and 617 sons of mothers without ICP using a questionnaire found that in general a mother's ICP does not affect her son's health.[61]

MATERNAL OUTCOME

In general, fetal delivery results in the resolution of symptoms in mothers. Anecdotal cases have a persistence of symptoms of cholestasis and eventually develop a progressive cholestatic disease and/or cholelithiasis.[61] These cases may be related to MDR3 deficiency with altered bile composition and risk to develop progressive familial intrahepatic cholestasis type 3.[62] This condition should be suspected in young women with a history of cholestasis of unknown origin who develop a severe ICP.[62] Progressive familial intrahepatic cholestasis may have a progressive course with chronic icteric or anicteric cholestasis, portal hypertension, and liver failure. Women who experienced ICP can develop also the low phospholipids–associated cholelithiasis, either before or after pregnancy.[63] Biliary symptoms usually appear in young adults before the age of 40 years; a family history is often reported and the oversaturated bile can cause intrahepatic hyperechogenic foci, sludge, or microlithiasis.[64] Moreover, biliary pain and even pancreatitis may recur after cholecystectomy. Some rare familial cases may have a low phospholipid–associated cholelithiasis and induction of cholestasis by a reduced dosage of estrogens compared with pregnancy, that is, oral contraceptive-induced cholestasis.[65] A recent large Swedish study with more than 11,000 patients showed that the risk of later hepatobiliary cancer and autoimmune-modiated and cardiovascular diseases is greater in women with ICP than in women without this diagnosis.[66] Recurrence of ICP ranges between 45% and 70%.[67]

TREATMENT

A recent metaanalysis including 9 randomized clinical trials demonstrated that ursodeoxycholic acid (UDCA) is effective in reducing pruritus and improving liver test results in patients with ICP and improves fetal outcome.[68] This study shows that UDCA is safe, well-tolerated, and decreases the prematurity rate and consequently the number of hospitalizations in intensive care units. A number of mechanisms of action may explain these effects, including the hydrophilic properties of UDCA, the improvement of both transport and secretion of bile acids by the liver by increasing the activity of canalicular transporters, and improving the bile acid transport across the placenta, thus decreasing exposure of the fetus to toxic bile acids.[69] A novel mechanism of action of UDCA has been explored in an elegant study determining the concentrations of bile acids and sulphated progesterone metabolites in maternal and fetal serum and placenta using high performance liquid chromatography–mass spectrometry/mass spectrometry.[70] The results of this study show that the ABCG2 export pump located at the apical membrane of trophoblast cells plays an important role in the placenta barrier for sulphated progesterone metabolites and bile acids, with the consequent protection of the fetus against the accumulation of these compounds in the maternal compartment.

Another metaanalysis of the literature including both nonrandomized and randomized, controlled studies, including a total of 836 ICP showed that UDCA, had decreased pruritus in 73% of randomized, controlled studies and in 100% of NRSs with available data.[71] Liver function tests were improved in 82% and 100%, respectively. Moreover, the use of UDCA was associated with lower rates of prematurity and less frequent use of neonatal intensive care unit.[71]

More recently, the Cochrane Collaboration published an updated review of interventions for treating ICP after the first published in 2011.[72] This review included 21 trials with a total of 1197 women, and assessed 11 different interventions resulting in 15 different comparisons. Compared with placebo, UDCA showed improvement in pruritus in 5 (228 women) out of 7 trials. Two trials (48 women) reported lower pruritus scores for S-adenosylmethionine (SAMe) compared with placebo, whereas 2 other trials of 34 women reported no differences between groups. UDCA was more effective improving pruritus than either SAMe or cholestyramine, however, combined UDCA + SAMe was no more effective than UDCA alone with regard to pruritus improvement. Overall, there were no differences in instances of fetal distress in the UDCA groups compared with placebo, but the difference was not significant. On the basis of these data, the authors conclude that large trials of UDCA to determine fetal benefits or risks are needed. Moreover, there was insufficient evidence to indicate that SAMe, guar gum, activated charcoal, dexamethasone, cholestyramine, salvia, and even Chinese agents (yinchenghao decoction, danxioling and yiganling, or yiganling alone or in combination) are effective in treating women with cholestasis of pregnancy.

Rifampicin, which has been used in the treatment of pruritus in cholestatic liver diseases for its complementary mechanism of action to UDCA,[73] has been administered in 27 women with ICP (28 affected pregnancies). In 14 pregnancies (54%), serum bile acids decreased after the introduction of rifampicin.[74] In 10 pregnancies (38%), there was a 50% decrease in serum bile acids.[73,74] Although these data should be considered as preliminary, they suggest that rifampicin may be used as a useful adjunct to the treatment with UDCA in women with severe ICP.

Indeed, the crucial point in the management of ICP is to ascertain the optimal gestational age that would minimize the risk of overall perinatal mortality. In a large cohort of women with ICP (with 1,604,386 singleton, nonanomalous pregnancies evaluated between 34 and 40 weeks' gestation) it was found that the risk of fetal, neonatal, or infant mortality was minimized by delivery at 36 weeks of gestation for those diagnosed beyond the gestation; therefore, preterm delivery at this gestational age may be optimal.[75]

SUMMARY

ICP is a peculiar disorder of pregnancy whose etiology is likely multifactorial. In the last decade, genetic defects in at least 6 canalicular transporters have been found to be associated with ICP. All the association studies with these candidate genes stress the complex variability of genotypes, the different penetrance, and the influence of several environmental factors. In some way, ICP could be regarded as a phenotypic manifestation of a complex genetic condition involving bile secretion or its regulation.

Increased maternal bile acids have been shown to be correlated with fetal complications, such as anoxia, prematurity, perinatal death, fetal distress and stillbirth. ICP is generally a benign condition for mothers; long-term sequelae include the gallstone risk and chronic liver disease in some cases, suggesting a link between ICP and genetic conditions leading to an altered bile composition. Moreover, a positive association between ICP and hepatitis C before and after the diagnosis has been evidenced. The current medical treatment for ICP is UDCA; by examining all available evidence from the more recent literature, UDCA is recommended in the management of ICP owing the possible benefits on pruritus, liver function tests, safety, and decreased rates of prematurity and fetal adverse effects.

REFERENCES

1. Williamson C, Geenes V. Intrahepatic cholestasis of pregnancy. Obstet Gynecol 2014;124:120–33.
2. Joshi D, James A, Quaglia A, et al. Liver disease in pregnancy. Lancet 2010;375: 594–605.
3. Arrese M, Reyes H. Intrahepatic cholestasis of pregnancy: a past and present riddle. Ann Hepatol 2006;5:202–5.
4. Qi HB, Shao Y, Wu WX, et al. Grading of intrahepatic cholestasis of pregnancy. Zhonghua Fu Chan Ke Za Zhi 2004;39:14–7.
5. Locatelli A, Roncaglia N, Arreghini A, et al. Hepatitis C virus infection is associated with a higher incidence of cholestasis of pregnancy. Br J Obstet Gynaecol 1999;106:498–500.
6. Paternoster DM, Fabris F, Palù G, et al. Intra-hepatic cholestasis of pregnancy in hepatitis C virus infection. Acta Obstet Gynecol Scand 2002;81:99–103.
7. Ropponen A, Sund R, Riikonen S, et al. Intrahepatic cholestasis of pregnancy as an indicator of liver and biliary diseases: a population-based study. Hepatology 2006;43:723–8.
8. Marschall H-U, Shemer EW, Ludvigsson JF, et al. Intrahepatic cholestasis of pregnancy and associated hepatobiliary disease: a population based cohort study. Hepatology 2013;58:1385–91.
9. Belay T, Woldegiorgis H, Gress T, et al. Intrahepatic cholestasis of pregnancy with concomitant hepatitis C virus infection, Joan C. Edwards SOM, Marshall University. Eur J Gastroenterol Hepatol 2015;27:372–4.
10. Hinoshita E, Taguchi K, Inokuchi A, et al. Decreased expression of an ATP-binding cassette transporter, MRP2, in human livers with hepatitis C virus infection. J Hepatol 2001;35:765–73.
11. Iwata R, Baur K, Stigier B, et al. A common polymorphism in the ABCB11 gene is associated with advanced fibrosis in hepatitis C but not in non-alcoholic fatty liver disease. Clin Sci (Lond) 2011;120:287–96.
12. Berg B, Helm G, Petersohn L, et al. Cholestasis of pregnancy. Clinical and laboratory studies. Acta Obstet Gynecol 1996;175:957–60.
13. Laatikainen T, Ikonen E. Fetal prognosis in obstetric hepatosis. Ann Chir Gynaecol Fenn 1975;64:155–64.
14. Reis H, Baez ME, Gonzalez MC, et al. Selenium, zinc and copper plasma levels in intrahepatic cholestasis of pregnancy, in normal pregnancies and in healthy individuals in Chile. J Hepatol 2000;32:542–9.
15. Reis H, Kauppila A, Korpela H, et al. Low serum selenium concentration and glutathione peroxidase activity in intrahepatic cholestasis of pregnancy. Br Med J 1987;294:150–2.

16. Wilkstrom Shemer E, Marshall HU. Decreased 1,25 dihydroxy vitamin D levels in women with intrahepatic cholestasis of pregnancy. Acta Obstet Gynecol Scand 2010;89:1420–3.
17. Gonzales M, Reyes H, Arrese M, et al. Intrahepatic cholestasis of pregnancy in twin pregnancies. J Hepatol 1989;9:84–90.
18. Rioseco A, Ivankovic M, Manzur A, et al. Intrahepatic cholestasis of pregnancy: a retrospective case-control study of perinatal outcome. Am J Obstet Gynecol 1994;170:890–5.
19. Savander M, Ropponen A, Avela K, et al. Genetic evidence of heterogeneity in intrahepatic cholestasis of pregnancy. Gut 2003;52:1025–9.
20. Heinonen S, Kirkinen P. Pregnancy outcome with intrahepatic cholestasis. Obstet Gynecol 1999;94:189–93.
21. Bull LN, van Eijk MJ, Pawlikowska L, et al. A gene encoding a liver-specific ABC transporter is mutated in progressive familial intrahepatic cholestasis. Nat Genet 1998;20:233–8.
22. Klomp LW, Vargos JC, van Mil SW, et al. Characterization of mutations in ATP8B1 associated with hereditary cholestasis. Hepatology 2004;40:27–38.
23. Mullenbach R, Bennet A, Tetlow N, et al. ATP8B1 mutations in British cases with intrahepatic cholestasis of pregnancy. Gut 2005;54:829–34.
24. Dixon PH, Wadsworth A, Chambers J, et al. A comprehensive analysis of common genetic variation around six candidate loci for intrahepatic cholestasis of pregnancy. Am J Gastroenterol 2014;109:76–84.
25. Noe J, Stieger B, Meier PJ. Functional expression of the canalicular bile salt export pump of human liver. Gastroenterology 2002;123:1659–60.
26. Jacquemin E, Cresteil D, Manouvrier S, et al. Heterozygous non-sense mutation of the MDR3 gene in familial intrahepatic cholestasis of pregnancy. Lancet 1999;353:210–1.
27. Dixon PH, Weerasekera N, Linton KJ, et al. Heterozygous MDR3 missense mutation associated with intrahepatic cholestasis of pregnancy: evidence for a defect in protein trafficking. Hum Mol Genet 2009;9:1209–17.
28. Floreani A, Carderi I, Paternoster D, et al. Hepatobiliary phospholipid transporter ABCB4, MDR3 variants in a large cohort of Italian women with intrahepatic cholestasis of pregnancy. Dig Liver Dis 2008;40:366–70.
29. Schneider G, Paus TC, Kullak-Ublick GA, et al. Linkage between a new splicing site mutation in the MDR3 alias ABCB4 gene and intrahepatic cholestasis of pregnancy. Hepatology 2007;45:150–8.
30. Sookian S, Castano G, Burguen A, et al. Association of the multidrug-resistance-associated protein gene (ABCC2) variants with intrahepatic cholestasis of pregnancy. J Hepatol 2008;48:125–32.
31. Kim I, Ahn SH, Choi M, et al. Differential regulation of the bile acid homeostasis by the farnesoid X receptor in liver and intestine. J Lipid Res 2007;48:2664–72.
32. Van Mil SW, Milona A, Dixon PH, et al. Functional variants of the central bile acid sensor FXR identified in intrahepatic cholestasis of pregnancy. Gastroenterology 2007;133:507–16.
33. Davit-Spraul A, Gonzales E, Jacquemin E. NR1H4 analysis in patients with progressive familial intrahepatic cholestasis, drug-induced cholestasis or intrahepatic cholestasis of pregnancy unrelated to ATP8B1, ABCB11 and ABCB4 mutations. Clin Res Hepatol Gastroenterol 2012;36:569–73.
34. Floreani A, Caroli D, Lazzari R, et al. Intrahepatic cholestasis of pregnancy: new insights into its pathogenesis. J Matern Fetal Neonatal Med 2013;26:1410–5.
35. He P, Wang F, Jiang Y, et al. Placental proteome alterations in women with intrahepatic cholestasis of pregnancy. Int J Gynaecol Obstet 2014;126:256–9.

36. Du Q, Pan Y, Zhang Y, et al. Placental gene-expression profiles of intrahepatic cholestasis of pregnancy reveal involvement of multiple molecular pathways in blood vessel formation and inflammation. BMC Med Genomics 2014;7:42–52.
37. Brites D, Rodrigues CMP, da Concejao Cardos M, et al. Unusual case of severe cholestasis of pregnancy with early onset, improved by ursodeoxycholic acid administration. Eur J Obstet Gynecol Reprod Biol 1998;76:165–8.
38. Chao TT, Sheffield JS. Primary dermatologic findings with early-onset intrahepatic cholestasis of pregnancy. Obstet Gynecol 2011;117:456–8.
39. Zamah AM, El-Sayed YY, Milki AA. Two cases of cholestasis in the first trimester of pregnancy after ovarian hyperstimulation. Fertil Steril 2008;90:1202.e7–10.
40. Zhou L, Qi H, Luo X. Analysis of clinical characteristics and perinatal outcome of early-onset intrahepatic cholestasis of pregnancy. Zhonghua Fu Chan Ke Za Zhi 2013;48:20–4.
41. Lehroff S, Pomeranz MK. Specific dermatoses of pregnancy and their treatment. Dermatol Ther 2013;26:274–84.
42. Kenyon AP, Piercy CN, Girling J, et al. Pruritus may precede abnormal liver function tests in pregnant women with obstetric cholestasis: a longitudinal analysis. BJOG 2001;108:1190–2.
43. Walker IA, Nelson-Piercy C, Williamson C. Role of bile acid measurement in pregnancy. Ann Clin Biochem 2002;39:105–13.
44. Glantz A, Marschall HU, Mattson LA. Intrahepatic cholestasis of pregnancy: relationships observed bile acid levels and fetal complication rates. Hepatology 2004;40:467–74.
45. German AM, Kato S, Carvajal JA, et al. Bile acids increase response and expression of human myometric receptor. Am J Obstet Gynecol 2003;189:577–82.
46. Israel EJ, Guzman ML, Campos GA. Maximal response to oxytocin of the isolated myometrium from pregnant patients with intrahepatic cholestasis. Acta Obstet Gynecol Scand 1986;65:581–2.
47. Brouwers L, Koster MP, Page-Christiaens GC, et al. Intrahepatic cholestasis of pregnancy: maternal and fetal outcomes associated with elevated bile acid levels. Am J Obstet Gynecol 2015;212:100.e1–7.
48. Milkiewicz P, Gallagher R, Chambers J, et al. Obstetric cholestasis with elevated gamma glutamyl transpeptidase: incidence, presentation and treatment. J Gastroenterol Hepatol 2003;18:1283–6.
49. Jansen PLM, Muller M. Genetic cholestasis: lessons from the molecular physiology of bile formation. Can J Gastroenterol 2000;14:233–8.
50. Kremer AE, Bolier R, Dixon PH, et al. Autotaxin activity has a high accuracy to diagnose intrahepatic cholestasis of pregnancy. J Hepatol 2015;62:897–904.
51. Martineau MG, Raker C, Dixon PH, et al. The metabolic profile of intrahepatic cholestasis of pregnancy is associated with impaired glucose tolerance, dyslipidemia, and increased fetal growth. Diabetes Care 2015;38:243–8.
52. Reid R, Ivery KJ, Rencoret RH, et al. Fetal complications of obstetric cholestasis. Br Med J 1976;1:870–2.
53. Henderson CE, Shah RR, Gottimukkala S, et al. Primum non nocere: how active management became modus operandi for intrahepatic cholestasis of pregnancy. Am J Obstet Gynecol 2014;124:189–96.
54. Bannister-Tyrrell M, Ford JB, Morris JM, et al. Intrahepatic cholestasis of pregnancy is not associated with stillbirth in an Australian maternity population. Eur J Obstet Gynecol Reprod Biol 2014;176:203–6.
55. Suri V, Jain R, Aggarwal N, et al. Useful of fetal monitoring in intrahepatic cholestasis of pregnancy: a prospective study. Arch Gynecol Obstet 2012;286:1419–24.

56. Lee RH, Kwok KM, Ingles S, et al. Pregnancy outcomes during an era of aggressive management for intrahepatic cholestasis of pregnancy. Am J Perinatol 2008; 25:341–5.

57. Oztekin D, Aydal I, Oztekin O, et al. Predicting fetal asphyxia in intrahepatic cholestasis of pregnancy. Arch Gynecol Obstet 2009;280:975–9.

58. Rook M, Vargas J, Caughey A, et al. Fetal outcomes in pregnancies complicated by intrahepatic cholestasis of pregnancy in Northern California cohort. PLoS One 2012;7:1–6.

59. Jin J, Pan S, Huang L, et al. Risk factors for adverse fetal outcomes among women with early-versus late-onset intrahepatic cholestasis of pregnancy. Int J Gynaecol Obstet 2015;128(3):236–40.

60. Hu Y, Ding Y-L, Yu L. The impact of intrahepatic cholestasis of pregnancy with hepatitis B virus infection on perinatal outcomes. Ther Clin Risk Manag 2014; 10:381–5.

61. Hamalainen ST, Turunen K, Kosunen E, et al. Men's health is not affected by their mothers' intrahepatic cholestasis of pregnancy. Am J Mens Health 2015. [Epub ahead of print].

62. Lucena J-F, Herrero JI, Quiroga G, et al. A multidrug resistance 3 gene mutation causing cholelithiasis, cholestasis of pregnancy, and adult biliary cirrhosis. Gastroenterology 2003;124:1037–42.

63. Davit-Spraul A, Gonzales E, Baussan C, et al. The spectrum of liver diseases related to ABCB4 gene mutations: pathophysiology and clinical aspects. Semin Liver Dis 2010;30:134–46.

64. Poupon R, Rosmorduc O, Boelle PY, et al. Genotype-phenotype relationships in the low-phospholipids-associated cholelithiasis syndrome: a study of 156 consecutive patients. Hepatology 2013;58:1105–10.

65. Pasmant E, Goussard P, Baranes L, et al. First description of ABCB4 gene deletions in familial low phospholipid-associated cholelithiasis and oral contraceptives-induced cholestasis. Eur J Hum Genet 2012;20:277–82.

66. Wilkstromer Shemer EA, Stephansson O, Thuresson M, et al. Intrahepatic cholestasis of pregnancy and cancer, immune-mediated and cardiovascular diseases: a population-based cohort study. J Hepatol 2015;63(2):456–61.

67. Hay JE. Liver disease in pregnancy. Hepatology 2008;47:1067–76.

68. Bacq Y, Sentilhes L, Reyes HB, et al. Efficacy of ursodeoxycholic acid in treating intrahepatic cholestasis of pregnancy: a meta-analysis. Gastroenterology 2012; 143:1492–501.

69. Erlinger S. Ursodeoxycholic acid in intrahepatic cholestasis of pregnancy: good, but can do better. Clin Res Hepatol Gastroenterol 2013;37:117–8.

70. Estiù MC, Monte MJ, Rivas L, et al. Effects of ursodeoxycholic acid treatment on the altered progesterone and bile acid homeostasis in the mother-placenta-foetus trio during cholestasis of pregnancy. Br J Clin Pharmacol 2014;79: 316–29.

71. Grand'Maison S, Durand M, Mahone M. The effect of ursodeoxycholic acid treatment for intrahepatic cholestasis of pregnancy on maternal and fetal outcomes: a meta-analysis including non-randomized studies. J Obstet Gynaecol Can 2014; 36:632–41.

72. Gurung V, Stokes M, Middleton P, et al. Interventions for treating cholestasis in pregnancy [review]. Cochrane Database Syst Rev 2013;(6):CD000493.

73. Marshall HU, Wagner M, Zollner G, et al. Complementary stimulation of hepatobiliary transport and detoxification systems by rifampicin and ursodeoxycholic acid in humans. Gastroenterology 2005;129:476–85.

74. Geenes V, Chambers J, Khurana R, et al. Rifampicin in the treatment of severe intrahepatic cholestasis of pregnancy. Eur J Obstet Gynecol Reprod Biol 2015; 189:59–63.
75. Puljic A, Kim E, Page J, et al. The risk of infant and fetal death by each additional week of expectant management in intrahepatic cholestasis of pregnancy by gestational age. Am J Obstet Gynecol 2015;212:667.e1–5.

Liver Transplantation for Cholestatic Liver Diseases in Adults

Vandana Khungar, MD, MSc[a], David Seth Goldberg, MD, MSCE[b],*

KEYWORDS

- MELD exceptions • Living donor transplantation • Cholestatic liver disease
- Waitlist mortality

KEY POINTS

- Cholestatic liver diseases are the indication for liver transplantation in 10% of patients in the United States.
- Post-transplant outcomes in patients with cholestatic liver diseases are as good as, if not better than, other forms of liver disease.
- Primary biliary cirrhosis and primary sclerosing cholangitis can recur after liver transplantation, and potentially affect long-term graft outcomes.

INTRODUCTION

Liver transplantation (LT) is a lifesaving therapy for patients with primary cholestatic liver disease, including primary sclerosing cholangitis (PSC) and primary biliary cirrhosis (PBC), as well as secondary forms of cholestatic liver disease, including those with cholestatic complications of LT needing a retransplant. These 3 processes are the focus of this as article because they are the most common forms of cholestatic liver disease necessitating LT. Patients with cholestatic liver disease can be transplanted for either complications of end-stage liver disease or for cholestatic disease-specific symptoms before the onset of end-stage liver disease. Patients with cholestatic liver diseases face unique complications compared with patients with other chronic liver diseases, and need to be regularly assessed for symptoms of cholestasis (ie, pruritus); laboratory abnormalities caused by cholestasis (most

Disclosures: Dr V. Khungar has nothing to disclose. Dr D.S. Goldberg receives research funding support from Intercept.
[a] Division of Gastroenterology, University of Pennsylvania, 3400 Spruce Street, 2 Dulles, Philadelphia, PA 19104, USA; [b] Division of Gastroenterology, University of Pennsylvania, Blockley Hall, 423 Guardian Drive, Room 730, Philadelphia, PA 19104, USA
* Corresponding author.
E-mail address: david.goldberg@uphs.upenn.edu

notably fat-soluble vitamins); and, for patients with PSC, development of hepatobiliary tumors and complications of concomitant inflammatory bowel disease (IBD), including colon cancer. Patient survival after LT for cholestatic liver diseases is generally better than for other indications, as discussed later.[1] Although an LT can be lifesaving for cholestatic liver diseases, one of the main challenges is the potential for recurrent disease that may necessitate retransplantation.

Other cholestatic diseases that may necessitate LT include total parenteral nutrition–induced cholestasis, biliary atresia, Alagille syndrome, progressive familial intrahepatic cholestasis, sarcoidosis, cystic fibrosis–associated liver disease, secondary sclerosing cholangitis, and fibropolycystic disease of the liver, which are rare outside the pediatric setting, and are not discussed in this article.

PRIMARY BILIARY CIRRHOSIS
Identifying Patients Most Likely to Need a Liver Transplant

Several mathematical models have been developed to estimate projected survival in PBC in order to determine optimal timing for LT. The Mayo risk score was developed in an attempt to predict time to transplant in patients with PBC. This model incorporates age, bilirubin level, albumin level, prothrombin time, peripheral edema, and presence or absence of diuretic therapy. When the score is greater than 7.8 it is thought that patients benefit from LT.[1] Two studies found that pretransplant disease severity as measured by the Mayo PBC risk score seemed to have a direct effect on survival following LT for PBC. Patients with higher risk scores had a tendency for worse outcomes regardless of the era of transplantation.[2,3] As expected, patients who were malnourished or chronically ill preoperatively had less favorable short-term outcomes after LT.[2] These data suggest that predictive risk models such as the Mayo PBC risk score may be able to predict the probability of poor outcomes following LT for PBC.

Indications for Transplantation

PBC has gone from the leading indication for liver transplantation in the 1980s to the sixth most common indication in 2006 because of effective medical therapy with UDCA.[4] It still remains the indication for LT in up to 5% of patients receiving an LT in the United States each year. Despite the effectiveness of UDCA, 30% of patients are incomplete responders and face the greatest risk of progressing to cirrhosis. Furthermore, because the disease is asymptomatic in some patients, PBC can be diagnosed at such a late stage that even effective medical therapy cannot stave off the need for LT.

Most patients with PBC who require an evaluation for LT have developed decompensation from cirrhosis and portal hypertension, including ascites, hepatic encephalopathy, variceal bleeding, or hepatocellular carcinoma (HCC). Patients with more-preserved liver function can also be considered for LT if they have intractable symptoms of PBC, including pruritus, chronic fatigue, or severe metabolic bone disease.[5] These indications are controversial because the current system of LT follows an urgency-based model that prioritizes patients using the Model for End-stage Liver Disease (MELD) score. Unless a living donor is available, patients with PBC without complications from portal hypertension have difficulty obtaining deceased donors because of their low MELD scores and the disparity in available deceased donors compared with the number of patients on the waiting list.[6–8] The other alternative is to apply for exception points for these patients, but these are not standard indications for exception points, and practices related to exception points vary from region to region.[9] Importantly, even though LT may be lifesaving for patients with decompensated cirrhosis from PBC, for those with symptoms such as fatigue from PBC there is the potential that fatigue attributable to PBC may not resolve with LT.[10]

Waiting List Mortality for Patients with Primary Biliary Cirrhosis

Until recently, information on the waiting list mortality among patients with PBC in the United States relied on small case series or older data. However, a recent study evaluated the waiting list outcomes for these patients by analyzing United Network for Organ Sharing (UNOS) data for all adults on the waiting list between 2002 and 2014. During this period, 16.5% of waitlisted patients with PBC died on the waiting list without receiving a liver transplant, compared with 12.4% with hepatitis C virus (HCV) and 8.5% with PSC. Importantly, the risk of waiting list mortality varied across the United States, but, despite this, patients with PBC had higher waiting list mortality than patients with PSC in the first 3 months after being waitlisted, and 40% higher overall. Compared with patients with PSC, patients with PBC died more often from cardiovascular causes.[11]

Model for End-stage Liver Disease Score Exceptions in Primary Biliary Cirrhosis

As mentioned earlier, since 2002, patients on the LT waiting list have been prioritized using the MELD score, an objective score to prioritize the sickest first. The MELD score is a good predictor of survival in patients with all forms of liver disease, although the Mayo PBC risk performs similarly to the MELD score in predicting survival in patients with PBC.[8] The MELD score is based on 3 parameters (serum creatinine level, bilirubin level, and international normalized ratio [INR]), and does not account for symptoms of liver disease that do not affect laboratory tests. For patients with PBC, this most commonly manifests as intractable pruritus. There are no standardized policies for granting exception points for patients with pruritus. Transplant centers may submit an application to their regional review board (RRB; there is 1 RRB within each of the 11 UNOS regions) to have the case reviewed on a case-by-case basis. There is variability among centers and regions in the use of such exceptions; however, given that they are related to quality of life, and not mortality, they are being approved less frequently, and in the future may be eliminated. As one example of geographic variability in exception points, a study published in 2011 by Argo and colleagues[9] examined regional differences in the use of symptom-based MELD exceptions, which specifically excludes those for HCC, which includes exceptions for symptoms such as the pruritus and fatigue commonly seen in patients with PBC. The investigators reviewed Organ Procurement and Transplantation Network (OPTN) data for waiting list registrants during the MELD allocation from February 27, 2002 to November 22, 2006. Although use of system-based exception varied widely across UNOS regions, it did not correlate with organ availability as estimated by the regional mean physiologic MELD at transplantation. There were no statistical differences between PSC and PBC, and cholestatic diseases were treated as 1 group in this analysis.

Living Donor Liver Transplantation for Primary Biliary Cirrhosis

Because the symptoms of PBC are not captured by the MELD score, living donor liver transplant (LDLT) is an attractive option for patients with PBC. Post-LDLT outcomes in PBC are excellent, with reported 5-year survival rates of 80%. No significant difference is seen in survival for deceased donor versus living donor transplants in patients with PBC.[12]

Posttransplant Outcomes in Primary Biliary Cirrhosis

Outcomes of LT in patients with PBC are excellent and in general better than for other indications for LT. In Western populations (United States and United Kingdom), 1-year, 3-year, 5-year, and 10-year survival rates posttransplantation were 93% to 94%, 90% to 91%, 82% to 86%, and 67% respectively. Graft survival in patients with PBC at 1, 3, 5, and 10 years was 85%, 83%, 57% to 81%, and 61%, respectively.[12,13] Patients with PBC, as with other autoimmune diseases, may need longer courses of steroid therapy or higher doses. Some patients are even kept on low doses of prednisone chronically. Those who received an LDLT were more likely to have corticosteroid withdrawal than those who received deceased donor transplants for PBC in a study of 1032 patients.[14] Nevertheless, there are no controlled trials that have identified the optimal immunosuppression regimen in these patients.

Recurrence rates of PBC posttransplant are estimated at 21% to 23% at 10 years and greater than 43% at 15 years.[15] Median time to recurrence is 3 to 5.5 years, although it can be as rapid as less than 1 year after transplant. Diagnosing recurrent PBC after LT can be difficult because antimitochondrial antibodies can remain positive after transplant without recurrent disease. Anti–parietal cell antibodies may be useful in the diagnosis of posttransplant PBC recurrence, but are not yet a definitive tool.[16] The diagnosis requires a liver biopsy with histologic features of portal inflammatory infiltrates, lymphoid aggregates, epithelioid granulomas, and bile duct damage. To date, no predictors of disease recurrence have been identified, but human leukocyte antigen mismatch and choice of immunosuppression may have affect recurrence rates. The treatment of posttransplant recurrent PBC is also unclear. Biochemical improvement can be seen with ursodeoxycholic acid but there is no clear evidence that it improves patient or graft survival or alters the natural history of disease recurrence.[17] Despite a high rate of posttransplant recurrence, graft loss caused by recurrent PBC occurs at a rate of 1% to 5.4%.[18]

Although patient and graft survival are often used as outcomes for LT, an important multicenter study by Gross and colleagues[10] answered the question of what the quality of life before and after liver transplantation for cholestatic liver disease is. Using the National Institute of Diabetes and Digestive and Kidney Diseases Liver Transplant Database Quality of Life Questionnaire, a validated and reliable instrument, 4 areas were assessed: liver-related symptoms, physical functioning, health satisfaction, and overall wellbeing. An increase in disease severity led to a worsened quality of life, but this was reversible with LT. Patients with PBC were compared with those with PSC and there were no significant differences in the following measures of QOL before LT or at 1-year follow-up: symptoms composite score, pain rating, function composite score, Karnofsky score, sick days, employment status, health rating, health satisfaction, life satisfaction, or happiness. All results were reported as composites for the 157 adult patients with PSC and PBC. Results were remarkable for significantly improved health-related quality-of-life ratings after LT compared with scores before LT, with improvements in symptoms, function, health satisfaction, and overall quality of life. Importantly, the health-related quality of life at 1 year after LT was not associated with pre-LT clinical factors, suggesting that a remarkable recovery can be made even by those who are very ill before transplant.[10,19]

Secondary Cholestatic Disease Posttransplantation

Cholestasis posttransplantation is a common occurrence; it can be extrahepatic, caused by mechanical obstruction of the main bile ducts, or intrahepatic, with a variety of causes. Cholestasis in the post-LT period usually remains subclinical, but, when severe, it is associated with irreversible liver damage, necessitating retransplantation.

The causes of cholestasis are best categorized by time of occurrence: early (within 6 months of LT) or late (>6 months post-LT). Common causes of intrahepatic cholestasis include ischemia/reperfusion injury, bacterial infection, acute cellular rejection, cytomegalovirus infection, small for size grafts, medication injury, intrahepatic biliary strictures, chronic rejection, hepatic artery thrombosis or stenosis, ABO blood group incompatibility, biliary cast syndrome, fibrosing cholestatic hepatitis C, cholangiopathy postdonation after cardiac death (DCD) donation, and recurrent disease (**Table 1**).

By contrast, extrahepatic cholestasis is usually related to biliary stones or anastomotic strictures. Extrahepatic cholestasis caused by anastomotic strictures typically requires interventions to reverse, which can be endoscopic retrograde cholangiopancreatography (ERCP) or percutaneous transhepatic cholangiogram depending on the location, presence of a duct-to-duct anastomosis versus Roux-en-Y, and accessibility of the biliary tract.

There has been a continued emphasis on increasing the use of DCD livers, which can provide good posttransplant graft and patient survival, but are frequently associated with biliary complications, most commonly ischemic cholangiopathy (diffuse intrahepatic strictures). These patients need to be relisted, and the challenge is obtaining high enough priority for retransplantation. A recent analysis of OPTN/UNOS data from 2002 to 2011 revealed that, because of the use of MELD exception points, DCD patients relisted for LT underwent retransplantation 71.4% of the time. Of those with an approved MELD exception, 85.2% underwent retransplantation, compared with 57% of those with an exception denied, and 69.4% of those not applying for an exception. Patients with an approved exception were 3.3 times more likely to undergo retransplantation. Clearly, standardization of exception points for DCD recipients requiring retransplantation is required.[20]

Table 1
Causes of posttransplant cholestasis

Early (6 mo)	Late (>6 mo)
Extrahepatic: • Stricture: anastomotic, compressive • Multiple strictures: HAT or ischemic • Bile leak • Cholangitis	Extrahepatic: • Stricture: anastomotic • Multiple strictures: HAT, ischemic, recurrent PSC • Choledocholithiasis
Intrahepatic: • Ischemia/reperfusion injury • ABO incompatibility • Hepatic artery thrombosis/stenosis • Acute cellular • Sepsis • Drug induced • Small for size • Posttransplant infections:– bacterial, fungal, CMV, HCV, HBV	Intrahepatic: • Intrahepatic biliary strictures • ABO incompatibility • Chronic rejection • Recurrent disease (PBC, PSC, HCV) • Drug induced • Acute cellular rejection • De novo AIH • De novo viral hepatitis

Abbreviations: AIH, autoimmune hepatitis; CMV, cytomegalovirus; HAT, hepatic artery thrombosis; HBV, hepatitis B virus.

PRIMARY SCLEROSING CHOLANGITIS
Indications for Transplantation

PSC is a chronic disease that leads to progressive fibrosis and stricturing of the biliary tract and the hepatic parenchyma, and frequently develops into biliary cirrhosis. Similar to other forms of chronic disease, LT is indicated for patients with PSC who develop complications of portal hypertension, which include ascites, hepatic encephalopathy, variceal hemorrhage, and/or spontaneous bacterial peritonitis.[21] In addition, patients with PSC who develop cirrhosis are at risk for developing HCC, although at much lower rates than other forms of chronic liver disease (eg, hepatitis C, nonalcoholic steatohepatitis).[22] In the small subset of patients with PSC who do develop HCC, indications for transplantation and increased waiting list priority (exception points) are based on the Milan criteria: (1) tumor less than or equal to 5 cm, or 2 or 3 tumors less than or equal to 3 cm.[23]

In contrast with other causes of chronic disease that almost uniformly require transplantation when complications of portal hypertension and/or HCC develop, PSC has 2 unique indications for LT: cholangiocarcinoma (CCA) and recurrent bacterial cholangitis. Although nearly all patients with chronic liver disease who are placed on a transplant waiting list have underlying cirrhosis, this is not a requirement for listing for LT. It is estimated that, among patients with PSC, from 25% to 50% of patients waitlisted for a liver transplant do not have radiographic and/or histologic evidence of cirrhosis,[24] and/or complications of portal hypertension (eg, ascites).[25]

The incidence of CCA is dramatically higher in patients with PSC compared with patients with other causes of liver disease, and/or the general population. Depending on the means of diagnosis (eg, radiographic diagnosis, postmortem), the lifetime risk of developing CCA in the setting of PSC ranges from 10% to 40% in patients with PSC.[26-29] Historically, CCA was deemed a contraindication to LT, but in a subset of patients with CCA (hilar CCA occurring most commonly, but not exclusively, in PSC), the posttransplant outcomes are good. Among patients with hilar CCA who undergo neoadjuvant chemoradiation and survive to undergo a liver transplant, the 5-year recurrence- free survival is 65%.[30] But hilar CCA, with or without PSC, should only be considered an indication for LT among patients who undergo the Mayo Clinic PSC protocol (discussed in detail earlier).[27-29]

The second indication for transplantation that is unique to patients with PSC (or rarely in patients with biliary strictures from diseases such as autoimmune cholangiopathy or congenital or acquired structural biliary anomalies) is recurrent bacterial cholangitis. Long-standing biliary inflammation leads to the development of biliary strictures and subsequent stasis, which places patients with PSC at an increased risk of recurrent bacterial cholangitis. Although the risk of bacterial cholangitis is influenced by the severity of disease, presence of a dominant stricture, and history of prior biliary manipulation (ie, endoscopic retrograde cholangiopancreatography with sphincterotomy), it is a common complication of PSC. Available data suggest that nearly 40% of patients with PSC waitlisted for a liver transplant in the United States have a history of at least 1 episode of bacterial cholangitis before waitlisting, with almost 30% of patients developing at least 1 subsequent episode while on the waiting list.[24] Recurrent cholangitis has been considered an indication for LT because of the potential for morbidity (eg, frequent hospitalizations, impaired quality of life) and hypothesized risk of mortality.

Patients with PSC may also develop complications from long-standing cholestasis, including refractory pruritus, weight loss, and metabolic bone diseases. These complications may lead to significant morbidity, use of medical care, and frequent hospitalizations. Although these complications impair a patient's quality of life; under the current urgency-based (sickest-first) system of LT, such patients have low waiting list priority in the absence of concomitant severe liver dysfunction, and thus are only considered for LT under extenuating circumstances and/or if a potential living liver donor were available.

Waiting List Mortality for Patients with Primary Sclerosing Cholangitis

In the United States, a patient's rank on the liver transplant waiting list is based on the MELD score. This score is a calculated value based on the patient's serum bilirubin level, creatinine level, and INR. The weighting of each of these laboratory values varies and depends on the scale of each value, such that small increases in a patient's serum creatinine yields greater increases in MELD scores than small changes in the serum bilirubin level.[31–34] Because most patients with PSC on the liver transplant waiting list, especially those without cirrhosis and portal hypertension, have disease that manifests with greater increases in their serum bilirubin levels, rather than the serum creatinine levels, many had speculated that, under the MELD system, patients with PSC would have less access to transplantation. Despite these concerns, since 2002 this has not been the case.[24,25] Compared with waitlisted patients in the United States from 2002 to 2009 with all other causes of liver disease, the adjusted risk of dying on the waiting list was significantly lower for patients with PSC (hazard ratio for waiting list mortality, 0.72; 95% confidence interval, 0.66–0.79; P<.001).[25] Several hypotheses exist to explain this phenomenon: (1) preferential use of LDLTs[35] in patients with PSC; (2) increased prioritization among the patients with recurrent bacterial cholangitis granted increased priority in the form of MELD exception points[36]; (3) cirrhosis and portal hypertension being less prevalent among waitlisted patients with PSC[24,25,37–39]; and (4) the low attributable risk of mortality caused by bacterial cholangitis among patients with PSC who develop this complication.[24]

Between February 2002 and March 2011, transplanted centers applied for MELD exception points in order to gain increased waiting list priority for more than 320 patients with PSC with bacterial cholangitis, based on the concern that bacterial cholangitis in patients with PSC increased the patient's risk of mortality, despite limited data to support this contention until recently. In a 10-year study from 2 large liver transplant centers, there were 171 patients waitlisted for a liver transplant with PSC, of whom 39% had a history of bacterial cholangitis before listing, and 28% had at least 1 episode of bacterial cholangitis while on the waiting list. Despite this highly prevalent condition, the waiting list mortality was not significantly different for patients with a history of recurrent bacterial cholangitis, and over this 10-year period no patients were removed from the waiting list for death or clinical deterioration caused by bacterial cholangitis.[24]

Model for End-stage Liver Disease Exception Points for Patients with Primary Sclerosing Cholangitis

As mentioned earlier, in select circumstances, CCA can be an indication for transplantation and increased waiting list priority, rather than a contraindication to transplantation. Because of the excellent posttransplant results from the Mayo Clinic in Rochester among patients with hilar CCA (with and without PSC), patients meeting specific criteria are eligible for exception points and increased waiting list priority. To be eligible for LT, patients must meet specific inclusion and exclusion criteria (**Table 2**), including the presence of perihilar CCA less than or equal to 3 cm without metastatic disease, and then must undergo neoadjuvant chemoradiation and staging to ensure the

Table 2
Inclusion and exclusion criteria for patients with cholangiocarcinoma being considered for the Mayo treatment protocol and MELD exception points

Inclusion Criteria	Exclusion Criteria
Intraluminal brush or biopsy showing evidence of positive tumor cells or cells strongly suspicious for CCA, or	Evidence of extrahepatic disease or regional lymph node involvement
Radiographic malignant-appearing stricture, and 1 of the following criteria:	Previous malignancy (excluding skin or cervical cancer) within the 5 y before diagnosis of CCA
Ca 19–9>100 U/mL in the absence of acute bacterial cholangitis	Previous abdominal radiotherapy
Polysomy on FISH	Uncontrolled infection before treatment
Well-defined mass on cross-sectional imaging	Prior attempt at surgical resection of the tumor leading to violation of the tumor plane
—	Any medical condition precluding transplantation
—	Any transperitoneal biopsy, including percutaneous and/or endoscopic ultrasonography-guided FNA

Abbreviations: Ca, cancer antigen; FISH, fluorescence in-situ hybridization; FNA, fine-needle aspiration.

absence of extrahepatic disease.[30] Patients who meet all of these criteria and undergo the protocol at a transplant center with a formalized treatment protocol that mirrors that derived at the Mayo Clinic may then be eligible for exception points on successful chemoradiation and tumor staging.[30]

Unlike CCA, there are no formalized protocols for awarding exception points for patients with PSC who experience recurrent bacterial cholangitis. These exception applications have been reviewed on a case-by-case basis, and, excluding UNOS region 9, which had a regional policy for awarding exception points, were at the discretion of members of each UNOS region's RRB. A consensus conference convened in 2006 recommended that exception points for recurrent cholangitis be restricted to patients with recurrent cholangitis complicated by bacteremia or other septic complications[40]; however, the criteria used in practice to award exception points have not been stringent.[36] Since publications of these guidelines, 158 patients had at least 1 exception approved for recurrent cholangitis, with 70% of such patients never having an episode of bacteremia or sepsis, or having only a single episode of cholangitis.[36] Importantly, three-quarters of patients receiving a MELD exception were transplanted.[36] The increased access to transplant for patients receiving exception points, with data lacking on the risk of mortality as a result of cholangitis, has led UNOS to develop more stringent criteria for awarding exception points to such patients.

Posttransplant Outcomes

Approximately 5% of all adult transplant recipients in the United States each year have PSC as the primary cause of liver disease necessitating a liver transplant. Despite this, approximately 14% of transplant recipients with PSC receive an LDLT, compared with 3.5% to 4% of transplant recipients with other forms of chronic liver disease.[35] When considering all liver transplant recipients (deceased donor or living donor), patients with PSC have posttransplant graft and patient survival that is not different than other transplant recipients; in the era before direct-acting antiviral therapies for hepatitis C, patients with PSC had superior posttransplant survival compared with these patients.[41] However, when considering only recipients of a living donor allograft in the United States from 2002 to 2013, patients with PSC transplanted at an experienced center (defined as having performed >15 LDLTs) had superior posttransplant graft and patient survival even after adjusting for other factors.[42]

Although patients with PSC have excellent posttransplant survival, they are at risk for recurrent PSC, which is estimated to occur in 15% to 35% of transplant recipients.[43] The wide range of the estimated risk of recurrent PSC rests in part on the challenges in diagnosing recurrent PSC, because it is considered a diagnosis of exclusion. Recurrent PSC has a similar radiographic, endoscopic, and/or histologic appearance to PSC before transplantation, but the features characteristic of PSC can also be seen in patients who have developed a hepatic artery stenosis/thrombosis, chronic ductopenic rejection, cytomegalovirus infections of the biliary tract, and/or received a transplant from a donor with an incompatible blood type or as a donation after cardiac death. For these reasons, the diagnosis of recurrent PSC is one of exclusion, and requires exclusion of conditions that can mimic recurrent PSC (**Table 3**).[43]

Management of immunosuppression in liver transplant recipients with PSC, unlike nonimmune causes, is more complex because of the increased risk of acute cellular rejection in patients with PSC. However, despite this increased risk there are no data showing the optimal regimen, in terms of the backbone of the immunosuppression regimen or the number of immunosuppressant medications that are needed. Furthermore, there are no data that have shown an association between a patient's posttransplant immunosuppression regimen and the risk of recurrent PSC, and whether long-term combination immunosuppression is needed.[44–46] In contrast with the lack of data on the relationship between posttransplant immunosuppression and rejection or recurrent PSC, there are data that suggest that choice of immunosuppression affects posttransplant activity of IBD in patients with PSC. Specifically, combination therapy with tacrolimus and mycophenolate mofetil has been associated with a significantly increased risk of worsening of IBD after transplantation, whereas combination cyclosporine and azathioprine was associated with fewer IBD flares.[47] In spite of these data, one-third of patients with PSC and IBD have worsening of IBD symptoms after LT.[48–50]

Table 3	
Diagnostic criteria for recurrent PSC following LT	
Inclusion Criteria	**Exclusion Criteria**
Confirmed diagnosis of PSC before LT	Hepatic artery stenosis or thrombosis on radiographic imaging or angiography
Cholangiography (MRCP or ERCP) performed ≥90 d after transplantation showing intrahepatic and/or extrahepatic biliary structuring, beading, and/or irregularity, or	Chronic ductopenic rejection on histologic evaluation of liver biopsy Isolated extrahepatic anastomotic strictures
Liver biopsy showing fibrous cholangitis and/or fibro-obliterative lesions, with or without biliary fibrosis or cirrhosis, and/or ductopenia	Donor and recipient ABO incompatibility Nonanastomotic strictures occurring before day 90 posttransplantation

Abbreviation: MRCP, magnetic resonance cholangiopancreatography.
Adapted from Graziadei IW, Wiesner RH, Batts KP, et al. Recurrence of primary sclerosing cholangitis following liver transplantation. Hepatology 1999;29(4):1050–6.

In addition, with regard to posttransplant outcomes and management in transplant recipients with PSC, there is the issue of management of posttransplant IBD. The basic underlying premise of medical management of IBD posttransplantation does not differ from IBD in other settings, with the goals of therapy focused on managing a patient's symptoms, and, when present, endoscopic abnormalities. However, one additional consideration is the potential for an increased risk of infections when biologic therapy (eg, infliximab) is added to standard posttransplant immunosuppression.[47-50] For this reason, some experts consider azathioprine as the preferred treatment option for patients with moderate to severe IBD, especially because azathioprine has been used in transplant recipients for more than 20 years, in combination with other immunosuppressant medications (eg, tacrolimus). Nevertheless, for patients who do not respond to azathioprine and/or have severe IBD (eg, fistulizing Crohn disease) biologic therapy should be considered, with close monitoring for infectious complications. The risk of developing colorectal cancer in patients with PSC and IBD persists after LT, thus continued colorectal surveillance every 1 to 2 years for patients transplanted with PSC and IBD should continue after LT.[48,51,52]

REFERENCES

1. Dickson ER, Grambsch PM, Fleming TR, et al. Prognosis in primary biliary cirrhosis: model for decision making. Hepatology 1989;10(1):1–7.
2. Markus BH, Dickson ER, Grambsch PM, et al. Efficiency of liver transplantation in patients with primary biliary cirrhosis. N Engl J Med 1989;320(26): 1709–13.
3. Neuberger JM, Gunson BK, Buckels JA, et al. Referral of patients with primary biliary cirrhosis for liver transplantation. Gut 1990;31(9):1069–72.
4. Lindor KD, Gershwin ME, Poupon R, et al. Primary biliary cirrhosis. Hepatology 2009;50(1):291–308.
5. Milkiewicz P. Liver transplantation in primary biliary cirrhosis. Clin Liver Dis 2008; 12:461–72.
6. Harnois DM, Yataco ML, Nakhleh RE. Recurrence of autoimmune hepatitis, primary biliary cirrhosis, and primary sclerosing cholangitis after transplantation. Clin Liver Dis 2014;3(4):90–2.
7. Duclos-Vallee JC, Sebagh M. Recurrence of autoimmune disease, primary sclerosing cholangitis, primary biliary cirrhosis, and autoimmune hepatitis after liver transplantation. Liver Transpl 2009;S2:S25–34.
8. Imam MH, Talwalkar JA. Transplantation for primary biliary cirrhosis. In: Busuttil RW, Klintmalm BGB, editors. Transplantation of the liver. Philadelphia: Elsevier; 2015. p. 159–66.
9. Argo CK, Stukenborg GJ, Schmitt TM, et al. Regional variability in symptom-based MELD exceptions: a response to organ shortage? Am J Transplant 2011;11(11): 2353–61.
10. Gross CR, Malinchoc M, Kim WR, et al. Quality of life before and after liver transplantation for cholestatic liver disease. Hepatology 1999;29(2):356–64.
11. Kaif M, Hasanin M, Singal A, et al. Patients with primary biliary cirrhosis have the highest wait-list mortality. Gastroenterology 2015;148:S-1032.
12. Kaneko J, Sugawara Y, Tamura S, et al. Long-term outcome of living donor liver transplantation for primary biliary cirrhosis. Transpl Int 2012;25(1):7–12.
13. Liberal R, Zen Y, Mieli-Vergani G, et al. Liver transplantation and autoimmune liver diseases. Liver Transpl 2013;19(10):1065–77.

14. Campsen J, Zimmerman M, Trotter J, et al. Liver transplantation for primary biliary cirrhosis: results of aggressive corticosteroid withdrawal. Transplant Proc 2009; 41(5):1707–12.
15. Sylvestre PB, Batts KP, Burgart LJ, et al. Recurrence of primary biliary cirrhosis after liver transplantation: histologic estimate of incidence and natural history. Liver Transpl 2003;9(10):1086–93.
16. Ciesek S, Becker T, Manns MP, et al. Anti-parietal cell autoantibodies (PCA) in primary biliary cirrhosis: a putative marker for recurrence after orthotopic liver transplantation? Ann Hepatol 2010;9(2):181–5.
17. Charatcharoenwitthaya P, Pimentel S, Talwalkar JA, et al. Long-term survival and impact of ursodeoxycholic acid treatment for recurrent primary biliary cirrhosis after liver transplantation. Liver Transpl 2007;13(9):1236–45.
18. Carrion AF, Bhamidimarri KR. Liver transplant for cholestatic liver diseases. Clin Liver Dis 2013;17(2):345–59.
19. Kim WR, Lindor KD, Malinchoc M, et al. Reliability and validity of the NIDDK-QA instrument in the assessment of quality of life in ambulatory patients with cholestatic liver disease. Hepatology 2000;32(5):924–9.
20. Maduka RC, Abt PL, Goldberg DS. Use of model for end-stage liver disease exceptions for donation after cardiac death graft recipients relisted for liver transplantation. Liver Transpl 2015;21(4):554–60.
21. Martin PDA, Feng S, Brown R, et al. Evaluation for liver transplantation in adults: 2013 practice guideline by the American Association for the Study of Liver Diseases and the American Society of Transplantation. Hepatology 2014;59(3): 1144–65.
22. Zenouzi R, Weismuller TJ, Hubener P, et al. Low risk of hepatocellular carcinoma in patients with primary sclerosing cholangitis with cirrhosis. Clin Gastroenterol Hepatol 2014;12(10):1733–8.
23. Mazzaferro V, Regalia E, Doci R, et al. Liver transplantation for the treatment of small hepatocellular carcinomas in patients with cirrhosis. N Engl J Med 1996; 334(11):693–9.
24. Goldberg DS, Camp A, Martinez-Camacho A, et al. Risk of waitlist mortality in patients with primary sclerosing cholangitis and bacterial cholangitis. Liver Transpl 2013;19(3):250–8.
25. Goldberg D, French B, Thomasson A, et al. Waitlist survival of patients with primary sclerosing cholangitis in the model for end-stage liver disease era. Liver Transpl 2011;17(11):1355–63.
26. Boonstra K, Weersma RK, van Erpecum KJ, et al. Population-based epidemiology, malignancy risk, and outcome of primary sclerosing cholangitis. Hepatology 2013;58(6):2045–55.
27. Gores GJ, Darwish Murad S, Heimbach JK, et al. Liver transplantation for perihilar cholangiocarcinoma. Dig Dis 2013;31(1):126–9.
28. Heimbach JK, Haddock MG, Alberts SR, et al. Transplantation for hilar cholangiocarcinoma. Liver Transpl 2004;10(10 Suppl 2):S65–8.
29. Ahrendt SA, Pitt HA, Nakeeb A, et al. Diagnosis and management of cholangiocarcinoma in primary sclerosing cholangitis. J Gastrointest Surg 1999;3(4):357–67 [discussion: 367–8].
30. Darwish Murad S, Kim WR, Harnois DM, et al. Efficacy of neoadjuvant chemoradiation, followed by liver transplantation, for perihilar cholangiocarcinoma at 12 US centers. Gastroenterology 2012;143(1):88–98.e3 [quiz: e14].
31. Merion RM, Schaubel DE, Dykstra DM, et al. The survival benefit of liver transplantation. Am J Transplant 2005;5(2):307–13.

32. Wiesner R, Edwards E, Freeman R, et al. Model for end-stage liver disease (MELD) and allocation of donor livers. Gastroenterology 2003;124(1):91–6.
33. Saab S, Wang V, Ibrahim AB, et al. MELD score predicts 1-year patient survival post-orthotopic liver transplantation. Liver Transpl 2003;9(5):473–6.
34. Kamath PS, Wiesner RH, Malinchoc M, et al. A model to predict survival in patients with end-stage liver disease. Hepatology 2001;33(2):464–70.
35. Goldberg DS, French B, Thomasson A, et al. Current trends in living donor liver transplantation for primary sclerosing cholangitis. Transplantation 2011;91(10):1148–52.
36. Goldberg D, Bittermann T, Makar G. Lack of standardization in exception points for patients with primary sclerosing cholangitis and bacterial cholangitis. Am J Transplant 2012;12(6):1603–9.
37. Somsouk M, Kornfield R, Vittinghoff E, et al. Moderate ascites identifies patients with low model for end-stage liver disease scores awaiting liver transplantation who have a high mortality risk. Liver Transpl 2011;17(2):129–36.
38. Goldberg DS, Olthoff KM. Standardizing MELD exceptions: current challenges and future directions. Curr Transplant Rep 2014;1(4):232–7.
39. Goldberg DS, Fallon MB. Model for end-stage liver disease-based organ allocation: managing the exceptions to the rules. Clin Gastroenterol Hepatol 2013;11(5):452–3.
40. Freeman RB Jr, Gish RG, Harper A, et al. Model for end-stage liver disease (MELD) exception guidelines: results and recommendations from the MELD Exception Study Group and Conference (MESSAGE) for the approval of patients who need liver transplantation with diseases not considered by the standard MELD formula. Liver Transpl 2006;12(12 Suppl 3):S128–36.
41. Thuluvath PJ, Guidinger MK, Fung JJ, et al. Liver transplantation in the United States, 1999-2008. Am J Transplant 2010;10(4 Pt 2):1003–19.
42. Goldberg DS, French B, Abt PL, et al. Superior survival using living donors and donor-recipient matching using a novel living donor risk index. Hepatology 2014;60(5):1717–26.
43. Graziadei IW, Wiesner RH, Batts KP, et al. Recurrence of primary sclerosing cholangitis following liver transplantation. Hepatology 1999;29(4):1050–6.
44. Egawa H, Ueda Y, Ichida T, et al. Risk factors for recurrence of primary sclerosing cholangitis after living donor liver transplantation in Japanese registry. Am J Transplant 2011;11(3):518–27.
45. Schreuder TC, Hubscher SG, Neuberger J. Autoimmune liver diseases and recurrence after orthotopic liver transplantation: what have we learned so far? Transpl Int 2009;22(2):144–52.
46. Kugelmas M, Spiegelman P, Osgood MJ, et al. Different immunosuppressive regimens and recurrence of primary sclerosing cholangitis after liver transplantation. Liver Transpl 2003;9(7):727–32.
47. Jorgensen KK, Lindstrom L, Cvancarova M, et al. Immunosuppression after liver transplantation for primary sclerosing cholangitis influences activity of inflammatory bowel disease. Clin Gastroenterol Hepatol 2013;11(5):517–23.
48. Joshi D, Bjarnason I, Belgaumkar A, et al. The impact of inflammatory bowel disease post-liver transplantation for primary sclerosing cholangitis. Liver Int 2013;33(1):53–61.
49. Moncrief KJ, Savu A, Ma MM, et al. The natural history of inflammatory bowel disease and primary sclerosing cholangitis after liver transplantation–a single-centre experience. Can J Gastroenterol 2010;24(1):40–6.
50. Singh S, Loftus EV Jr, Talwalkar JA. Inflammatory bowel disease after liver transplantation for primary sclerosing cholangitis. Am J Gastroenterol 2013;108(9):1417–25.

51. Engels EA, Pfeiffer RM, Fraumeni JF Jr, et al. Spectrum of cancer risk among US solid organ transplant recipients. JAMA 2011;306(17):1891–901.
52. Vera A, Gunson BK, Ussatoff V, et al. Colorectal cancer in patients with inflammatory bowel disease after liver transplantation for primary sclerosing cholangitis. Transplantation 2003;75(12):1983–8.

Moving?

Make sure your subscription moves with you!

To notify us of your new address, find your **Clinics Account Number** (located on your mailing label above your name), and contact customer service at:

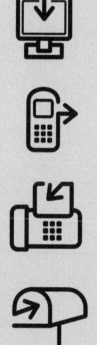

Email: **journalscustomerservice-usa@elsevier.com**

800-654-2452 (subscribers in the U.S. & Canada)
314-447-8871 (subscribers outside of the U.S. & Canada)

Fax number: **314-447-8029**

Elsevier Health Sciences Division
Subscription Customer Service
3251 Riverport Lane
Maryland Heights, MO 63043

*To ensure uninterrupted delivery of your subscription, please notify us at least 4 weeks in advance of move.